Bridging The Gap

A Textbook for Medical Interpreters

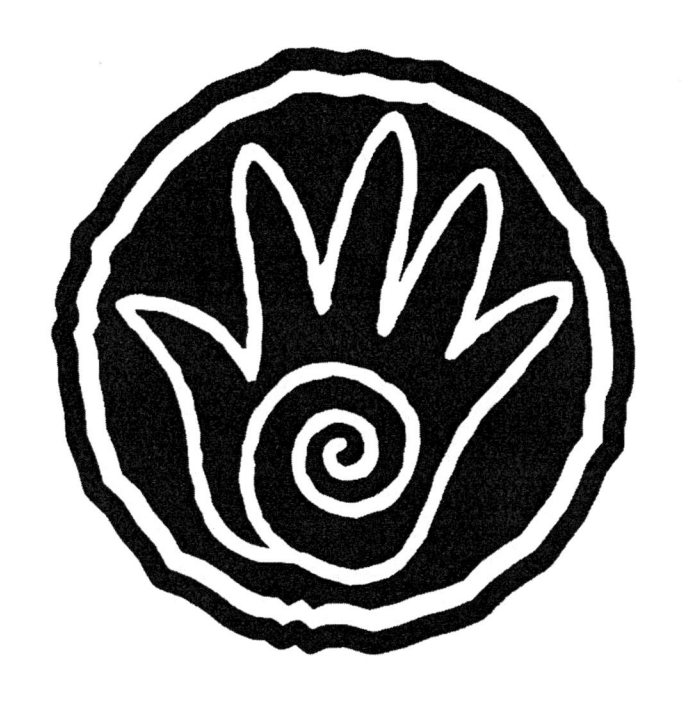

The Cross Cultural Health Care Program

The Cross Cultural Health Care Program actively protects this copyright.

Bridging The Gap: A Textbook for Medical Interpreters
is not in the public domain.

All rights reserved. No part of this book may be reproduced or transmitted in any form or by any means, graphic, electronic, or mechanical, including photocopying, recording, taping or by any information storage or retrieval system, without permission in writing from the Cross Cultural Health Care Program.

This textbook is intended for use by students who attend an authorized *Bridging the Gap* interpreter training by a licensed training agency. It should not be used as the basis or guide for any other interpreter training.

© 2014 The Cross Cultural Health Care Program
(206) 860-0329 | www.xculture.org

Acknowledgements

Updated and revised by

Barry Fatland
Gabrielle Knight

Special thanks to the following for their contributions to making this textbook a reality:

Barry Fatland
Gabrielle Knight
Adrian Hodos,
Rebecca Lee
Mikaela Louie
Elizabeth Rondon, CHI, CMI
Cynthia Roat
Bookda Gheisar,
Robert Putsch, MD
Ira SenGupta
Rose Long
Nimisha Ghosh Roy

CCHCP Board of Directors (2014)

Dwight Wheaton, Esq.
Robert Kaplan, Esq.
Dale Morris
Kathy Salmonson
Tom Byers
Patricia Dawson, MD, PhD
Vinayak Karnataki, MBA
Rob Anderson

Preface

The Cross Cultural Health Care Program (CCHCP) was established in 1992 in Seattle, Washington with a grant from the W.K. Kellogg Foundation. From the beginning, the organization's goal has been to bridge the gap between underserved communities and services to improve their health and well-being.

An independent non-profit since 2002, CCHCP has become a leader in providing training and resources to overcome language and cultural barriers in health and human services. Each year, CCHCP trains interpreters, providers, and trainers in health and human services locally and nationally. Widely acknowledged as the creator of the premier 40-hour medical interpreter training program in the nation, CCHCP is a pioneer in many other areas of cultural and linguistic competence. Published resources span a series of nationally respected medical glossaries, ethnic profiles of refugee and immigrant communities, training manuals, videos and research reports.

The first edition of *Bridging The Gap: A Basic Training for Medical Interpreters* was originally developed by CCHCP in 1995 at the request of and with funding from the U.S. Public Health Service, Region X, in response to the lack of training available for medical interpreters working in migrant clinics in the Pacific Northwest. The Georgia State Office of Rural Health and Primary Care as well as the W.K. Kellogg Foundation also provided funding for the first edition.

The original course was developed over the course of nine months. Original contributing authors were Cynthia Roat, Bookda Gheisar, Robert Putsch, MD and Ira SenGupta. The authors began by reviewing interpreter training materials developed in other parts of the U.S. and Canada. Content areas were identified with additional help from the Training Committee of the Society of Medical Interpreters (SOMI) in Seattle.

As goals and objectives were developed, an advisory committee was formed to give input into the process and review the final document. The community members on this advisory committee provided vital concepts and approaches found in the first edition. The members of the board included:

- Allen Apodaca, *Northwest Regional Primary Care Association*
- Liliana Bastres, *Clackamas County Health Department*
- Zulema Borges, *The Society of Medical Interpreters*
- Sharon Doyle; *Institute for Training and Development, Seattle Central Community College*
- Emma Federov, *Refugee Health Advocacy Project*
- Maria Garcia, *U.S. Public Health Service, Region X*
- Carolina Lucero, *SeaMar Community Clinic, Home Care Division*
- Andy Pascua, *Yakima County Diversity Initiative*
- Lucina Sigüenza, *U.S. Public Health Service, Region X*
- Irina Stevenson, *The Society of Medical Interpreters*
- Martha Wagner, *Washington State Department of Social and Health Services.*

The original 40-hour course, developed specifically for Spanish language interpreters, was first taught in December 1995 and revised based on the experience from that training. Recognizing the need to train interpreters of other languages, a 40-hour and a 24-hour version for multicultural interpreter groups was adapted from the original curriculum in early 1996. After the 40-hour *Bridging The Gap* course was offered locally and nationally over several years, the course was revised in 1997, 1998 and 1999.

During this time, many changes have occurred in the field of medical interpreting. Some notable changes include the emergence and acceptance of medical interpreter codes of ethics and the development of national interpreter certification programs. Many states have already begun to mandate their own criteria for licensing interpreters. CCHCP also recognized the need to provide interpreters with professional resources, access to relevant exercises, and understandable lessons. These changes in the field of medical interpreting prompted CCHCP to update and publish *Bridging The Gap: An Interactive Textbook for Medical Interpreters.*

Rose Long, then director of the CCHCP Interpreter Training Program, and Nimisha Ghosh Roy, CCHCP program developer and coordinator, collaborated in the development of this interactive textbook that was published in April of 2010.

The following organizations granted permission for the publication of their materials in the curriculum:
- International Medical Interpreters Association *(IMIA Code of Ethics)*
- King County Public Health Department (*Preventing the Spread of Influenza*, used for a sight translation practice exercise)
- National Council on Interpreting in Health Care *(NCIHC Code of Ethics)*
- California Interpreting Association *(CHIA Code of Ethics)*
- National Health Law Program, *(HIPAA and Language Services in Health Care* and *Health Care Interpreters: Are They Mandatory Reporters of Child Abuse?)*
- Territorial Government of the Northwest Territories, Canada, (*Handbook for Interpreters in Health*, used to develop Part B: Medical Terminology for Medical Interpreters)

In 2014, the textbook was updated and revised by Gabrielle Knight and Barry Fatland. CCHCP employees Adrian Hodos and Elizabeth Rondon also contributed new content.

About this Curriculum

The goal of this course is to help develop:

- a theoretical framework to understand the work and role of medical interpreters;
- professional criteria to help interpreters choose how to deal with situations effectively;
- concrete skills dealing with interpretation, culture, and advocacy that will allow interpreters to respond effectively to each situation.

The curriculum is written with the guiding philosophy that the patient-provider relationship is of the utmost importance in a health care encounter. It is within the power of the medical interpreter to ensure the success of that relationship. A *Bridging The Gap* trained interpreter empowers the patients he/she serves while respecting the patient's autonomy.

A goal of the training is to develop the community competence of interpreters. A *Bridging The Gap* trained interpreter is pro-active in continuing to learn about the community he/she serves. A part of developing community competence in the *Bridging The Gap* curriculum is developing an awareness and understanding of health disparities. A *Bridging The Gap* trained interpreter understands that he/she is a part of the system that continuously strives to eliminate health inequalities.

A unique aspect of this curriculum is its treatment of culture as an integral part of communication and therefore an important aspect of the interpreter's work. Culture is a crucial element in communication and health care bringing alive this quote from CCHCP's Executive Director, Ira SenGupta: "Every single human interaction is cross-cultural."

Developing cultural competence is a long-term and ongoing process. It is important to build a culturally competent framework from which to address the needs of multicultural communities. CCHCP's philosophy is informed by Cross et al.'s definition of cultural competence, which is:

> "Cultural competence is a set of congruent behaviors, attitudes and policies that come together in a system or agency or among professionals, enabling effective work to be done in cross-cultural situations."

As we recognize these basic cultural frameworks, it is equally important to note the many differences between individuals who come from the same community. To be culturally competent, we need to learn specific information about a community as well as simultaneously treat each person as a unique individual who is not necessarily representative of his or her whole group. This delicate balance is not easy to achieve in the diverse society we live in; however, it is a goal worth working for.

How to Use This Textbook

The Curriculum Structure

Bridging the Gap: A Basic Textbook for Medical Interpreters is divided into two parts: (1) Interpreter Skills for Medical Interpreters; and (2) Medical Terminology. Interpreter Skills for Medical Interpreters focuses on the theoretical framework and concrete skills needed by medical interpreters. Medical Terminology is dedicated to the study of basic English medical terminology. This can be used in conjunction with the bilingual medical glossaries that are included as part of the curriculum.

The curriculum is designed to be hands-on and interactive. Trainees are encouraged to bring their own life experiences and knowledge to the classroom, in order to foster a collaborative group learning environment.

Important Concepts and Vocabulary

The text box on the first page of each lesson provides an overview of the important vocabulary and concepts highlighted in the lesson. Two different types of textboxes are present in the manual. One highlights important concepts, policies, and institutions. The other type of text box provides definitions of important vocabulary, correlating the bold vocabulary words in the main body of the text.

In Part 2, Medical Terminology, the vocabulary words are presented at the beginning of each chapter and defined throughout the text. We encourage students to utilize their bilingual medical glossaries, as well as the definitions included throughout the section on medical terminology.

Contents

Part 1: Interpreting Skills 1

   Section 1: Interpreting Skills 3

      Lesson 1: Roles of the Interpreter 5

      Lesson 2: Codes of Ethics For Medical Interpreters 14

      Lesson 3: Modes of Interpreting 47

      Lesson 4: Being a Conduit 51

      Lesson 5: Clarifying 66

      Lesson 6: Managing the Flow of the Session 86

      Lesson 7: Memory Development 99

      Lesson 8: Sight Translation 108

   Section 2: Culture and its Impact on Interpreting 121

      Lesson 9: Introduction to Culture 123

      Lesson 10: Cultural Bumps 129

      Lesson 11: Culture of Biomedicine 139

      Lesson 12: The Culture Broker Role 159

   Section 3: Navigating the Health Care System 165

      Lesson 13: The United States Health Care System 167

      Lesson 14: Defining the Advocate Role 180

      Lesson 15: Effective Advocacy 187

   Section 4: Professional Development 195

      Lesson 16: Professional Conduct and Self-Care 197

      Lesson 17: Telephonic and Video Remote Interpreting 205

      Lesson 18: Resources for Professional Growth 211

Part 2: Medical Terminology 229

   Section 1: Learning Medical Terminology 231

   Section 2: Body Systems Terminology 241

   Section 3: Medical Terminology Study Tools 308

Part 1

Interpreting Skills

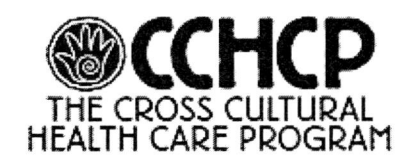

CCHCP
THE CROSS CULTURAL
HEALTH CARE PROGRAM

Section 1

Interpreting Skills

Lesson 1

ROLES OF THE INTERPRETER

GOAL

Identify barriers to effective communication in interpreted sessions and describe the roles of the interpreter in overcoming these barriers.

KNOWLEDGE OUTCOMES

- Identify the basic purpose of an interpreter

- Identify four barriers to understanding that can occur in a medical interview between an English-speaking provider and a limited-English-speaking patient

- Identify four interpreter roles

- Identify the ways in which an interpreter can overcome barriers that occur in a medical interview by selecting appropriate roles

- Understand the principle of incremental intervention

- Understand how medical interpreting differs from other types of interpreting

Vocabulary

Adversarial environment

Advocate

Barriers of register

Clarifier

Collaborative environment

Conduit

Cultural barriers

Cultural broker

Facilitation

Incremental intervention

Interpreter

Limited English proficiency (LEP)

Linguistic barriers

Source language

Systemic barriers

Target language

Translator

> **How are professionally trained interpreters different than bilingual staff?**
>
> In 1980, an 18-year-old named Willie Ramirez was admitted to a Florida hospital in a comatose state. There was no trained medical interpreter present. Mr. Ramirez's friends and family members, who did not speak English well, used the word "intoxicated" to explain Mr. Ramirez's condition to the doctors. They believed that "intoxicated" meant the same thing as *intoxicado* in Cuban Spanish. They thought that Mr. Ramirez was unwell because of something he had eaten, not realizing that the word "intoxicated" has strong connotations with drug and alcohol use. Due this miscommunication, doctors believed that Mr. Ramirez was suffering from a drug overdose and did not order a neurological consult for two days. Mr. Ramirez became quadriplegic due to a misdiagnosed brain hemorrhage. It was later determined that, had the brain hemorrhage been treated promptly, Mr. Ramirez would not have become quadriplegic. The lawsuit that followed resulted in a settlement of approximately $71 million.
>
> **Brainstorm**
> How could a trained medical interpreter have affected the outcome of this tragic story?

Introduction

For many people, language and cultural differences become a significant barrier to accessing quality health care from mainstream medical providers. Meanwhile, providers are finding their practices serving more and more **limited English proficiency (LEP)** patients every year. Separated by a language and cultural gap that makes healing very challenging, both patients and providers are turning to a professional who holds the keys to communication: the trained medical interpreter. Medical interpreters can be:

- part-time or full-time professional interpreters employed by health care providers for face-to-face or remote interpreting services
- qualified bilingual medical assistants, receptionists, or other staff who leave their regular jobs to interpret as needed (dual-role interpreters)
- freelance or contract interpreters who provide on-call professional interpretation in a variety of settings, including health care

Medical interpretation requires a great deal of skill, and successful interpreting requires much more than speaking two languages. Trained medical interpreters develop special skills to facilitate effective communication in health care settings, where clarity and accuracy are essential and sometimes a matter of life and death. This lesson will develop a clear image of an interpreter's purpose, the potential roles of an interpreter, and when each role is appropriate.

The Purpose of a Medical Interpreter

The basic purpose of the medical interpreter is to facilitate understanding in communication between people who are speaking different languages. **Facilitation** implies that the interpreter is active, rather than passive. Understanding implies that the interpreter's goal is not to simply repeat words, but to ensure that the message was understood. Communication is the exchange of information between the patient and their health care provider. Communication refers to the meaning of the words that are spoken. Speaking refers to the fact that **interpreters** deal with *spoken* language. Those who render *written* messages from one language to another are called **translators**.

While this course deals mainly with spoken language interpreters, there are also Sign Language interpreters who work in medical settings.

The purpose of an interpreter can go beyond facilitating communication to include facilitating equal access to health services for limited English proficiency patients. This will be discussed in the section on advocacy.

Notice what this definition of an interpreter's purpose does *not* include:

- the interpreter is not a social worker
- the interpreter is not a patient's emotional support system
- the interpreter cannot act as a bridge with the wider English-speaking community outside of the health care setting
- the interpreter cannot guarantee good medical outcomes or even guarantee that both patient and provider will be happy with the medical interview

Barriers to Communication

Four types of communication barriers can affect patient-provider encounters:
- **linguistic** barriers
- barriers of **register**
- **cultural** barriers
- **systemic** barriers

Vocabulary
Barrier: an obstacle
Facilitation: the act of making something easier
Interpreter: a person who deals with *spoken* communication between two or more languages
Limited English proficiency (LEP): Not speaking or understanding English fluently. A person who does not speak or understand English fluently is also referred to as someone who is **Limited English proficient.**
Linguistic: related to language
Source language: the language that an interpreter or translator is interpreting or translating *from*
Systemic: affecting an entire system, as opposed to a specific part
Target language: the language that an interpreter or translator is interpreting or translating *to*
Translator: a person who deals with *written* communication between two or more languages

Linguistic barriers

Differences in spoken language can create linguistic barriers. For example:
- the patient and provider speak entirely different languages
- the patient and provider may speak a little of each other's language, but not enough to ensure appropriate communication in a medical setting

Barriers of register

Differences in the level of formality or complexity of language can create barriers of **register**. For example:

- use of very complex language when speaking to someone who does not have the same level of education or language proficiency
- use of complicated medical terminology with someone who is not familiar with it (i.e. gastralgia vs. stomachache)

> **Vocabulary: Register**
>
> In the context of interpreting, "register" refers to the level, complexity, and style of the language used. "High register" language is more complex and may be more difficult to understand, especially to those with a limited formal education or limited fluency. "Low register" language is simpler and usually easier for most people to understand. Consider the following examples:
> **High register:**
> "This medication will alleviate the pyrexia and myalgia. Your symptoms will improve significantly."
> **Low register:**
> "This medicine will help the fever and muscle aches. You will feel much better."

Cultural barriers

Differences that lead to conflicting expectations of behavior, affecting both the meaning of the communication and the quality of the care can create cultural barriers. For example:

- different cultural beliefs about health and healing
- different cultural beliefs about doctors' authority and patients' autonomy

Systemic barriers

Differences in health care systems, racism, and difficulties navigating the health care system can create systemic barriers. For example:

- lack of understanding about how health care systems work
- systemic racism which affects the quality of care provided

> **The Four Interpreter Roles**
>
> **Conduit/message conveyer**
>
> **Clarifier**
>
> **Culture broker**
>
> **Advocate**

Interpreter Roles

In overcoming these barriers to effective communication, the interpreter may take on one of four roles:

Conduit: As a conduit, the interpreter is simply saying in the **target language** what the speaker said in the **source language**.

Clarifier: as a clarifier, the interpreter makes something that was said more clearly understandable. As a clarifier, the interpreter has to intervene in the conversation and speak with their own voice.

Culture broker: As a culture broker, the interpreter becomes more invasive, offering an explanation of a cultural framework. This diverts the attention of the provider from the patient to the interpreter.

Advocate: As an advocate, the interpreter speaks on behalf of the patient and is very much the focus of the interaction. This represents the most invasive role of the interpreter.

In fulfilling the role of a conduit, clarifier, culture broker, or advocate, it would be easy for the interpreter to become the focus of the interaction. However, interpreters must respect the patient's right to make their own decisions and the importance of the patient-provider relationship. Interpreters must facilitate accurate communication between the patient and the provider, but not take control of it.

Choosing an Appropriate Role

We have described four potential roles for the medical interpreter. The interpreter must be able to flow from role to role, depending on the interaction between patient and provider. The interpreter must often switch between different roles as potential misunderstandings arise and are resolved. The most appropriate role for the interpreter is the *least invasive role* that will assure effective communication and care.

The Incremental Intervention pyramid on the following page represents the amount of time that medical interpreters should spend in any one role. The largest portion of the pyramid is the bottom, which means that an interpreter spends most of their time in the conduit role. As you go up the pyramid, the roles become increasingly invasive. The interpreter stays less in the background and becomes more the center of attention.

We are concerned with the interpreter being invasive, because in any interpreted

---

Interpreter Roles And Barriers To Communication

Linguistic barrier: differences in spoken language
Conduit: Repeats what is said in the target language without adding, omitting, editing, or polishing any part of the message. The interpreter adopts this role unless he or she perceives a clear potential for misunderstanding.

Barrier of register: differences in the level of language used
Clarifier: checks for understanding; may ask the provider to lower the register; makes word pictures of terms that have no linguistic equivalent.

Cultural barrier: differences in beliefs around health and illness
Culture broker: provides a cultural framework for understanding the message being interpreted.

Systemic barrier: differences in understanding the health care system
Advocate: takes action on behalf of the patient outside the bounds of an interpreted session when the needs of the patient are not being met due to systemic barriers.

communication, there are three relationships that have been established:

1) Patient - Provider
2) Patient - Interpreter
3) Provider - Interpreter

The patient-provider relationship is the most important because the other relationships exist only so that this one can occur. The interpreter provides the means for the development of the crucial patient - provider relationship and must take care to support, and not undermine, that relationship. The more invasive a role the interpreter takes, the greater the risk of getting in the way of the patient-provider relationship. However, if an interpreter takes a role that is too limited, misunderstandings may occur that not only undermine the patient's relationship with the provider but may even endanger the patient's life.

Incremental Intervention

The idea of interpreters moving from role to role as necessary, but always staying as much in the background as possible, is called **incremental intervention**. Using the idea of incremental intervention, the interpreter strives to keep their presence as unobtrusive as possible, while remaining aware of potential barriers to communication. When they perceive such barriers, they step into a more obtrusive role as needed to ensure effective communication, then they step back into a less obtrusive role.

Incremental Intervention Pyramid

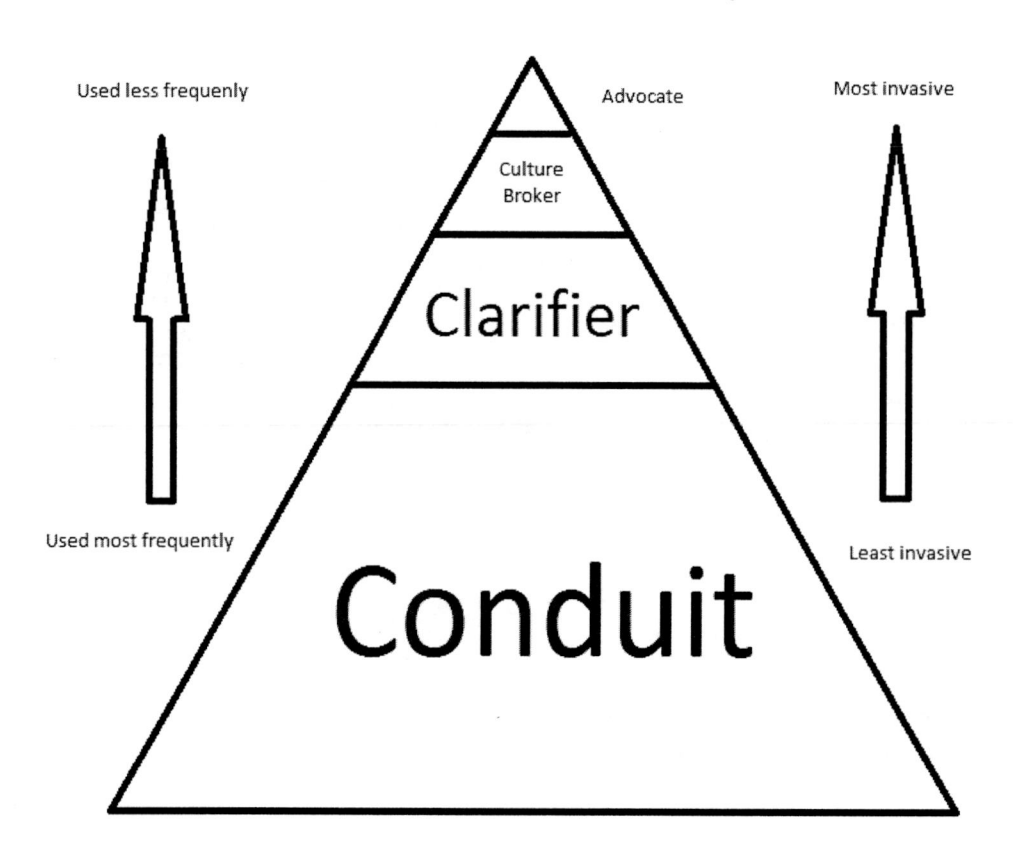

Pyramid from top to bottom: Advocate, Culture Broker, Clarifier, Conduit.

Left arrow (upward): Used less frequently at top, Used most frequently at bottom.
Right arrow (upward): Most invasive at top, Least invasive at bottom.

Roles of the Interpreter

Incremental Intervention	
*Pyramid: Advocate / Culture Broker / Clarifier / **Conduit** (highlighted)*	The interpreter starts the appointment in the conduit role, only relaying what is being said. Then he/she notices that the patient looks confused.
*Pyramid: Advocate / Culture Broker / **Clarifier** (highlighted) / Conduit*	The interpreter shifts into the clarifier role and asks for permission to check if the patient understood. The patient didn't understand.
*Pyramid: Advocate / Culture Broker / Clarifier / **Conduit** (highlighted)*	The interpreter shifts back into the conduit role, interpreting the patient's answer back to the doctor and the doctor's subsequent explanation to the patient.
*Pyramid: Advocate / **Culture Broker** (highlighted) / Clarifier / Conduit*	A bit later, the patient makes reference to an important cultural belief that the doctor misses. The interpreter shifts into the culture broker role to add cultural context.
*Pyramid: Advocate / Culture Broker / Clarifier / **Conduit** (highlighted)*	As the doctor asks for more information from the patient, the interpreter shifts back into the conduit role and interprets that question to the patient. In this way, the interpreter works to assure understanding in communication, while trying to stay as much in the background as possible.

Interpreter Roles in Other Settings

The same roles that are acceptable for a medical interpreter are *not* acceptable roles for a legal or business interpreter. In most courtrooms, the only role allowed is that of conduit (and clarifier, to the degree to which word pictures must be used when linguistic equivalency does not exist). Checking for comprehension, culture brokering, and advocacy are not permitted.

Consider the nature of the relationships involved. In a legal proceeding, each participant has a different role and a different objective:

- the judge's role is to determine the truth
- the defendant's objective is to be set free
- the role of the lawyer for the defense is to ensure a "not guilty" verdict
- the role of the lawyer for the prosecution is to ensure a "guilty" verdict

All the participants do not have the same objective. This is an adversarial environment. In this environment, generally some participants will achieve their objective, and some participants will not. Throughout the process, the interpreter needs to be careful not to influence the outcome. *In adversarial environments, the interpreter's role is limited and he or she must remain neutral or detached.*

On the other hand, consider the people involved in a medical setting:

- the provider's objective is for the patient to get well
- the patient's objective is to get well and stay well
- for the occasional family members that may be present, their goal is also for the patient to get well and stay well
- the interpreter's objective is to help all achieve their common objectives

Everyone involved in the medical encounter wants the same thing: the patient's good health. This is a collaborative environment, where everyone is working together for the same result. In collaborative environments, the interpreter may take a more flexible role.

In medical interpreting, the interpreter must be prepared to take a wider role than that of the court or business interpreter. The expanded roles described in this lesson are appropriate for medical interpreters but not necessarily for legal interpreters. Professional interpreters should always be aware of the setting in which they are working and the implications that the setting has for their role.

Summary

Health care facilities and providers are serving an ever-increasing population of LEP patients, which necessitates the use of language services. Trained interpreters assist patients and providers to communicate and understand important medical information and treatment.

Following the principle of incremental intervention, the interpreter can use the four basic roles to ensure effective communication between patient and provider, without being obtrusive. However, not all roles are appropriate in all environments. Interpreters need to understand when and how to use each role in a medical setting. This will be covered in the following lessons.

Knowledge Check

Test your knowledge of the material covered in Lesson 1.

What are different types of jobs an interpreter may perform?

What is the basic purpose of a medical interpreter?

What is the difference between translation and interpretation?

What are the four main barriers to communication that may affect communication between patient and provider?

What are the four interpreter roles?

How do the four interpreter roles correspond to the four barriers to communication?

What is "incremental intervention"?

Explain how each interpreter role is increasingly invasive into the patient-provider relationship.

Why is it important for the interpreter to be as unobtrusive as possible in an interpreted encounter?

What is a collaborative environment, and how does it affect the roles an interpreter may take on?

What is an adversarial environment, and how does it affect the roles an interpreter may take on?

Lesson 2
CODES OF ETHICS FOR MEDICAL INTERPRETERS

GOAL

Understand how to use a code of ethics for interpreters in health care.

KNOWLEDGE OUTCOMES

- Identify seven common values found in the three main codes of ethics for interpreters in health care

- Refer to the code of ethics when making decisions about difficult or complicated real-life situations

- Gain a basic understanding of relevant regulations, such as HIPAA and mandatory reporting guidelines

Vocabulary
Alert and oriented
Child abuse
Code of ethics
Disclosure
Domestic abuse
Elder abuse
Ethics
HIPAA privacy law
Imminent danger
Mandatory reporting
Standards of practice
Threats of violence/danger to self and others

Codes of Ethics

> You are interpreting for a mother and her five year old son who has an ear infection. The doctor asks the mother, "Have you treated your son's ear infections with Aural Acutic before? Do you know how to administer this medication?"
>
> You ask the doctor for clarification, "The interpreter would like to make sure you said ORAL, right?" The doctor says, "Yes, I said aural," and then you continue to interpret the conversation.
>
> The next day you interpret for a provider who also prescribes Aural Acutic. As the provider demonstrates to the patient how to put the medicine directly into the ear you suddenly realize your mistake: You interpreted the type of medication as an 'oral' medication, instead of an 'aural' medication.
>
> **Brainstorm**
>
> How would you respond to the situation described here?
> What principles would you use to guide your response?
> What decision would you make?

Introduction

As previously discussed, the basic purpose of the interpreter is to facilitate understanding in communication between people speaking different languages. This is the overarching principle that guides medical interpretation. In order to support clear, effective communication and to protect the rights of both the interpreter and the patient, some very basic rules have been developed that govern the way medical interpreters work. These rules, or guidelines, are known as a **code of ethics.**

The code of ethics is there to help the professional make a decision when faced with a difficult situation. A code of ethics is not a definitive 'how to' solve the difficult dilemmas faced by a medical interpreter, but rather a guide for when difficult decisions must be made.

This lesson will discuss what ethics are, why they are necessary, and how to apply the code of ethics to real life examples. This lesson discusses three widely-used codes of ethics from the International Medical Interpreters Association (IMIA), the National Council on Interpreting in Health Care (NCIHC), and the California Healthcare Interpreting Association (CHIA). We will discuss the common values found in each of these codes of ethics.

What Are Ethics, and Why Are They Important?

When considering the case study at the beginning of this lesson, your decision was probably based on morals and values that are important to you. Your understanding of what is appropriate and inappropriate guided you towards making the right

> **Vocabulary**
>
> **Ethics:** the principles that help us know what appropriate behavior is
>
> **Code of ethics:** a guideline to help a professional make decisions about what to do, especially in difficult situations

decision. When we discuss 'ethics' we are discussing the broad rules that help us know what is appropriate and what inappropriate behavior is. These broad rules, when assembled together in a document, are known as a code of ethics.

The code of ethics represent a set of guidelines that help each professional do their work in the most effective way possible. The code doesn't give definitive answers, or a 'how to;' instead, it provides guidelines. It represents the shared goals, values, and expectations for the members of a profession.

Each person has beliefs and personal values they use when making a decision. A code of ethics is a formalized set of principles for appropriate behavior. Instead of relying on individual beliefs and preferences of what is acceptable, a code of ethics provides a standard that professional medical interpreters can use to hold themselves and each other accountable. When your supervisors or fellow interpreters are not readily available, knowing the code of ethics will help you to make decisions confidently on your own.

All health care interpreters, regardless of their personal values and beliefs, have a common goal: to facilitate understanding in communication between people who are speaking different languages. Whichever code of ethics you choose to follow, you will practice the values and principles that support the achievement of the common goal.

Core Values of Medical Interpreter Codes of Ethics

In this lesson, we will present the seven common values that can be found in three widely-used codes of ethics for medical interpreters. These three codes of ethics are from the International Medical Interpreters Association (IMIA), the National Council on Interpreting in Health Care (NCIHC), and the California Healthcare Interpreting Association (CHIA). The full text of each of these codes of ethics can be found at the end of this chapter.

Understanding Common Values in The Codes of Ethics

This section will discuss how each of the seven values can be applied in the practice of medical interpreting.

Accuracy
The interpreter will accurately convey the content and spirit of the message by using the most effective mode of interpretation in a way that takes into consideration its

---

Seven Common Values

The seven common values that are found in the IMIA, NCIHC, and CHIA Code of Ethics are, in alphabetical order:

- Accuracy
- Advocacy
- Confidentiality
- Cultural competence
- Impartiality
- Professionalism
- Respect

cultural context. As an interpreter, you must:

- repeat everything that the patient or provider says, even if it seems irrelevant, rude, or unnecessary
- interpret meaning, not words
- correct errors as soon as you realize they were made

Advocacy

The interpreter will engage in patient advocacy when the patient's health, well-being, or dignity is at risk. Advocacy is undertaken after careful thought and analysis of the situation. Advocacy is done on behalf of an individual to support good health outcomes. As an interpreter, you may:

- advocate on behalf of a patient or group to correct mistreatment or abuse, or to protect the patient from serious harm
- advocate according to the established procedures of the institution

Confidentiality

Interpreters will maintain confidentiality of all assignment-related information within the treating team, while observing relevant requirements regarding disclosure. As an interpreter, you must:

- follow applicable confidentiality laws, such as HIPAA
- only share information learned while interpreting with members of the treating team, unless you have the patient's consent, or it is required by law

- not share information with the patient's family members regardless of cultural norms
- be aware of applicable laws that apply to mandated reporting for abuse or violence
- only share experiences for purposes of professional development if and when all identifying information is removed
- avoid situations that expose you to confidential information (for example, avoid being alone with the patient)
- clearly explain that your role includes interpreting everything said during the session(s) by everyone present
- encourage the patient not to disclose information in confidence to you

Cultural Competence

The interpreter will continually develop awareness of his/her own culture and other cultures encountered in their professional duties. The interpreter will explain cultural differences/practices to patients and health care providers when appropriate and necessary to facilitate effective communication. As an interpreter, you must:

- understand that culture is a central factor in all communication, and that understanding cultural context is necessary to interpret meaning accurately
- be aware of your own culture
- possess enough understanding of patient and biomedical culture to

facilitate communication across cultures, and to identify potential cultural barriers that may be hindering clear communication

Impartiality

The interpreter strives to maintain impartiality. Impartiality means that the interpreter does not interject personal opinions, nor counsel or advise patients. The interpreter does not project personal biases or beliefs. As an interpreter, you must:

- refrain from accepting an assignment when family or close personal relationships affect impartiality
- remain emotionally detached from the content of the message, and withdraw if unable to do so
- not judge the content of the message or any of the parties in the interaction
- respect patients' right to make their own decisions and avoid counseling or advising patients
- keep in mind that being impartial does not mean being uncaring

Professionalism

At all times, the interpreter will act in a professional and ethical manner, according to the standards of the profession. As an interpreter, you must:

- monitor your own performance and behavior to ensure that your actions will not interfere with the flow of communication between the patient and the provider
- not take on other roles while interpreting, even if you fulfill other roles in the health care setting at other times
- recognize and state your limitations in any given interaction
- avoid potential conflicts of interest and personal involvement
- adhere to the policies of the institution where you are interpreting when offered a gift from a patient
- refrain from using your position to gain favors from clients
- strive to continually further your knowledge and skills

Respect

The interpreter treats all parties with respect. As an interpreter, you must:

- treat everyone with courtesy and dignity
- respect the autonomy and expertise of all parties in the encounter

Confidentiality and Privacy Laws

To adhere to the value of confidentiality in the code of ethics, the interpreter will maintain confidentiality of all assignment-related information within the treating team, while observing relevant requirements regarding disclosure.

The Health Insurance Portability and Accountability Act (HIPAA) became law in 1996. The main goal of the HIPAA Privacy Law is to make sure that patients' health information is properly protected. This act describes some of the requirements that health care workers, including medical interpreters, are required to follow regarding **disclosure** of a patient's health information.

As a medical interpreter, it is important that you are familiar with the privacy rights of the patient. However, as an interpreter, you do not need to counsel the patient about their rights.

A patient's identifying health information, such as birth date, phone number, and social security number, as well as any information about their health or treatment that would allow another person to identify them, is protected by the HIPAA Privacy Law.

In general, health care providers can share a patient's health information with family, friends or others involved in the patient's care or payment for the patient's care if the patient does not object. See the text box on the following page for more information about HIPAA.

> **Vocabulary**
>
> **Disclosure:** the act of making information known

Understanding HIPAA

The HIPAA Privacy Law can be difficult to understand without seeing how it works in a real-life context. The following are some things that healthcare providers and interpreters can and can't do under HIPAA (Department of Health and Human Services).

It is acceptable to share a patient's health information when:

The patient does not object

- An emergency room doctor may discuss a patient's treatment in front of their friend if the patient has asked the friend to come into the treatment room.
- The hospital may discuss the patient's bill with the patient's family member who accompanies the patient to the hospital and has questions about the charges.
- The doctor may talk to the patient's family member who is driving the patient home from the hospital about keeping the patient's foot raised during the ride home.
- The doctor may discuss the drugs that need to be taken with the patient's health aide who has come with the patient to the appointment.

A patient is not alert and oriented

- A surgeon who did emergency surgery with the patient may tell their spouse about the patient's condition (by phone or in person) while the patient is unconscious.
- A pharmacist may give a patient's prescription to a friend sent for the pick-up by the patient.

It is *not* acceptable to share a patient's health information when:

- The patient asks the provider not to provide health information to anyone else.
- The patient's friends or family members ask the interpreter about the patient's condition.

Remember, you may be unaware that you are violating HIPAA unintentionally. Consider the following examples of HIPAA violations:

- An interpreter leaves her interpreting documentation forms in her/his car while she goes shopping. Someone breaks into her car and steals the invoices, which contain her patient's name, date of birth and other identifying pieces of information.
- An interpreter is talking to his/her supervisor in the elevator after a difficult interpreting session. They are careful not to use the patient's name. However, a nurse who works in the hospital overhears the conversation, and, based on the details of their conversation, knows which patient is being discussed.

Codes of Ethics

> **Mandatory Reporting**
>
> Health care workers may be required to report different types of abuse or danger, including:
>
> **Child abuse:** physical or emotional maltreatment or sexual molestation of a child. More information can be found at: www.childwelfare.gov
>
> **Elder abuse:** action or neglect which causes harm or distress to an older person. More information can be found at: https://ncea.acl.gov/
>
> **Domestic abuse:** physical, sexual, or emotional mistreatment of one partner by another in an intimate relationship. More information can be found at: www.acf.hhs.gov/blog/category/domestic-violence
>
> **Threats of violence/danger to self and others:** when a person threatens to harm themselves or others
>
> **Imminent danger:** something harmful that is about to happen
>
> **Mandatory reporter:** a professional who is required by law to report certain information, which would otherwise be considered confidential

Confidentiality and Mandatory Reporting Laws

There are laws in most states that require professionals to report issues that would otherwise be considered confidential. These professionals are known as **mandatory reporters.** In most states, health care workers are considered mandatory reporters. Whether or not an interpreter is considered a mandatory reporter depends on the definitions used within the laws of a specific state. The laws that do require interpreters to report abuse generally use terms such as "any person," "every person," and "hospital personnel." When researching the laws pertinent in your state, be sure to fully understand the definitions of each term used.

The laws describing who is considered a mandatory reporter and their specific responsibilities vary by state. It is very important to learn about your state's laws regarding mandatory reporting. Failure to report may be considered a misdemeanor and may be associated with penalties and fines.

Summary

As an interpreter, you will likely encounter many situations in which you will need to use your judgment to determine what to do. The codes of ethics cannot provide a definitive solution for every situation you may encounter. However, they are a guide to help you decide what to do. Additionally, understanding applicable privacy laws, as well as mandatory reporting laws, can help you make informed, ethical decisions.

The best teacher of ethics is your own experience. In your work as an interpreter, you will continue to learn and grow as you use the code of ethics to guide your practice.

Skill Development

The skill-building section of this lesson includes case studies for you to practice applying the code of ethics and standards of practice to real-life situations.

You can also use your own experiences, as well as the case studies to stimulate discussion about the application of the code of ethics to your medical interpreting practice.

Ethical decision making

The following are some steps to follow for ethical decision-making.

Step 1: Ask questions to determine whether there is a problem.

Step 2: Identify and clearly state the problem.

Step 3: Identify the ethical principles that might apply and determine which are the most important and relevant.

Step 4: Clarify your own personal values and beliefs that are related to the problem.

Step 5: Consider all alternative and possible actions and determine the benefits and risks of each.

Step 6: Make a decision and carry out the chosen action.

Step 7: Evaluate the outcome and consider what might be done differently next time.

Ethics Case Studies

ETHICS CASE STUDY #1

You are interpreting for a young man. As you wait with the patient for the doctor, the patient confides in you that he thinks he has a sexually transmitted disease. He is very upset. He says he has had sexual relations with a woman other than his wife, and he is very afraid that his wife may find out.

When the doctor comes in to examine the patient, he listens to the patient's symptoms, then asks the young man if he has had any sexual partners other than his wife. The young man lies: he says no. The doctor leaves the room to get some materials. When the doctor is gone, the patient admits that he lied, and asks you what he should do.

- What is the conflict?
- What are the options you have? What decisions can you make?
- Which of the seven common values in the interpreter codes of ethics can you use to guide your decision making?

ETHICS CASE STUDY #2

You are interpreting for a patient who is from an area of your country that you are not from. The patient speaks a dialect of your language that you find very difficult to understand. The first few times that the patient uses a word you don't understand, you stop him to ask for clarification. However, after the fifth or sixth time, the doctor is obviously getting annoyed. You start to feel a bit guilty (after all, this is your own language!) and try to guess on a few of them. Suddenly you realize that you may have made a serious mistake in interpreting some of the patient's symptoms.

- What is the conflict?
- What are the options you have? (What decisions can you make?)
- Which of the seven common values in the interpreter codes of ethics can you use to guide your decision making?

Ethics Case Studies

ETHICS CASE STUDY #3

You are interpreting for a young woman during a visit with her obstetrician. The doctor has just suggested the patient undergo a procedure known as amniocentesis. She briefly explains the procedure to the patient and then leaves you with some informational brochures about the procedure and asks you to translate them for the patient.
You know that a member of your community had an amniocentesis performed and suffered from the complications. You are quite familiar with the risks of this procedure. When the doctor leaves, the patient turns to you and says, "I don't understand this procedure at all. What should I do?"

- What is the conflict?
- What are the options you have? (What decisions can you make?)
- Which of the seven common values in the interpreter codes of ethics can you use to guide your decision making?

ETHICS CASE STUDY #4

You and another Arabic speaking staff interpreter are enjoying a quick break by the nurses' station. You are both engaged in an animated discussion in your native language about the upcoming election. A nurse comes by with a question for you. You both stop the discussion and you politely answer the nurse in English. As she walks away, you both resume your conversation in Arabic.
The nurse walks away feeling frustrated and concerned that you were both speaking about her. She shares her experiences with the other English speaking nurse on duty. They both agree that they have had the same experiences and are equally frustrated. You hear one of them comment, "They are good interpreters, but they should speak English! After all, it's what we all speak here!!"

- What is the conflict?
- What are the options you have? (What decisions can you make?)
- Which of the seven common values in the interpreter codes of ethics can you use to guide your decision making?

Ethics Case Studies

ETHICS CASE STUDY #5

You have interpreted various times for an elderly woman who had a difficult health problem. She is extremely grateful for your help and has brought you a gift of some traditional food that she made. You explain that you are paid for your work and that she does not owe you anything, but she insists she will be very offended if you do not accept her gift.

What would you do if she had brought you a gift of some gold jewelry? What would you do if she invited you to her granddaughter's wedding?

- What is the conflict?
- What are the options you have? (What decisions can you make?)
- Which of the seven common values in the interpreter codes of ethics can you use to guide your decision making?

ETHICS CASE STUDY #6

Your patient has been scheduled for a follow-up appointment in 3 months. You know the doctor has given him a prescription for only one month's worth of insulin. What should you do?

- What is the conflict?
- What are the options you have? (What decisions can you make?)
- Which of the seven common values in the interpreter codes of ethics can you use to guide your decision making?

Ethics Case Studies

ETHICS CASE STUDY #7

You are interpreting for a group of fifteen women who had recently come to the United States from a Somali refugee camp who are attending a free nutrition class at the clinic. The instructor spends a lot of time explaining the nutritional value of cooking with olive oil, which the women seemed to understand. At the end of the class, the instructor provides the women with a meal cooked in olive oil to taste and the Somali women adamantly refuse to eat it.

Confused, the instructor asks you, "Will you eat this food cooked in olive oil?" You don't have a problem eating food cooked in olive oil. What should you do?

- What is the conflict?
- What are the options you have? (What decisions can you make?)
- Which of the seven common values in the interpreter codes of ethics can you use to guide your decision making?

Exploring case studies from your own experience

Consider the following guidelines if you are planning to share case studies from your own experience (Andrews):

- How did you know it was an ethical dilemma?
- What was the setting like? (who, what, where, when)
- What were the different perspectives of the participants?
- What were the conflicting beliefs?
- Could you have used additional information? Where could you have gotten the information?
- How did you resolve the dilemma?
- What would you do differently next time?

Codes of Ethics: Resources

In this lesson you have been introduced to a number of resources that will help you to become more comfortable and familiar with the IMIA, NCIHC, and CHIA codes of ethics. Other resources that will be useful for further study include:

- **Appendix A: IMIA Code of Ethics**
- **Appendix B: NCIHC Code of Ethics**
- **Appendix C: CHIA Ethical Principles for Healthcare Interpreters**
- **Appendix D:** *HIPAA and Language Services in Health Care* from the National Health Law Program
- **Appendix E:** *Health Care Interpreters: Are They Mandatory Reporters of Child Abuse?* from the National Health Law Program

In addition to these resources, you also have your own background knowledge and experience, as well as those that your peers have shared during this training.

Regardless of the code of ethics you choose to follow, use these resources to continue your study of ethics in medical interpreting.

Appendix A:

International Medical Interpreters Association (IMIA) Code of Ethics

1. Interpreters will maintain confidentiality of all assignment-related information.

2. Interpreters will select the language and mode of interpretation that most accurately conveys the content and spirit of the messages of their clients.

3. Interpreters will refrain from accepting assignments beyond their professional skills, language fluency, or level of training.

4. Interpreters will refrain from accepting an assignment when family or close personal relationships affect impartiality.

5. Interpreters will not interject personal opinions or counsel patients.

6. Interpreters will not engage in interpretations that relate to issues outside the provision of health care services unless qualified to do so.

7. Interpreters will engage in patient advocacy and in the intercultural mediation role of explaining cultural differences/practices to health care providers and patients only when appropriate and necessary for communication purposes, using professional judgment.

8. Interpreters will use skillful unobtrusive interventions so as not to interfere with the flow of communication in a triadic medical setting.

9. Interpreters will keep abreast of their evolving languages and medical terminology.

10. Interpreters will participate in continuing education programs as available.

11. Interpreters will seek to maintain ties with relevant professional organizations in order to be up-to-date with the latest professional standards and protocols.

12. Interpreters will refrain from using their position to gain favors from clients.

Appendix B:

National Council on Interpreting in Health Care (NCIHC) Code of Ethics for Interpreters in Health Care

1. The interpreter treats as confidential, within the treating team, all information learned in the performance of their professional duties, while observing relevant requirements regarding disclosure.

2. The interpreter strives to render the message accurately, conveying the content and spirit of the original message, taking into consideration its cultural context.

3. The interpreter strives to maintain impartiality and refrains from counseling, advising or projecting personal biases or beliefs.

4. The interpreter maintains the boundaries of the professional role, refraining from personal involvement.

5. The interpreter continuously strives to develop awareness of his/her own and other (including biomedical) cultures encountered in the performance of their professional duties.

6. The interpreter treats all parties with respect.

7. When the patient's health, well-being, or dignity is at risk, the interpreter may be justified in acting as an advocate. Advocacy is understood as an action taken on behalf of an individual that goes beyond facilitating communication, with the intention of supporting good health outcomes. Advocacy must only be undertaken after careful and thoughtful analysis of the situation and if other less intrusive actions have not resolved the problem.

8. The interpreter strives to continually further his/her knowledge and skills.

9. The interpreter must at all times act in a professional and ethical manner.

Appendix C:

California Healthcare Interpreters Association (CHIA) Ethical Principles for Healthcare Interpreters

1. Interpreters treat all information learned during the interpreting as confidential.

2. Interpreters are aware of the need to identify any potential or actual conflicts of interest, as well as any personal judgments, values, beliefs or opinions that may lead to preferential behavior or bias affecting the quality and accuracy of the interpreting performance.

3. Interpreters strive to support mutually respectful relationships between all three parties in the interaction (patient, provider and interpreter), while supporting the health and well-being of the patient as the highest priority of all healthcare professionals.

4. Interpreters conduct themselves in a manner consistent with the professional standards and ethical principles of the healthcare interpreting profession.

5. Interpreters transmit the content, **spirit** and cultural context of the original message into the target language, making it possible for patient and provider to communicate effectively.

6. Interpreters seek to understand how diversity and cultural similarities and differences have a fundamental impact on the healthcare encounter. Interpreters play a critical role in identifying cultural issues and considering how and when to move to a **cultural clarifier** role. Developing **cultural sensitivity** and **cultural responsiveness** is a life-long process that begins with an introspective look at oneself.

Appendix D

National Health Law Program HIPAA and Language Services in Health Care

(Youdelman, National Health Law Program)

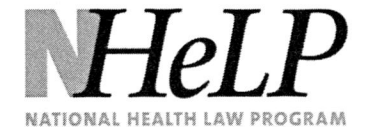

NHeLP — NATIONAL HEALTH LAW PROGRAM

HIPAA AND LANGUAGE SERVICES IN HEALTH CARE[1]

In 1996, the Health Insurance Portability and Accountability Act (HIPAA) became law and began to reshape how patients and health care providers think about the privacy of patient information. For interpreters who work in health care settings, it is important to understand how the patient privacy requirements of HIPAA affect their work and conduct.

It was not until April 2003, that the regulations outlining health privacy protections became fully operational. The "privacy rule" provides a set of minimum national standards that limit the ways that health plans, pharmacies, hospitals, clinicians, and others (called "covered entities") can use patients' personal medical information. As stated by the Department of Health and Human Services, "A major goal of the Privacy Rule is to assure that individuals' health information is properly protected while allowing the flow of health information needed to provide and promote high quality health care and to protect the public's health and well-being."[2]

The regulations protect medical records and other individually identifiable health information, whether it is on paper, in computers or communicated orally. The responsibility to abide by HIPAA binds the covered entity not only to ensure that its own staff protect patient privacy but also that anyone who it "controls" (such as volunteers) and with whom it contracts (called "business associates") follows these regulations. Thus, interpreters who work in health care settings – whether as an employee, independent contractor or volunteer – are generally required to uphold the HIPAA privacy regulations.

The purpose of this memo is to explain HIPAA and its application to interpretation provided in health care settings.

1. Who is covered by the HIPAA privacy rule?

HIPAA regulates the conduct of covered entities. The nature and extent of an individual's obligations under HIPAA depend on the person's relationship to the covered entity. An interpreter in a health care setting may be:
- a "member of the workforce" of a covered entity;
- a "business associate" of a covered entity; or
- a person approved by the patient – neither of the above but approved by the patient to interpret.

As different situations arise, the nature of the interpreter's relationship to a covered entity becomes increasingly important. While some overlap exists, different HIPAA expectations attach to members of the covered entity's workforce, business associates, and a "person approved by the patient." It is likely that an interpreter may be subject to different rules at different times, varying as the interpreter provides services for a variety of health care providers.

Member of the workforce. The HIPAA privacy rule applies directly only to "covered entities".[3] Covered entities include health plans,[4] health care clearinghouses,[5] and certain health care providers.[6] All members of a covered entity's "workforce" are required to abide by the HIPAA privacy rule. Being a member of the "workforce" is not limited to employees but also includes volunteers and trainees. Basically, any person whose conduct, when performing work for a covered entity, is under the direct control of the entity is subject to the privacy rule. It does not matter whether a person is actually paid by the covered entity.[7] This would include, for example, interpreters employed (full or part-time) by a hospital or other health care provider, volunteer interpreters coordinated through a covered entity's volunteer program, and other interpreters who are under the "control" of the covered entity.

Business Associates. In general, a "business associate" is a person or organization that performs functions for, or provides services to, a covered entity that involve the use or disclosure of individually identifiable health information.[8] The privacy rule requires that the covered entity ensure that its contract or other arrangement[9] with the business associate include specified written safeguards to protect individually identifiable health information used by, or disclosed to, its business associates. In addition, a covered entity may not authorize its business associates to make any use or disclosure of protected health information that would violate the privacy rule.

The business associate must ensure that all of its agents, including subcontractors who have access to protected information, agree to implement reasonable and appropriate safeguards to protect it. A business associate would include, for example, both a language agency and an individual interpreter who contracts directly with a covered entity. For the language agency, each of its agents – the interpreters themselves – would be bound to uphold the privacy rule through their relationship with the business associate.

Person approved by the patient. The privacy rule allows other individuals to have access to a patient's health information *with the patient's consent.* This includes a family member, other relative, or a close personal friend of the individual, or any other person identified by the individual. To these "persons approved by the patient," the covered entity may disclose protected health information directly relevant to the person's involvement with the patient's care or payment related to the patient's health care if the covered entity: obtains the individual's agreement; *or* provides the individual with the opportunity to object to the disclosure and the individual does not express an objection; *or* reasonably infers from the circumstances, based on the exercise of professional judgment, that the individual does not object to the disclosure.

Thus, an interpreter brought by a patient to a clinical visit would be allowed to interpret and have access to a patient's protected health information even if not a member of a covered entity's workforce or acting as a business associate. The "person approved by the patient" category could also include, but only if the patient consents, an *ad hoc* interpreter such as another patient or person in the facility (who is not a member of the workforce or a business associate). Because in this situation the patient has consented and the interpreter is neither a member of the covered entity's workforce nor a business associate, the interpreter is not bound by the privacy rule. But if the patient is concerned about disclosing certain information to an ad hoc interpreter, the patient has the right not to consent. If the patient does not object, the covered entity may reasonably believe consent has been given and disclose the patient's information. The patient may ask the covered entity to provide an interpreter who would be subject to the protections of the HIPAA privacy rule.

2. **How do I know if the "member of the workforce" or "business associate" rules apply to me?**

It depends on the situation and it can be difficult to determine whether someone is a member of a covered entity's workforce or a business associate. In practical terms, the HIPAA rules must be observed by both members of the workforce (since the rules must be enforced by the covered entity) and business associates (through their contract with the covered entity). The only practical difference relates to HIPAA-required training – a covered entity is responsible for training all members of its workforce about HIPAA requirements. A business associate does not have the same responsibility (unless required by the contract between the covered entity and business associate).

Since payment is not the deciding factor (see definition of "member of the workforce" in Q.1 above), determining whether someone is a member of the workforce depends in part on the nature of the interpreter's work at the covered entity. If the interpreter is under the regular control of the covered entity, then she is a member of the workforce. For example, if a language agency sends the same interpreter to the same covered entity on a regular basis (for example, the same two days each week for the same hours) and the covered entity controls the interpreter's work conditions (e.g. assigning where the interpreter works, when breaks are taken, etc.), the interpreter is more likely to be considered a member of the workforce than if the interpreter worked at a different covered entity each day with hours and responsibilities more closely controlled by the business associate.

It is likely that only a retrospective review would determine that an interpreter should be considered a member of the workforce. This might occur, for example, pursuant to a complaint investigation by HHS' Office for Civil Rights. If OCR determined the interpreter was a member of the workforce, the interpreter should have received training from the covered entity. If no training was provided, the interpreter would not be subject to any penalties, but the covered entity might be found in violation of HIPAA.

3. **What patient information is protected under HIPAA?**

An interpreter who is a member of a covered entity's workforce or a business associate must abide by the privacy rule and not disclose certain protected information about a patient. Generally, the privacy rule protects all "individually identifiable health information" held or transmitted by a covered entity or its business associate. It does not matter what format the information is in – electronic, paper, or oral. "Individually identifiable health information" is information created or received by a covered entity, including demographic data, which identifies the individual (or could reasonably be thought to identify the individual) and relates to:

- the individual's past, present or future physical or mental health or condition;
- the provision of health care to the individual; or
- the past, present, or future payment for the provision of health care to the individual.[10]

Individually identifiable health information includes many common identifiers such as name, address, birth date, and Social Security Number. This information is protected and may only be disclosed in certain circumstances (see Q. 4 below).

There are no restrictions on the use or disclosure of "de-identified" health information. De-identified health information neither identifies nor provides a reasonable basis for believing it could identify an individual.

In certain circumstances, a person's primary language may constitute individually identifiable health information and be prohibited from disclosure. For example, if there are a relatively small number of foreign language speakers in a community, disclosing a person's language and one other characteristic (such as age) might be sufficient to identify that person and thus disclosure would be prohibited.

4. **When can an interpreter disclose protected patient information?**

A major purpose of the privacy rule is to define and limit the circumstances in which an individual's protected health information may be used or disclosed. *Member of the workforce.* Interpreters who are members of a covered entity's workforce may not use or disclose protected health information, except:

- as the privacy rule permits or requires; or
- as the individual who is the subject of the information (or the individual's personal representative) authorizes in writing.

A member of the workforce should consult the privacy policy of the covered entity to determine the interpreter's role in disclosing information. While a covered entity must disclose information in certain circumstances, and may disclose information in others, the covered entity may restrict the persons who can make the disclosure. For example, the covered entity may not allow the interpreter to provide the information before obtaining clearance or may only allow certain individuals to disclose this information.

If a covered entity's privacy policy permits the interpreter to disclose this information, these are the rules that apply. A covered entity *must* disclose protected health information in only two situations:

- to individuals (or their personal representatives) when they request access to, or an accounting of disclosures of, their protected health information; and
- to the federal Department of Health and Human Services when it is undertaking a compliance investigation or review or enforcement action.

A covered entity *may* – but is not required to – disclose protected health information in the following circumstances[11]:

- in connection with treatment, payment, and health care operations[12];
- if the individual gave "informal permission", that is the individual had an opportunity to object to the disclosure and did not;[13]
- incidental to an otherwise permitted use and disclosure – as long as the covered entity has adopted reasonable safeguards as required by the privacy rule, and the information being shared is limited to the "minimum necessary";
- public interest and benefit activities – there are specific recognized activities[14] such as when required by law or for public health activities;
- and providing a limited data set for the purposes of research, public health or health care operations – limited protected health information may be provided to researchers without a patient's permission.

If an emergency or an individual's incapacity prevents a patient from agreeing or objecting to the use or disclosure, the covered entity may, in the exercise of professional judgment, determine whether the disclosure is in the best interests of the individual. If **so**, the entity may disclose only the protected health information that is directly relevant to the person's involvement with the individual's health care.

Whenever possible, a patient should be asked prior to disclosing information. But if this is impossible or impractical, whether an interpreter can disclose patient information depends on a number of factors. If the disclosed information is health information, and germane to the person's care, then it can be disclosed (unless the patient said otherwise), assuming the interpreter is viewed as part of the health team (which should be the case). This is allowed under the provision above that allows disclosure "in conjunction with treatment." If the information is not germane to treatment, then it should not be disclosed at all. How the information was obtained from or about the client should not matter.

Business Associate. The contract between a covered entity and a business associate may not permit the business associate to disclose any information that a covered entity may not. Thus, a business associate and its agents are subject to the same requirements as a covered entity. An interpreter should review the covered entity's privacy policy to understand any limits placed on the interpreters' disclosure of information (see above under "member of the workforce" for more information on what must and may be disclosed). The contract between the covered entity and business associate may also impose additional requirements on the business associate, so it may be important for the interpreter to review those requirements as well.

Person approved by the patient. An interpreter who is neither a member of a covered entity's workforce nor working for a business associate is not bound by the privacy rule. However, the interpreter may have independent ethical and confidentiality responsibilities – pursuant to either a Code of Ethics or other governing law or principles – that prohibit an interpreter from disclosing confidential or personal information about a patient.

5. **Can an interpreter disclose information the patient discloses related to child/elder abuse or threatened violence to him/herself?**

Any time an interpreter learns of this type of information in the course of interpreting, it is the interpreter's responsibility to interpret the information (just as any other information provided by the client would be interpreted). The provider should then address the situation and may be required to report the information pursuant to state mandatory reporting laws. If the interpreter learned of the information outside of the interpreting encounter (for example, while speaking with the client in the waiting room), whether the interpreter must disclose this information to the provider or others depends on state law[15] and the applicable interpreter's code of conduct, regardless of HIPAA.

6. **What information should patients receive about the HIPAA privacy rule?**

An interpreter may be asked to explain a HIPAA "privacy notice" to a patient. This notice generally explains a covered entity's privacy practices. A covered entity should give it to a patient the first time a patient is seen. If the patient receives health care services from an organized health care arrangement – such as a managed care organization or group practice – she may receive a single notice of the policies that apply throughout the system.

Member of the workforce. A covered entity that has a "direct treatment relationship" (such as a hospital or individual physician, but not a laboratory) with an individual must make a good faith effort to obtain written acknowledgement from her of receipt of the privacy practices notice. If a translation of the privacy notice is not available, an interpreter who is a member of the workforce likely will be responsible for providing a sight translation of the document and requesting written acknowledgement.

It is questionable whether providing an English privacy notice to an LEP individual would constitute "good faith" on the part of the covered entity. The determination will probably depend on the circumstances, but this would certainly not be a preferred practice.

Business Associate. The business associate does not have a responsibility to distribute a privacy notice to patients. The contract between the covered entity and business associate may require the business associate and its agents to provide a sight translation of a privacy notice to assist the covered entity in meeting its HIPAA obligations.

Person approved by the patient. These interpreters do not have a responsibility to provide any notice but may be asked by the covered entity to provide a sight translation of a privacy notice.

7. **Are all interpreters required to attend HIPAA training? If so, who is responsible for providing the training?**

Member of the workforce. Yes. The privacy rule requires covered entities to train all workforce members on its privacy policies and procedures, as necessary and appropriate for them to carry out their functions.[16] Because knowledge of what information can and cannot be disclosed is integral to the function of an interpreter, training would be necessary. Thus, for an interpreter who is a member of a covered entity's workforce, the covered entity must provide HIPAA training. If an interpreter does not receive training, the covered entity could be found in violation of HIPAA.

Business Associate. Not by law. The privacy rule does not impose specific requirements on business associates regarding training of its agents. The covered entity could, however, include a provision in its contract with a business associate to require training of the interpreters. Or the business associate could have its own internal policy to train its agents regarding HIPAA since its contract with the covered entity must include written safeguards to protect individually identifiable health information used by, or disclosed to, the business associates.

8. **What are the implications of the HIPAA privacy rule on the use of interpreters who have not signed an agreement of confidentiality with either the interpreter agency that sent them or the covered entity where they are interpreting?**

Member of the workforce. A covered entity may require its staff to sign an agreement of confidentiality or may require compliance with HIPAA as a condition of employment.

Business Associate. A covered entity must sign a contract with a business associate that ensures confidentiality as required by the privacy rule. If the business associate (either an interpreter who has a direct relationship/contract with a covered entity or a language agency) refuses to sign, the covered entity would be violating HIPAA and should not use the interpreter/agency. A business associate may also be required, pursuant to its contract with a covered entity, to have its agents – the interpreters – sign a confidentiality agreement. If no requirement is included in the contract, the business associate is not required to do so by HIPAA. The business associate may have its own internal requirement for its agents to sign confidentiality and/or other agreements.

Persons approved by the patient. HIPAA does not address these interpreters. Interpreters who provide services through a community based organization or other resource may have independent requirements addressing confidentiality.

9. **If an interpreter believes that the privacy rules are being violated, is it the interpreter's responsibility to mention it to the health care provider or otherwise report the violation?**

An interpreter would only have to report a suspected violation if a specific policy applying to the interpreter requires it. However, an interpreter may affirmatively *choose* to report a violation to the covered entity and/or the HHS Office for Civil Rights.

Member of the workforce. Reporting would depend on the policies of the covered entity. The interpreter should review the entity's written HIPAA policy and proceed accordingly.

Business Associate. There is no requirement for a business associate to report possible violations (unless the contract with the covered entity requires it). The covered entity must ensure that a business associate does not materially breach its contract. If a material violation does occur, the covered entity must take reasonable steps to cure the breach or terminate the contract with the business associate. The business associate may have its own internal procedures that require reporting.

Person approved by the patient. No requirements exist for a covered entity to train other interpreters. Since the patient had to consent to the other person serving as an interpreter, the covered entity does not have any responsibility to ensure this interpreter maintains the patient's confidentiality according to the privacy rule.

Person approved by the patient. There is no responsibility to report suspected violations.

10. **Often interpreters are asked to call patients to provide information about appointments, medications, or lab results. Is it a HIPAA violation to leave a message on an answering machine or with a family member?**

No, it is not a violation of the privacy rule to leave a message on an answering machine or with a family member *unless* the patient has requested a restriction on the communication of information. Even then, a covered entity does not have to agree to any restriction on the otherwise permissible communication of information. However, if it does agree to a restriction, it cannot violate the restriction except in an emergency where the restricted protected health information is needed to provide emergency treatment. A business associate would be required to uphold any restriction agreed to by the covered entity.

An interpreter who works for a covered entity or business associate should check whether the patient requested a limitation (which should be noted in the patient's record).

11. **Does HIPAA require that health care providers provide language services or, for larger entities, have a Language Services Department?**

No. The requirement to provide language services arises from Title VI of the Civil Rights Act of 1964. However, the privacy rule requires that covered entities distribute a privacy notice to their patients and make a good faith effort to obtain written acknowledgement from patients of receipt of the notice. It is difficult to imagine how a covered entity could meet this requirement without providing a limited English proficieny individual with either a translated privacy notice or an oral interpretation of it.

12. **Does monitoring of interpreting for quality assurance purposes violate HIPAA?**

Generally, the answer is no. If the covered entity hires a quality assessor to evaluate either members of its workforce or business associates, it would have to ensure the assessor abides by HIPAA, just like any other business associate. If a covered entity's business associate (such as a language agency or interpreter) conducts its own quality assessment, the business associate must ensure all of its agents as well as secondary business associates uphold its privacy requirements (pursuant to its contract with the covered entity). Thus, if the quality assessment monitor is employed by the language agency or working pursuant to a contract with the language agency, the monitor is bound to uphold HIPAA and there is no violation.

The only situation where a violation could occur is if an interpreter who is a business associate of a covered entity submits to quality monitoring requested by a third party (not the covered entity or a business associate) that does not have an obligation to abide by HIPAA. For example, an interpreter may be asked to undergo third party monitoring by a language agency for whom the interpreter works part-time. If the entity requesting monitoring does not have its own responsibility to uphold HIPAA, any monitor hired by the language agency would not be subject to HIPAA and could release a patient's protected information. An interpreter should ensure that any monitoring of her work is conducted by a person or entity which is also obligated to keep patient information confidential pursuant to HIPAA.

13. **Many interpreters keep detailed appointment books or schedules that include patient information (e.g. patient name, phone number, medical record number, date of birth, physician's name). Is this a HIPAA violation?**

No, keeping records does not violate HIPAA. This is allowed because the interpreter – either a member of a covered entity's workforce or a business associate – is collecting this information so that it can perform services on behalf of a covered entity. But the interpreter must be careful to keep the information confidential as required by HIPAA.

14. **Some interpreters must report patient information about an interpretation session to obtain payment. However, patients are never told that this information is being collected or reported. Is this practice in compliance with HIPAA?**

Yes, this complies with HIPAA because the interpreter is using the information for a management and administrative purpose of receiving payment for her services.[17] However, the covered entity or business associate must obtain reasonable assurances from those processing the information that the information will be kept confidential and will not be further disclosed unless required by law.

15. **What if a state's privacy law is different than HIPAA?**

In general, state laws that are contrary to the privacy rule are preempted by the federal requirements, which means that the federal requirements will apply.[18] "Contrary" means that it would be impossible for a covered entity to comply with both the state and federal requirements, or that the provision of state law impedes accomplishing the full purpose of HIPAA.[19]

But the privacy rule provides exceptions to the general rule of federal preemption. Thus, contrary state laws remain in effect if they:

- relate to the privacy of individually identifiable health information and provide *greater* privacy protections or rights with respect to such information;
- provide for the reporting of

disease or injury, child abuse, birth, or death, or for public health surveillance, investigation, or intervention; or
- require certain health plan reporting, such as for management or financial audits.

States may also, in certain circumstances, apply to HHS for an exception.[20]

[1] This report was made possible through the generous support of The California Endowment. [2] HHS Office for Civil Rights, *OCR Privacy Brief: Summary of the HIPAA Privacy Rule*, at 1, available at http://www.hhs.gov/ocr/privacysummary.pdf. [3] 45 C.F.R. § 106.103. [4] Health plans include: a group health plan as defined in the Public Health Service Act (PHSA) if the plan has 50 or more participants or is administered by an entity other than the employer who established and maintains the plan; a health insurance issuer as defined in the PHSA; a health maintenance organization as defined in the PHSA; Part A or Part B of Medicare and Medicare supplemental policies; Medicaid; a long-term care policy, including most nursing home fixed indemnity policies; an employee welfare benefit plan covering two or more employers; the health care program for active military personnel and the Civilian Health and Medical Program of the Uniformed Services; the veterans health care program; the Indian Health Service program; and the Federal Employees Health Benefit Plan. 42 U.S.C. § 1171(5), *see also* 45 C.F.R. § 106.103. [5] Health care clearinghouses are defined as public or private entities that process or facilitate the processing of nonstandard data elements of health information into standard data elements. 42 U.S.C. § 1320d, Social Security Act (SSA) § 1171, *see also* 45 C.F.R. § 106.103. [6] Health care providers are only covered if they electronically transmit health information in connection with certain transactions, like claims. Health care providers are defined as including providers of services (hospitals, critical access hospitals, skilled nursing facilities, comprehensive outpatient rehabilitation facilities, home health agencies, hospice programs, or for limited purposes regarding services provided in a teaching facility, a fund), providers of medical or other health services (defined in 42 U.S.C. § 1395x(s), SSA § 1861) and any other person furnishing health care services or supplies. *See* 45 C.F.R. § 106.103. [7] 45 C.F.R. § 160.103.

[8] *Id.*

[9] The rule requires a covered entity to have a contract or "other arrangement" with a business associate to ensure compliance with the privacy rule. It remains unclear, however, what would constitute an allowable "other arrangement." 45 C.F.R. §§ 164.502, 162.504. [10] 45 C.F.R. § 160.103. [11] The privacy rule contains much more detailed information describing these reasons. *See* 45 C.F.R. § 164.502(a)(1). [12] These terms are defined in the privacy rule. [13] Informal permission may be obtained by asking the individual outright, or by circumstances that clearly give the individual the opportunity to agree, acquiesce, or object (where the individual is incapacitated, in an emergency situation, or not available, covered entities generally use their professional judgment to determine if the use and disclosure is in the best interests of the individual). 45 C.F.R. §§ 164.510, 164.512. [14] *See* 45 C.F.R. § 164.512. [15] For more information on whether interpreters are mandated to report child abuse, *see* National Health Law Program, *Health Care Interpreters: When Are They Mandated to Report Child Abuse?*, available at http://www.healthlaw.org/pubs/200312.interpreter.html. For information on state reporting requirements on domestic violence, *see* Family Violence Prevention Fund, *National Consensus Guidelines on Identifying and Responding to Domestic Violence Victimization in Health Care Settings, Appendix J*, available at http://endabuse.org/programs/healthcare/files/Consensus.pdf. [16] 45 C.F.R. § 164.530. [17] 45 C.F.R. §§ 164.501 (defining "payment"), 164.506(c). [18] 45 C.F.R. § 160.203. [19] 45 C.F.R. § 160.202. [20] 45 C.F.R. §§ 160.203-205.

Appendix E

National Health Law Program Health Care Interpreters: Are They Mandatory Reports of Child Abuse?

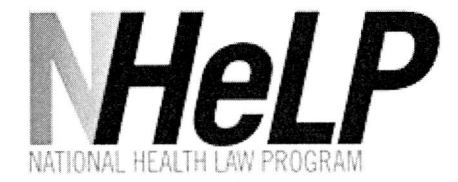

(Youdelman, National Health Law Program)

I. Introduction

As the nation continues to diversify and more health care providers are using interpreters to communicate with their patients, one issue that arises is whether interpreters are covered by mandatory child abuse reporting laws. Members of some professions are mandated by state law to report known and suspected cases of child abuse seen within the course of their employment.[2] While most states require health care workers to report child abuse, the laws are not clear if interpreters in health care settings fall within the parameters of the health care profession. It is important that interpreters know whether or not they fall within a state's mandatory reporter category, as they could be liable for not reporting cases of child abuse. Failure to report cases of abuse is a misdemeanor in many states.

II. Are Health Care Interpreters Mandatory Reporters?

Individuals who are required to report usually have direct contact with children. Some state statutes are very explicit in how they define health care workers, while others are not. Depending on the wording and interpretation of a statute, an interpreter may or may not fall into this designation and be a mandatory reporter. Although interpreters generally work in clinical settings with a practitioner who is usually required to report, interpreters cannot assume that the practitioner will report a child abuse case. The wording of a mandatory reporting statute may independently require the interpreter to report.

Whether an interpreter has a duty to report suspected or known child abuse depends on the laws of a particular state. Those who must report pursuant to state reporting laws generally fit into four categories. The state breakdown is as follows:[3]

· Four states[4] require "any person" or "every person" to report

· Thirty-three states[5] require health care workers or "hospital personnel" to report

· Thirteen states[6] require "any person" or "every person" and health care workers to report[7]. Texas requires "any person" or "every person" and "professionals" to report[8] Ten states (including those with the highest LEP populations) were examined to ascertain whether interpreters are required to report child abuse observed in health care settings.[9] None of the reporting statutes in those states specifically requires interpreters to report. However, three states have adopted statutes that require *all* persons to report suspected abuse regardless of their profession. Four states require "hospital personnel" to report, which may sometimes include interpreters (see below). Two of the ten states have adopted both the catchall "any person" provision, and a specific health care worker provision. One state has an "any person" as well as a "professional" provision. Only one state clearly did not require health care interpreters to report child abuse.

a. **The "Any Person" or "Every Person" Requirement**

Three of the ten states we examined require "any person" or "every person" to report suspected cases of child abuse. These states are Florida, New Jersey, and North Carolina. For example, in New Jersey, the statute states that "any person having reasonable cause to believe that a child has been subjected to child abuse or acts of child abuse shall report...."[10] Thus, a health care interpreter would be required to report child abuse, regardless of the context within which she learned of the abuse.

Although Florida has an "any person" requirement, the state additionally requires health care workers to give their name when making a report of child abuse. Individuals who are not health care workers (or members of certain other professions listed in the statute) are allowed to report anonymously.[11]

b. **The "Health Care Worker" Requirement**

Of the ten states we examined, California, Illinois, Massachusetts, and New York require some categories of health care workers to report suspected cases of child abuse.

New York requires "hospital personnel engaged in the admission, examination, care or treatment of persons" to report child abuse and neglect.[12] Thus, whether or not health care interpreters fall into this category depends on whether (1) they are hospital "personnel;" and (2) they are engaged in the "admission, examination, care or treatment of persons." For example, a full time interpreter employed by a hospital would likely be considered hospital "personnel," while an interpreter who independently contracted with a hospital might not be. If interpreters are hospital personnel, the second question is whether they are engaged in "admission, examination, care or treatment." If an interpreter is used to communicate with LEP patients in the hospital admissions process, they are likely to be considered mandatory reporters.

Illinois and Massachusetts have statutory language that requires reporting from similar personnel, with the only difference being that hospital personnel engaged in *admissions* are not included.[13]

California exhaustively lists every profession that is required to report, but does not list interpreters or include a category as broad as "health care worker," as do the three states above.[14] While California's statute also requires child abuse reporting by persons who are currently licensed under a section of the Business and Professions Code;[15] interpreters are not among those so licensed. Therefore, health care interpreters are not mandated to report child abuse.

c. The "Any Person" and a "Health Care Worker" Requirement

A state with an "any" or "every" person mandatory reporting provision obviously requires all interpreters to report child abuse because they definitely fall within the catch-all "any"/"every" person. Of the states examined, New Mexico and Maryland have adopted the "any person" requirement, augmented by a specific requirement for certain types of health care workers to report child abuse. While Maryland has also adopted the "any person" requirement, it also has a separate requirement for health practitioners.[16] Maryland's statutory definition of health practitioner does not encompass interpreters, yet the "any person" requirement obligates interpreters to report cases of child abuse. New Mexico's health care worker provision is limited to physicians, residents and interns, although interpreters would be included under the "every person" provision.[17]

d. The "Any Person" and "Professional" Requirement

Like the states above which have a health care worker requirement in addition to an "any person" requirement, Texas requires "any person" as well as "professionals" to report child abuse.[18] In Texas, interpreters are obligated to report any suspected case of child abuse under the "any person" requirement.

Other states may use "professional" instead of "health care worker" and thus an examination of the Texas requirement may be helpful. The Texas statute defines a professional as "an individual who is licensed or certified by the state or who is an employee of a facility licensed, certified, or operated by the state and who, in the normal course of official duties or duties for which a license or certification is required, has direct contact with children."[19] Currently, Texas has no licensure or certification requirement for interpreters; however, an interpreter falls into this category if they are *employed* by a hospital or other licensed facility. The question will therefore be the meaning of "employee" and it is likely independent contractors would be excluded under this provision.

III. Other Important Components of Mandatory Reporting Laws

There are several other important components regarding failure to report and protections for good faith reporting. Interpreters need to know these requirements because a failure to report can have negative repercussions.

Failure to report a suspected case is a misdemeanor in six of the states we examined –California, Florida, Illinois, New Mexico, New York and Texas.[20] In Illinois, a first violation is a misdemeanor and any subsequent failure to report is considered a felony.[21] Massachusetts fines non-reporters up to $1000.[22] In New Jersey, a person is deemed a "disorderly person" for failing to report child abuse.[23] North Carolina and Maryland have no punishment for non-reporting.

Finally, most states give immunity from civil and criminal liability to mandatory reporters who report in good faith. If a health care interpreter suspects child abuse and reports it, but later the child abuse charge is determined to be unfounded, the interpreter cannot be held liable for reporting what he/she believed to be abuse. All ten states examined here give this immunity.

IV. Conclusion

To determine whether health care interpreters are required to report child abuse in a state, one should examine the state's child abuse and neglect statute regarding mandatory reporting. The National Clearinghouse on Child Abuse and Neglect Information has produced a chart with citations to every state's child abuse laws. The chart is also useful as a quick guide for the individuals and/or professions who must report child abuse and neglect.[24]

Checklist: What to look for in a state mandatory reporting statute:

- Is there an "any person" requirement clause?

If yes, then all health care interpreters have a mandatory reporting duty, and you need not go any farther.

If no, check if another provision may apply to interpreters

- Is there a health care worker, health personnel or hospital personnel requirement clause?

If yes, then look to see if a health care interpreter would fit within such a profession. If the terms are not defined within the clause, look for a definitions provision, usually in an earlier subsection of the statute or in cases decided by the courts in your state.

- Is the interpreter considered a hospital "employee" or "personnel," as opposed to an independent contractor or an employee of an interpreter service?

If yes, the interpreter must report

If no, check if another provision may apply to interpreters

- Is the interpreter engaged in the activities covered by the statute – e.g. admission, examination, care or treatment of patients?

If yes, the interpreter must report

If no, check if another provision may apply to interpreters

- Look for other relevant provisions:

Is there punishment for non-reporting?
Is there immunity for good faith reporting?

[1] This report was made possible through the generous support of The California Endowment.

[2] There may be a similar reporting requirement for elder abuse, but that is beyond the scope of this paper.

[3] For a breakdown of all states, *see* National Clearinghouse on Child Abuse and Neglect Information, *Statutes At-a-Glance, Mandatory Reporters of Child Abuse and Neglect* (Feb. 2002), *available at* http://www.calib.com/nccanch/pubs/sag/manda.pdf.

[4] Florida, New Jersey, North Carolina and Wyoming. *See* http://www.calib.com/nccanch/pubs/sag/manda.pdf.

[5] Alabama, Alaska, Arizona, Arkansas, California, Colorado, Connecticut, District of Columbia, Georgia, Hawaii, Illinois, Iowa, Kansas, Louisiana, Maine, Massachusetts, Michigan, Minnesota, Missouri, Montana, Nevada, New York, North Dakota, Ohio, Oregon, Pennsylvania, South Carolina, South Dakota, Vermont, Virginia, Washington, West Virginia, and Wisconsin. *See* http://www.calib.com/nccanch/pubs/sag/manda.pdf.

[6] Delaware, Idaho, Indiana, Kentucky, Maryland, Mississippi, Nebraska, New Hampshire, New Mexico, Oklahoma, Rhode Island, Tennessee, and Utah. *See* http://www.calib.com/nccanch/pubs/sag/manda.pdf.

[7] Although it may seem redundant and illogical, many state statutes contain a provision requiring health care workers or professionals to report child abuse *in addition to* having a provision requiring "any" or "every" person to do so. Why this is so and how it originated is beyond the scope of this paper.

[8] Other states from the thirteen that have an "any" or "every" person and health care worker requirement may fit into this category, but that is beyond the scope of this paper and not available from the chart cited above.

[9] The chosen states were California, Florida, Illinois, Maryland, Massachusetts, New Jersey, New Mexico, New York, North Carolina, and Texas.

[10] N.J. STAT. ANN. § 9:6-8.10 (West 2002).

[11] FLA. STAT. ANN. §39.201(1)(b) (West 2003).

[12] N.Y. SOC. SERV. LAW § 413(1) (McKinney 2003).

[13] 325 ILL. COMP. STAT. 5/4 (2001 & Supp. 2003); MASS. ANN. LAWS ch. 119, § 51A (Law. Co-op 2003).

[14] CAL. PENAL CODE § 11165.7 (West 2003).

[15] CAL. PENAL CODE § 11165.7(21) (West 2003).

[16] MD. CODE ANN., FAM. LAW §§5-704-705 (2002).

[17] N.M. STAT. ANN. § 32A-4-3(A) (Michie 2002).

[18] TEX. FAM. CODE ANN. § 261.101 (Vernon 2002).

[19] TEX. FAM. CODE ANN. § 261.101(a)-(b) (Vernon 2002).

[20] *See* CAL. PENAL CODE § 11166(b) (West 2003); FLA. STAT. ANN. § 39.205 (West 2003); 325 ILL. COMP. STAT. 5/4 (2001 & Supp. 2003); N.M. STAT. ANN. § 32A-4-3(F) (Michie 2002); N.Y. SOC. SERV. LAW § 420 (McKinney 2003); TEX. FAM. CODE ANN. § 261.109 (Vernon 2002).

[21] 325 ILL. COMP. STAT. 5/4 (2001 & Supp. 2003).

[22] MASS. ANN. LAWS ch. 119, § 51A (Law. Co-op 2003).

[23] N.J. STAT. ANN. § 9:6-8.14 (West 2002). A disorderly persons offense is a petty offense and is not a crime. N.J. STAT. ANN. § 2C:1-4 (West 2003).

[24] National Clearinghouse on Child Abuse and Neglect Information, *Statutes At-a-Glance, Mandatory Reporters of Child Abuse and Neglect* (Feb. 2002), *available at* http://www.calib.com/nccanch/pubs/sag/manda.pdf.

© 1999-2009 Pro Bono Net. All rights reserved.

Lesson 3

MODES OF INTERPRETING

GOAL

Understand when each mode of interpreting is appropriate in a health care setting.

KNOWLEDGE OUTCOMES

- Identify and demonstrate the four modes of interpreting
- Understand when it is appropriate to use each mode

Vocabulary
Consecutive interpreting mode
Sight translation
Simultaneous interpreting
Summarization

> Different modes of interpreting are used in different settings. Picture how interpreters are used in each of these settings:
>
> At large meetings, conferences, or presentations with participants who don't all understand the same language, interpreters, as well as those for whom they are interpreting, often wear headsets. The interpreter does not wait for the speaker to pause before beginning to interpret, and instead interprets as the speaker continues to speak.
>
> During one-on-one interactions, or in small groups, interpreters usually wait for the speaker to finish speaking, then they interpret in the pause that follows.
>
> **Brainstorm**
> Why do you think interpreters work differently in these settings?
> What are the factors that affect the way the interpreter works?

Introduction

When we discuss the "**modes** of interpreting," we are discussing the different methods and approaches used in interpreting. Interpreters use different modes of interpreting under different circumstances. In this lesson, we will discuss four modes of interpreting: **consecutive**, **simultaneous**, **sight translation**, and **summarization**. We will also discuss when and how these modes are used in medical interpreting.

Consecutive Interpreting

Consecutive interpreting is when the interpreter interprets after the speaker is done speaking. The speaker says a few sentences, then waits for the interpreter to interpret before continuing. Consecutive interpreting is sometimes known as "pause" interpreting, because the speaker pauses to wait for the interpretation of what they said.

Application in a medical setting: Consecutive interpreting is the most commonly used mode in medical interpreting. For a medical interview with three people (doctor, patient, and interpreter), this mode of interpreting is less confusing than the simultaneous mode.

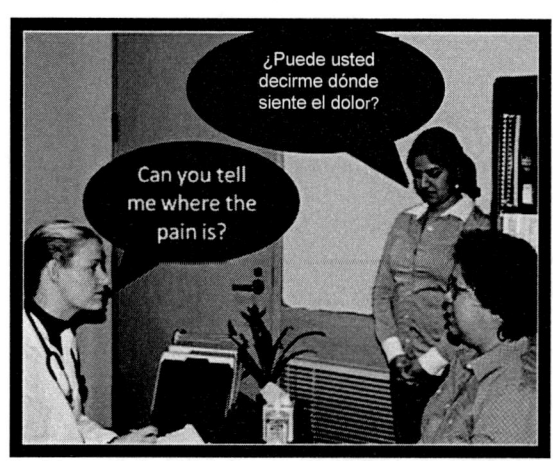

In this example of consecutive interpreting, after the provider speaks, the interpreter interprets and then waits for the patient to respond.

Sight Translation

Sight translation is when an interpreter reads a text written in one language (the source language), and verbally renders the text into another language (the target language). The interpreter does not provide a written translation of the document in question.

Application in a medical setting: Medical interpreters are often asked to provide sight translation spontaneously when they are in their primary role as a medical interpreter. This mode is used to interpret written information in oral form to either the patient or the provider

Ideally, health care institutions would provide professional written translations of all vital documents. However, this is not always the case, so interpreters may be asked to sight translate such documents.

Simultaneous Interpreting

In simultaneous interpreting, the interpreter interprets while the speaker is speaking, with a 3-4 second delay. This technique is most commonly used in legal or conference settings. It is used infrequently in medical settings.

Application in a medical setting: In medical interviews, simultaneous interpreting tends to be distracting and confusing. However, it can be useful in a mental health setting, if the patient launches into an emotional narrative or description that cannot be interrupted, or in cases where time is critical, such as a medical emergency.

> **Vocabulary**
>
> **Consecutive:** following in succession
>
> **Mode:** the way in which something is done
>
> **Simultaneous:** occurring at the same time
>
> **Summarization:** giving a brief statement of the main points of something

Summarization

Summarization occurs when one person speaks at length, or when two or more people speak at the same time, and the interpreter summarizes the important points at the end.

Application in a medical setting: Summarization is generally not recommended in a medical setting because of the great potential for errors and omissions. In fact, some professional medical interpreters do not consider it a mode of interpretation at all. Summarization should not be used as a technique for editing material that the interpreter feels is irrelevant.

The only time that summarization may be appropriate in a medical setting is when the doctor engages in a highly technical discussion with another health care provider in front of the patient but is not speaking to the patient.

For example, in a teaching hospital, the anesthesiologist may take the time to explain important technical steps in

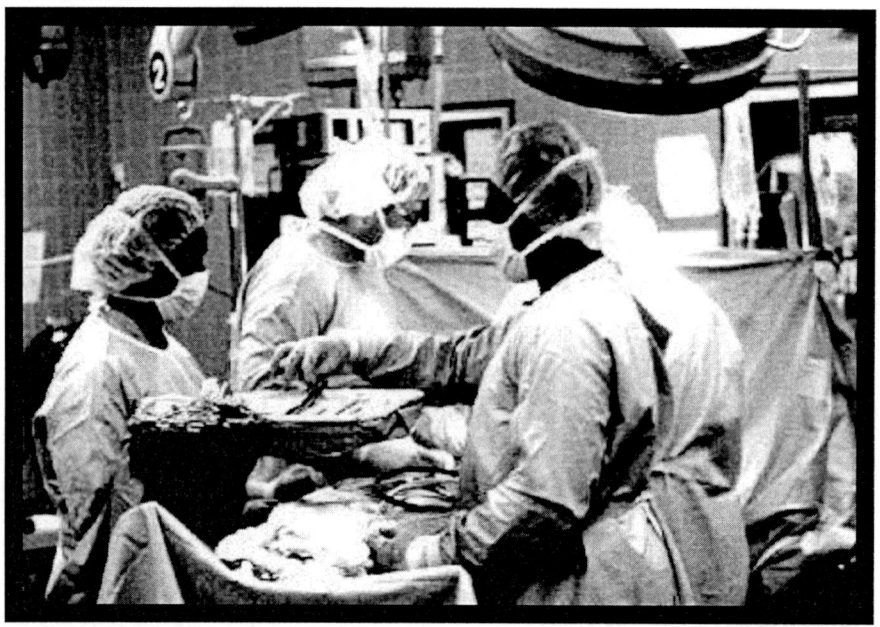

When interpreting for a family member watching a surgery, the interpreter may not need to interpret every word and medical term said by the providers. It may be sufficient to summarize after key parts of the surgery. *(Center for Disease Control (n.d))*

administering anesthesia for the benefit of medical students that are attending the surgery. The details of technical steps may not be relevant to the patient. It would be sufficient in this situation for the interpreter to summarize the information for the patient at the end of the explanation. Summarization may also be appropriate when interpreting for family members watching a surgery.

Summary

In summary, the four modes include consecutive interpreting, sight translation, simultaneous interpreting, and summarization. In medical interpreting, the most common mode used is consecutive interpreting.

Sight translation is also common in medical settings, due to the number of forms and handouts patients are asked to deal with. Simultaneous interpretation is useful in a limited number of specific situations, and summarization is generally discouraged in the medical setting, except in very specific situations. Interpreters must know not only what the modes are, but when it is appropriate to use each mode.

Lesson 4

BEING A CONDUIT

GOAL

Understand and demonstrate the characteristics of interpreting in a conduit role.

KNOWLEDGE OUTCOMES

- Identify the four specific guidelines for the conduit role of interpreting

- Identify when and why first person interpreting is preferred

- Understand the difference between a literal interpretation and an accurate interpretation

Vocabulary
Accurate interpretation
Conduit
First person
Idiom
Inflection
Literal interpretation
Non-verbal communication
Reported speech
Second person
Third person
Tone
Volume

Introduction

The basic purpose of the medical interpreter is to facilitate understanding in communication between people speaking different languages. In order to fulfill that purpose, the interpreter may sometimes have to switch between specific roles as the need arises.

This lesson will discuss the techniques involved in the most basic of those roles: the role of the **conduit**. Another term for the conduit role is "message conveyer." This is an accurate description of the conduit role. The basic purpose of the conduit role is to interpret everything that is said as faithfully and as accurately as possible. Add nothing; omit nothing; change nothing.

Four Guidelines for the Conduit Role

- The interpreter interprets in the first person.

- The interpreter interprets pauses, "ums," sighs, meaningful gestures, and everything that adds meaning to the communication.

- The interpreter gives an accurate interpretation, not a literal interpretation.

- The interpreter reflects tone, inflection, and volume.

Guidelines for Conduit Interpreting

The interpreter interprets in the first person.

If the patient says: "My stomach hurts," the interpreter interprets, "My stomach hurts." The interpreter does *not* say: "The patient says that her stomach hurts." (This is called reported speech.)

In general, the use of first person is better than the use of reported speech because it:
- reinforces the primary relationship between the provider and patient
- helps the interpreter to stay in the background, and not be the focus of attention
- helps the interpreter to focus on repeating exactly what was said
- shortens the communication and avoids confusion as to who is speaking

Using first person may seem uncomfortable at first, but it will become more natural with practice. Using first person is an established norm among professional interpreters. However, there are some exceptions to when the first person should be used. See the text box on the following page for more information.

The interpreter gives an accurate interpretation, not a literal interpretation.

Interpreters focus on transmitting meaning, not words. Even though a **literal interpretation** is one that interprets accurately word for word, it can sometimes give the wrong meaning. An interpreter's responsibility is to make sure

Being a Conduit

that he/she provides an accurate message; one that transmits the meaning of the words, if not the exact words themselves. Consider the following examples:

Patient: (In Spanish) *"El dolor comenzó ayer. No. Miento. Comenzó anteayer."*

Interpreter: (Providing a literal interpretation) "The pain started yesterday. No. I'm lying. It started the day before yesterday."

Patient: (In Spanish) *""El dolor comenzó ayer. No. Miento. Comenzó anteayer."*

Interpreter: (Providing an **accurate interpretation**) "The pain started yesterday. No. I mean, it started the day before yesterday."

Another example in Spanish is the verb *mandar.*

Patient (In Spanish) *"¿Mande?"*

Interpreter: (Providing a literal interpretation) "Order me?"

Patient: (In Spanish) *"¿Mande?"*

Interpreter: (Providing an accurate interpretation) "Excuse me?"

Exceptions to using first person interpreting

There are some situations where using the first person does not contribute to the clarity of the conversation. In these situations, using the first person can confuse the patient about who is speaking. These include:

- if the patient is disoriented, mentally ill, or otherwise shows confusion about who is speaking; or
- if the patient speaks a language whose grammatical structure makes it inappropriate to use first person (See below.)

In some languages, the use of the word "I" depends on who is speaking and to whom. The age and gender of the person speaking, and who is being spoken to, affect both the "I" and the verb form that follows.

When a young woman doctor needs to tell an older woman patient: "I think you need an X-ray"

In Vietnamese it should be interpreted as:
Cháu nghi' rang bác cân chup hinh quang tuyên x.
("Humble young woman thinks that respected aunty needs an X-ray.")

When an older male doctor needs to tell a younger woman patient: "I think you need an X-ray"

In Vietnamese it should be interpreted as:
Tôi nghi rang co cân chup hinh quang tuyên x.
("I think that young miss needs an X-ray.")

If the interpreter in this case is not also a young woman or older male like the doctor, translating this phrase in the first person would be profoundly disrespectful and therefore might get in the way of communication.

Some interpreters solve this problem by using the first person to interpret what the patient says to the doctor, but using reported speech ("The doctor said...") to communicate the doctor's words to the patient.

Bridging the Gap: A Textbook for Medical Interpreters

> ### Vocabulary
>
> **Literal interpretation**: interpreting what is said word for word, whether or not it makes sense in the target language
>
> **Accurate interpretation**: interpreting the meaning of the words in a way that makes sense in the target language
>
> **Non-verbal communication**: gestures, body language, facial expressions, and other cues that provide meaning without using spoken words
>
> **Tone**: the quality or pitch of a person's voice
>
> **Inflection**: the way that a phrase or word is spoken or emphasized
>
> **Volume**: the loudness of the speaker's voice

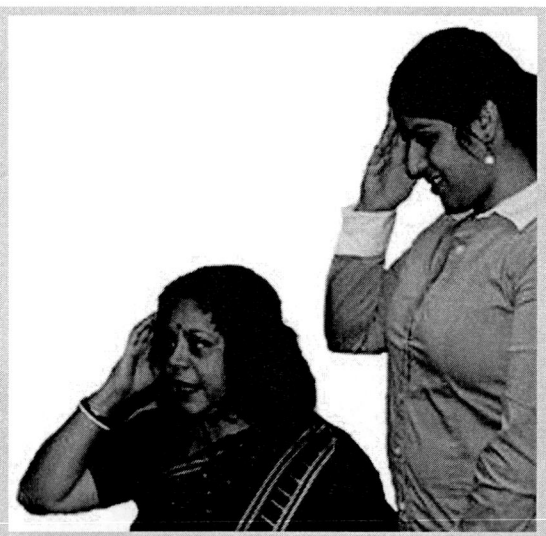

The interpreter incorporates meaningful gestures used by the patient during the interpretation.

The interpreter interprets pauses, "ums," sighs, meaningful gestures, and everything that adds meaning to the communication.

Non-verbal communication has a significant impact on the meaning of what is said. It is important to incorporate the speaker's gestures along with their words.

The interpreter reflects tone, inflection and volume.

The interpreter must include all the information that carries meaning in the message. This includes the **tone**, **inflection** and **volume** of the speaker.

Think of the difference between a person asking: "What?" in a neutral tone, "WHAT?!" in an angry tone, or "What?" in a sad tone. All three words are the same, but the meaning of the message is different.

As you reflect the speaker's tone, inflection and volume, be aware of how your interpretation comes across. In order to avoid giving the impression of mocking the speaker, adopt a tone and volume that is a little less than that of the speaker.

Summary

Medical interpreters use the conduit role more than any other role. As a conduit (or message conveyor), it is important to interpret everything that is said, as faithfully and accurately as possible.

Interpreters should strive to speak in the first person, except where it might hinder communication. Interpreters should be sure to provide an accurate interpretation, keeping in mind that this may not be the same as a literal interpretation. They should also be sure to interpret all non-verbal communication that adds meaning to what is said. The following skill development section includes interpreting practice exercises to help you further understand the conduit role through practice.

How to use the Interpreting Exercises

Each Interpreting Exercise is a written scenario and requires three people to play three roles:

1. Hospital Staff and Providers - who speak only in English
2. Patient - who speaks only in a non-English language
3. Interpreter - who interprets the conversation

- If possible, work in groups where all three participants speak the same target language.
- If there are not enough people who speak the same target language, the role-plays are still useful.
- Remember that for the purpose of the role-plays, the provider only speaks and understands English, and the patient only speaks and understands the target language.

Interpreting Exercise #1

This scenario is for three people.

Receptionist: (In English) "Good morning. How may I help you?"

Interpreter: (Interpret previous statement into target language)

Patient: (In target language) "Yes, I have an appointment with, um, doctor…what was his name? I don't remember. Well, you know, a tall man with a mustache.

Interpreter: (Interpret previous statement into English)

Receptionist: (In English) "Do you have your appointment card with you? I can check the computer. (Pause) OK, you'll be seeing Dr. Gambino today. He's running a little behind, but he should be with you soon. Tell me, are you still working at the restaurant?"

Interpreter: (Interpret previous statement into target language)

Patient: (In target language) "No, I was laid off about three weeks ago. Now I'm looking for work, but I can't find any."

Interpreter: (Interpret previous statement into English)

Receptionist: (In English) "I'm sorry to hear that. Well, have a seat and Dr. Gambino's nurse will call you shortly."

Interpreter: (Interpret previous statement into target language)

Interpreting Exercise #2

This scenario is for three people. Switch roles so that a different group member is now playing the interpreter.

Provider: (In English) "Hello, I'm Grace, Dr. Gambino's nurse. How are you feeling today?"

Interpreter: (Interpret previous statement into target language)

Patient: (In target language) "Pleased to meet you. Well, I'm not feeling very well. Those pills that the doctor gave me made me sick."

Interpreter: (Interpret previous statement into English)

Provider: (In English) "I'm sorry to hear that. Tell me what happened. And what pills were you taking?"

Interpreter: (Interpret previous statement into target language)

Patient: (In target language) "Those little white ones. They made me nauseous. I couldn't sleep all night, tossing and turning. At about six in the morning, I finally slept a little."

Interpreter: (Interprets previous statement into English)

Provider: (In English) "I'll make a note of it in the chart. Well, let me just take your blood pressure and your pulse. Oh sorry, my hands are cold! (Pause.) OK, 140 over 70. Well, just have a seat and the doctor will be right in."

Interpreter: (Interpret previous statement into target language)

Interpreting Exercise #3

Switch roles again so that each person will have had a chance to play the interpreter.

Receptionist: (In English) "Did Dr. Gambino want to see you back?"

Interpreter: (Interpret previous statement into target language)

Patient: (In target language) "Yes, I need an appointment in ... what did the doctor say? I think he said in six weeks."

Interpreter: (Interpret previous statement into English)

Receptionist: (In English) "OK, let me check the doctor's schedule... hmmm, let's see now... how about June 27th at 3:00?"

Interpreter: (Interpret previous statement into target language)

Patient: (In target language) "Don't you have anything earlier? That's when the kids get home from school. Around 10:00 would be good. By then I have the housework done and I'm free to come."

Interpreter: (Interpret previous statement into English)

Receptionist: (In English) "How about 10:20? Here is your appointment card. We'll see you on the 27th."

Interpreting Exercise #4

This scenario is for three people. Switch roles so that a different group member is now playing the interpreter.

Provider: (In English) "Hello. May I see your prescription and your insurance card, please?"

Interpreter: (Interpret previous statement into target language)

Patient: (In target language) "Let's see, here's the prescription, but I don't have insurance."

Interpreter: (Interpret previous statement into English)

Provider: (In English) "OK. Well, this medicine isn't very expensive. It's only $13.25. Do you want to go ahead and buy it here?"

Interpreter: (Interpret previous statement into target language)

Patient: (In target language) "OK, why not? Do I pay for it now?

Interpreter: (Translated the previous statement into English)

Provider: (In English) "No, you pay when you pick it up. I see on the computer that you don't have any drug allergies. So, this medicine is an antibiotic. You take one pill three times a day with food, until they are all gone."

Interpreter: (Interpret previous statement into target language)

Interpreting Exercise #5

This scenario is for three people. Only the patient and provider should have their books open.

Provider: (In English) "Good afternoon. Are you here for a blood test or a urine test?"

Interpreter: (Interpret the previous statement into the target language)

Patient: (In target language) "Well, I think it's for a blood test. Let's see, the doctor gave me these papers."

Interpreter: (Interpret the previous statement into English)

Provider: (In English) "Thank you. Yes, this is for a blood test. Sit down in the blue chair, please, and roll up your sleeve."

Interpreter: (Interpret the previous statement into the target language)

Patient: (In target language) "I don't like having blood drawn. You're not going to take much, are you? It's just that I have to go to work after this, and if you take a lot, I'll be too weak to work."

Interpreter: (Interpret the previous statement into English)

Provider: (In English) "Don't worry. I won't take so much blood that you feel weak. Your body will replace this blood in just a few hours. Now, make a fist please."

Interpreter: (Interpret the previous statement into the target language)

Interpreting Exercise #6

This scenario is for three people. Switch roles so that each person will have had a chance to play the interpreter.

Provider: (In English) "We've already pre-registered you over the phone, so I just have a few more questions. Who should we contact in case of emergency?"

Interpreter: (Interpret previous statement into target language)

Patient: (In target language) "My brother. He lives at 2437 Grant Avenue, and his telephone number is 998-6034."

Interpreter: (Interpret the previous statement into English)

Provider: (In English) "OK. And what kind of work are you doing now?"

Interpreter: (Interpret previous statement into target language)

Patient: (In target language) "I work cleaning houses with a company called 'Mary's Maids.' I have a card here somewhere."

Interpreter: (Interpret the previous statement into English)

Provider: (In English) "Thank you. And could you tell me, do you have commercial insurance? If not, we do have a discount program, if you would like to apply."

Interpreter: (Interpret previous statement into target language)

Interpreting Exercise #7

This scenario is for two people. There is a provider and an interpreter. Both group members may or may not speak the same target language. Only the provider should have his/her book open.

Discharge instructions after an ear operation

Provider: (In English) "Okay, the surgery is finished and everything looks great. Now I need to give you some instructions so you can take care of your ear. I want you to listen carefully; these instructions are important."

Interpreter: (Interpret previous statement into target language)

Provider: (In English) "First, keep your ear and the area behind your ear dry. You may wash your hair only if you keep the ear dry."

Interpreter: (Interpret previous statement into target language)

Provider: (In English) "The best way is to have someone help you as you lean over the sink. Keep a dry towel or cloth over the ear."

Interpreter: (Interpret previous statement into target language)

Provider: (In English) "There is a cotton ball in your ear canal. Leave it there; however, if it comes out, do not put another one in."

Interpreter: (Interpret previous statement into target language)

[Continued on next page.]

Interpreting Exercise #7 continued
(Discharge instructions after an ear operation)

Provider: (In English) "It is common to bleed a little from the ear after surgery. If you do bleed, you may place a cotton ball in the bowl of your ear, but remember, don't put it all the way down into the ear canal!"

Interpreter: (Interpret previous statement into target language)

Provider: (In English) "You will probably hear popping noises in your ear. Also, you may feel dizzy and feel some pain in your ear or neck when you chew."

Interpreter: (Interpret previous statement into target language)

Provider: (In English) "These are normal symptoms and may last for several weeks. However, if you develop a fever greater than 101°F, you should call our office."

Interpreter: (Interpret previous statement into target language)

Provider: (In English) "Here is a prescription for antibiotics. Take one pill daily after your evening meal. We'll see you back here for a follow-up exam in 2 weeks."

Interpreter: (Interpret previous statement into target language)

Interpreting Exercise #8

This scenario is for two people. There is a provider and an interpreter. Both group members may or may not speak the same target language. Only the provider should have his/her book open. Switch roles so that a different person is now playing the interpreter

Instructions on taking birth control pills

Provider: (In English) "Here are your birth control pills. You must take them in the correct way in order for them to be effective. So listen carefully to the instructions, okay?"

Interpreter: (Interpret previous statement into target language)

Provider: (In English) "Start taking the first pill on the first day of your menstrual period. Take one pill every day after that, until the package is all gone. Take your pill at the same time every day."

Interpreter: (Interpret previous statement into target language)

Provider: (In English) "You may find that your period is longer or shorter than usual, or you may not have periods at all while you are on the pill."

Interpreter: (Interpret previous statement into target language)

Provider: (In English) "If you miss one pill, take the pill you missed as soon as you remember it. Then take another pill at the usual time. It's okay to take two pills in one day if this happens."

Interpreter: (Interpret previous statement into target language)

[Continued on next page.]

Interpreting Exercise #8 continued
Instructions on taking birth control pills

Provider: (In English) "If you miss two or more pills, do not take any more pills from this package. Instead, use condoms or another form of birth control until you start your next period. At that time you can start a new package of pills."

Interpreter: (Interpret previous statement into target language)

Provider: (In English) "If you have missed any pills or if you think you might be pregnant, call the clinic. We may recommend you get a pregnancy test."

Interpreter: (Interpret previous statement into target language

Provider: (In English) "Also, please call us if you have any unusual symptoms, such as stomach or chest pain, shortness of breath, dizziness, or headache."

Interpreter: (Interpret previous statement into target language)

Provider: (In English) "Of course, if you have any questions, you can call our 24-hour Nurse Line and ask the nurse on duty to help you. We are always here if you need help!"

Interpreter: (Interpret previous statement into target language)

Lesson 5

CLARIFYING

GOAL

Understand when and how to intervene in the provider/patient dialogue with the purpose of clarifying the communication.

KNOWLEDGE OUTCOMES

- Identify circumstances that require intervention
- Learn guidelines to follow when intervening
- Use strategies for overcoming challenges of high register in communication
- Use strategies for interpreting words/phrases with no linguistic equivalence
- Learn guidelines for interpreting phrases with symbolic meaning
- Use strategies to check understanding

Vocabulary
Clarify
Idiom
Intervene
Linguistic equivalence
Symbolic meaning
Transparent communication
Word pictures

Clarifying

> **Brainstorm**
>
> When should an interpreter shift from the conduit role to the clarifier role?

Introduction

We have already seen that the most fundamental role of the interpreter is that of the conduit: interpret everything that is said, as faithfully and as accurately as possible. Add nothing, omit nothing, and change nothing.

However, sometimes the role of the conduit is not enough to overcome communication barriers. Sometimes, the interpreter may have to interrupt the provider - patient dialogue with a comment or a question. This is called **intervening**. Interpreters should only interrupt the dialogue between patient and provider for the purpose of **clarifying** the communication.

The interpreter should allow the primary conversation to occur between the patient and provider. The role of the clarifier is more invasive than the conduit role and should not be used as frequently as the role of the conduit. This lesson will introduce a variety of strategies and guidelines for successful intervention and clarification.

Guideline for Clarifying

The role of the clarifier can be summarized in this basic guideline: Interpret what is said faithfully, but in such a way that the listener can understand; check for understanding.

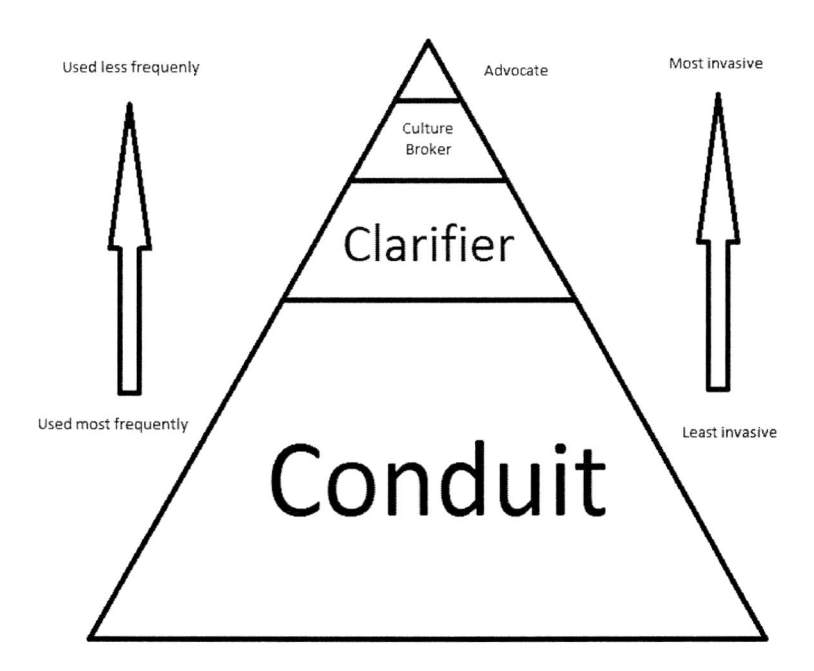

When Intervention Is Necessary

The interpreter may need to intervene in the patient-provider communication when:

- the interpreter needs to have the speaker repeat what he/she said
- the interpreter needs to ask the speaker to use shorter sentences
- the speaker is not pausing enough to allow for interpretation

When there is a linguistic or cultural concern that is causing misunderstanding, the interpreter will have to intervene and take additional steps to clarify the communication. Intervention and clarification may be required when:

- anyone uses language that the interpreter does not understand
- the interpreter suspects, due to non-verbal cues, that the patient does not understand what the provider is saying
- anyone uses a term that must be explained or put in a cultural context to be understood
- a cultural difference is causing a misunderstanding

There may be other instances where the interpreter has to intervene and clarify as well. Next, we will discuss how to intervene.

How to Intervene

Intervening can be difficult for a number of reasons. Trained interpreters are aware that they should be as unobtrusive as possible. However, intervening requires you to come out of the background and speak with your own voice. Additionally, providers are people of authority, and it requires a good deal of self-confidence to interrupt them.

An interpreter needs to be able to intervene effectively. Ineffective intervention can cause a breakdown in the relationship between the patient and provider, as well as undermine the patient or provider's trust in the interpreter.

The example on the following page illustrates ineffective intervention.

Vocabulary

Intervene: come between; interrupt

Clarify: make something more easily understood

Transparent communication: communication where everyone is aware of what is being said

---

Clarifying

Intervention Example #1

As you read through the following example, think about what the interpreter could have done differently to improve the communication between the patient and the provider.

Provider: (In English) Mrs. Dheer, what a pleasure to see you! How are you?"

Interpreter: (Interprets the provider's statement into target language)

Patient: (In target language) "I'm well, doctor. Very busy with so many activities at the temple and at my son's school. And you? How is your baby?

Interpreter: (Interprets the patient's statement into English)

Provider: (In English) Oh, he's fine, just starting to crawl and getting into everything. I'm sure you know! Well, we got the results back from the fine needle biopsy we did last week.

Interpreter: (In English) Um...I don't know how to say that in my language.

Provider: (In English) Well, a fine needle biopsy is a procedure where we use a very thin needle to take a small sample of breast tissue to evaluate in the laboratory, looking for abnormal cells.

Interpreter: (In English) You don't mean she has cancer, do you? Oh no, how terrible! This is going to be a terrible shock to her! What a pity, she's so young! We'll need to handle this very carefully. Telling her could kill her!

Patient: (In target language, very worriedly to the interpreter) Listen, what did the doctor say? I have cancer, right? Oh dear, what am I going to do?

Interpreter: (In target language) Don't worry Mrs. Dheer! The thing is, they found something kind of serious and you'll probably need more tests. But don't worry, there are a lot of support groups that can help you face this. I can give you some names.

Provider: (In English, to the interpreter) Excuse me, what are you telling her? I'd appreciate it if you would just interpret what I say.

Interpreter: (In English) So, is it cancer? What should I do now? (Patient is crying and looking from the interpreter to the doctor with a worried look)

Provider: (In English) Now I'm confused! Are you asking me or is the patient asking me? This is unacceptable!

Intervening Successfully

As you can see from the previous example, ineffective intervention can quickly cause a breakdown in communication. It can also undermine the patient's trust in the interpreter and the provider, as well as the provider's trust in the interpreter.

An interpreter intervenes when there is a linguistic or cultural concern that is causing a misunderstanding, or when the interpreter does not understand what is being said. A good intervention is quick, smooth, and effective in either resolving a problem or bringing it to the provider's attention.

Following these guidelines can help you learn to intervene effectively:

Stay calm. Some interpreters become uncomfortable or even emotional when they have to intervene. Patients pick up on the interpreter's discomfort and may also become worried or emotional. It is important to stay calm at all times.

Make sure the intervention is transparent. Transparent communication simply means that one speaker knows what the interpreter is discussing with the other speaker. For example, if the provider uses a term that has no linguistic equivalent in the target language, you should let the provider know that you will need to explain this term. This way, the provider understands why you are speaking for so long.

Do not make assumptions. An interpreter should not assume that he/she knows what the patient is thinking or

Guidelines for Effective Intervention

- Stay calm.
- Be transparent.
- Don't make assumptions.
- Use third person while intervening.
- Return to conduit interpreting as soon as possible.

Vocabulary

Transparent communication: communication where everyone is aware of what is being said

feeling. If you suspect a problem, confusion, or a concern, ask the person if you are correct. Instead of assuming that a patient does not understand something, it would be better to check with the patient to see if she understood.

Go back to conduit interpreting as quickly as possible, and let the provider resolve the problem. Sometimes an interpreter's intervention solves a problem directly; for example, by asking for a clarification of a word. Sometimes, however, the intervention serves to show that a problem exists; for example, when you ask a patient if he understood, and he says, "No." It is best to simply interpret the response to the provider and let the provider decide how to handle the situation. If you decide to suggest a course of action that would help the situation, it is best to phrase it as a suggestion, and allow the provider to make a decision about how to proceed.

Clarifying

Intervention Example #2

As you read through this example again, notice how the interpreter's use of effective intervention supports, rather than hinders, communication between patient and provider.

Provider: (In English) Mrs. Dheer, what a pleasure to see you! How are you?

Interpreter: (Interprets the provider's statement into target language)

Patient: (In target language) "I'm well doctor. Very busy with so many activities at the temple and at my son's school. And you? How is your baby?

Interpreter: (Interprets the patient's statement into English)

Provider: (In English) "Oh, he's fine, just starting to crawl and getting into everything. I'm sure you know! Well, we got the results back from the fine needle biopsy we did last week."

Interpreter: (In target language) "The interpreter will ask the provider for clarification of a term."

(In English) "This is the interpreter speaking. The interpreter does not know how to interpret 'fine needle biopsy' and requests that you explain the term using simpler language."

The interpreter stays calm.
The interpreter remains transparent by letting the patient know she is going to request clarification.
The interpreter switches from first person to third person and makes it clear who is speaking.

Provider: (In English) Well, a fine needle biopsy is a procedure where we use a very thin needle to take a small sample of breast tissue to evaluate in the laboratory, looking for abnormal cells.

Interpreter: (In target language) "Well, we got the results back from the test we did last week. In this test, we used a very thin needle to take a small sample of breast tissue to evaluate in the laboratory to look for abnormal cells."

Patient: (In target language) "I see. And what were the results?

At this point, the interpreter can step back into the Conduit role and continue interpreting the conversation between the patient and the provider. The interpreter kept the focus on the dialogue between the patient and the provider, and can quickly return to the Conduit role.

© 2014 Cross Cultural Health Care Program

> **Intervention Example #3**
>
> Imagine that the provider is telling a patient how to take some birth control pills. The interpreter senses that the patient is lost. The intervention might sound like this:
>
> **Interpreter:** (In English) "The interpreter is concerned that Mrs. Nguyen does not understand and would like to check."
>
> *The interpreter stays calm.*
>
> *The interpreter provides transparent communication by making sure the provider knows what she is doing before addressing the patient.*
>
> *The interpreter switches from first person to third person. She clearly identifies who is speaking.*
>
> **Provider:** "Oh! Okay, go ahead."
>
> **Interpreter:** (In Vietnamese) "Mrs. Nguyen, speaking as the interpreter, I want to know if you understand what the doctor is saying. Is it clear how to take the birth control pills?"
>
> *The interpreter makes no assumptions, but verifies her suspicion that Mrs. Nguyen does not understand.*
>
> **Patient:** (In Vietnamese) "No, it isn't clear! This is very confusing!"
>
> **Interpreter:** (In English) "No, it isn't clear! This is very confusing!"
>
> *The interpreter goes back to conduit interpreting as quickly as possible and allows the provider to make a decision about how to handle the confusion.*

Strategies for Overcoming Challenges of High Register

Register refers to the level of formality or complexity of the language a person chooses to use. High register speech is very formal and complex. To lower the register of speech means to take something that was said in a complex way and say it in a simpler way.

Sometimes providers use high register speech that a patient may not understand. For example, a doctor might say, "That wound will require extensive observation." To lower the register would be to say, "The wound will have to be watched for a long time."

> **Using a Lower Register**
>
> Consider the following example of a patient with kidney stones:
>
> **Provider:** (In English) To help relieve the pain, you must consume oral fluids. This will help facilitate the passage of the stones into the bladder.
>
> **Interpreter:** (In English) The interpreter would like to ask the provider to repeat the instruction in a simpler language."
>
> **Provider:** (In English) To make the pain less you must drink a lot of water and other liquids. This will help the stones to come out of your body while you are urinating.
>
> After clarifying, the interpreter can go back to the conduit role.

Clarifying

There are some strategies that may be useful for when the provider is using language that is very formal or complex. You will need to choose the appropriate strategy depending on your experience and skill level. The strategies are:

Interpret using the same complicated level of language and watch for patient understanding.

Ask the provider to speak in simpler language.

Lower the register without changing essential meaning. This strategy should *only* be used if the interpreter is very experienced and very familiar with the subject matter being discussed. We discourage less experienced interpreters from using this strategy, as it can easily cause more misunderstanding than it was intended to solve.

Interpreting Words and Phrases with No Linguistic Equivalence

When a word has no linguistic equivalence, it means there is no word that means exactly the same thing in another language. When the provider or patient uses words that have no equivalent word in either English or the target language two useful strategies include:

- ask the provider to explain the word or concept
- use a word picture

Usually, the best strategy is to ask the provider to explain the word or concept. Alternatively, the interpreter can use word pictures. A word picture is a description of what something means. When the phrase in question is a technical medical term, it is recommended that the interpreter inform the provider of exactly what they are going to say to make sure that they do not change the meaning.

For example, suppose the provider used the word "glaucoma," for which there is no word in the patient's language. The interpreter, thinking she knows what

Vocabulary

Idiom: a phrase or expression whose meaning cannot be understood from the meaning of its individual words

Linguistic equivalence: when words or concepts can be expressed equally well in different languages

Symbolic meaning: when words or phrases mean something other than their literal definition

Word picture: a description of what something means

Using Word Pictures

When the speaker uses a word that has no equivalent meaning in the target language, the speaker "sees" a picture in their mind associated with that word. The interpreter then creates a "word picture" to demonstrate the meaning of the word to the listener. See the examples below.

Biopsy: A test in which a small piece of skin or tissue is taken to be examined in a laboratory.

"Sobador" [Spanish]: A *sobador* is a traditional healer who uses manipulation and massage of bones to heal.

Ambulance: A car that takes sick or injured people to the hospital in an emergency.

© 2014 Cross Cultural Health Care Program

glaucoma is, might substitute the phrase "an eye infection." However, glaucoma is not an eye infection, but an increase in pressure inside the eye. If she had informed the provider what she was going to do, the provider would have been able to catch the errors. It might sound like this:

Doctor: (In English) "I'm afraid you have glaucoma."

Interpreter: (In English) "This is the interpreter speaking: there is no word for glaucoma in the target language. I will say that the patient has an eye infection."

Doctor: (In English) "No, that would be incorrect. Tell her that she has high pressure inside her eye."

Interpreting Idioms

If a literal translation of a word or phrase does not make sense, then most likely it is a word or phrase that has **symbolic meaning.** These phrases are sometimes called **idioms.** If idioms are being used, the interpreter could:

- use an equivalent idiom in the target language

Interpreting Idioms
Here are three examples of idioms and suggestions on how to interpret them.

Idiom	Meaning of idiom	How to interpret
(English) This one is hard to call.	This English phrase comes from sports, where a referee must make a "call" about a certain play. It means that a decision is hard to make.	The interpreter could say in their target language: "This decision is hard to make." Or, the interpreter could use an equivalent idiom in the target language, if one exists.
(Spanish) "Río que suena, piedras lleva." Literal translation: "The river that makes noise must be carrying rocks."	The meaning of this phrase is that if there is a sign that something is there, most likely, it is actually there.	In English, the idiom that corresponds to this Spanish phrase might be "Where there's smoke, there's fire."
(Vietnamese) "Gan chua goi Phat bang Anh." Literal translation: "Living near the temple, you will call Buddha your older brother."	In Vietnamese culture, claiming to be a relative of the Buddha would be extremely arrogant. The meaning of this phrase is that becoming too friendly and familiar with something will lead one to be arrogant about it.	An accurate English idiom that conveys the meaning of this phrase would be "Familiarity breeds contempt."

- interpret the underlying meaning, not the exact words
- ask the provider to avoid using idioms (if they use them frequently)
- ask for clarification if the intended meaning is unclear

Checking for Understanding

An important aspect of acting as a Clarifier is to constantly check for provider and patient understanding. The interpreter must always be aware of non-verbal cues that indicate a lack of understanding. Two common indicators of this are puzzled expressions or distracted eye contact (looking all over the room instead of focusing on the speaker).

If the interpreter suspects that someone is confused, they should stop the interview to intervene and clarify. They might say to the provider, "The interpreter would like to ask if the patient has understood." The provider now knows that the interpreter is going to check to see if the patient needs clarification.

The best way may be to simply ask the patient directly, "Do you understand?" However, this question may not always provide the correct information. Patients might answer the question "Do you understand?" with a nod or "yes" to avoid the embarrassment of admitting that they did not understand at all.

Besides asking directly if the patient understands, the interpreter could ask the patient to repeat instructions in their own words. Some providers know this technique as "teach-back".

If the patient really is confused, the interpreter should communicate that to the provider so that the provider can explain. The interpreter should avoid trying to provide an explanation. If the provider consistently uses complicated language, the interpreter should intervene and directly request that the provider use simpler language.

Summary

Remember, the main guideline for the role of the clarifier is:

Interpret what is said faithfully but in such a way that the listener can understand; check for understanding.

When clarifying, be sure to take your own level of skill and knowledge into account. Remember that an interpreter should always take on the least intrusive role possible, while facilitating effective communication. Whenever possible, use your intervention skills to bring a potential misunderstanding to the provider's attention and allow the provider to resolve the issue.

Skill Development

Clarifying and Intervening Exercises

In the following exercises, you will practice intervening and clarifying as discussed in this lesson.

As you analyze the interpretation after each scenario, be sure to focus on the following:

- Did the interpreter intervene appropriately? Did they follow the guidelines on how to intervene?

- Did the interpreter shift into the clarifier role when high register, phrases with no linguistic equivalent or idioms were used?

- Did the interpreter use appropriate strategies to clarify the communication?

Beginning skill level: Before doing these exercises, each member of the group should identify and individually make a list of words or concepts that might require intervening and clarifying. Look for instances of high register, lack of linguistic equivalency and the use of idioms. Then, role-play through the scenario, allowing the interpreter to practice intervening at the points discussed. Use available resources (such as medical glossaries) to define terms, if necessary.

Advanced Skill Level: If you and your group members are at an advanced interpreter skill level, the group members playing the provider and patient should role-play through the scenario with the interpreter interpreting. The interpreter will have to make decisions about when to intervene in the dialogue and how to clarify the communication as they hear the conversation for the first time.

Interpreting Exercise #1

This scenario is for three people. Remember, only the patient and provider should have their books open. The interpreter should request clarification as needed using the skills discussed in this lesson.

The patient is a three-year-old boy who is here for a follow-up visit after the doctor removed a splinter from the bottom of his foot. The mother is very worried.

Provider: (In English) "Last week I instructed you to do hot soaks three times a day and give him Tylenol for the pain. Have you been complying with my instructions?"

Interpreter: (Interpret previous statement into target language)

Patient: (In target language) "Yes, Doctor, I did what you told me. But on Friday, I saw that it was really red and hot, so I called on Saturday to see if I should bring him in and they said they'd call to let me know, but they never called."

Interpreter: (Interpret previous statement into English)

Provider: (In English) "Well, I'm not sure what to make of your son's foot, Mrs. Dominguez. I thought I had removed the splinter last week, but, I must say I'm concerned about this inflammation and the amount of drainage. I'd like to get an X-ray just to make sure there's nothing left inside."

Interpreter: (Interpret previous statement into target language)

Patient: (In target language) "Well, I think that there must be something still inside. You see how he's walking crooked? He doesn't want to step on it. And all this because he went out for one moment without his shoes. My goodness, I just don't know what to do with this boy! He's terrible, he never obeys me. I tell him that the Boogey Man is going to get him if he doesn't pay attention to me, but it doesn't help."

Interpreter: (Interpret previous statement into English)

Provider: (In English) "Yes, well, three-year-olds can be a handful. If there is something still in that foot, I'll have to refer him to the surgeons at the children's hospital, where they specialize in pediatric cases like this."

Interpreter: (Interpret previous statement into target language)

© 2014 Cross Cultural Health Care Program

Interpreting Exercise #2

This scenario is for **three or four** people. Switch roles so that a different group member is now playing the interpreter. If there are three people participating, one person can play both the patient and the daughter.

The patient is a sixty-seven-year-old woman who has come to the optometrist for a routine eye exam. The doctor has detected glaucoma and has asked the patient's adult daughter to come in to discuss the findings.

Provider: (In English) "I need to tell you that I found very elevated pressure in your left eye. This is a sure sign of glaucoma. Now, we can control glaucoma with eye drops, but if left untreated, this condition will lead to blindness in the long run."

Interpreter: (Interprets previous statement into target language)

Daughter: (In target language) "Oh no Mother, how terrible! How can that be? She has never complained about anything."

Interpreter: (Interprets previous statement into English)

Provider: (In English) "Actually, glaucoma is painless and symptomless and really can't be detected without a professional eye exam. Before we start you on treatment, I'd like to check your visual fields, to see if there's been any damage to the optical nerve, which I suspect there has been."

Interpreter: (Interprets previous statement into target language)

Patient: (In target language) "Is this disease what makes my eye burn and itch so much?"

Interpreter: (Interprets previous statement into English)

Provider: (In English) "No, ma'am, like I said, glaucoma doesn't have symptoms that you'd feel. That itching is probably due to seasonal allergies or dry eyes from sun exposure."

Interpreter: (Interprets previous statement into target language)

Interpreting Exercise #3

This role-play is for three people. Switch roles again so that each person will have had a chance to play the interpreter.

The patient is a young man who twisted his knee playing soccer.

Provider: (In English) "So, the nurse tells me you twisted your knee playing soccer. Let's see what we've got here. Hmmm, well now, does that hurt?"

Interpreter: (Interprets previous statement into target language)

Patient: (In target language) "Ouch!!! Yes, it really hurts! And can't you see how it's all swollen? Yesterday, I could hardly walk. Oh, my God!"

Interpreter: (Interprets previous statement into English)

Provider: (In English) "Well, it appears that the anterior ligament may be compromised. If it's ripped, we may have to intervene surgically. I'm going to give you a prescription for an anti-inflammatory to see if we can't get that swelling down, as well as something for the pain. And let's make you an appointment to get that X-rayed."

Interpreter: (Interprets previous statement into target language)

Patient: (In target language) "OK. And, well, it's not that I'm lazy, but, could you give me some letter for my boss so I could get a few days off? I just can't work like this."

Interpreter: (Interprets previous statement into English)

Provider: (In English) "Of course, I'll have the nurse type up a work release."

Interpreter: (Interprets previous statement into target language)

Interpreting Exercise #4

This scenario is for three people. Only the patient and provider should have their books open.

The patient is a 56-year-old man who is being seen in a surgery clinic in preparation for a gall bladder surgery.

Provider: (In English) "Hello, how are we feeling today? Ready for your surgery?"

Interpreter: (Interprets previous statement into target language)

Patient: (In target language) "Yes, doctor, but I do have a bit of a cold. I don't know if that could be a problem."

Interpreter: (Interprets previous statement into English)

Provider: (In English) "No, as long as you don't have a fever, you'll be A-OK. Now, I want to make sure you understand what we've got in mind for you. We're going to remove your gall bladder because of the gall stones. I hope we can do the procedure laparoscopically, but we may have to resort to the old method which involves a major incision."

Interpreter: (Interprets previous statement into target language)

Patient: (In target language) "How long will I be hospitalized? Will I be given general anesthesia?"

Interpreter: (Interprets previous statement into English)

Provider: (In English) "If we do the laparoscopy, we'll have you in and out quick as a whistle, after just one night. If we have to make a major incision, though, we'll have to keep you around for a bit longer, maybe up to a week. As for the anesthesia, yes, you'll have a general, given through an I.V."

Interpreter: (Interprets previous statement into target language)

Interpreting Exercise #5

This scenario is for three people. Switch roles so that a different group member is now playing the interpreter.

The patient is a 30-year-old man who has a persistent itchy rash.

Provider: (In English) "So, tell me how the rash has been? Still itching? Did the pills I gave you help at all?"

Interpreter: (Interprets previous statement into target language)

Patient: (In target language) "When I was taking both kinds of pills, I felt fine, but I ran out of one kind of pill and I stopped taking the others so often because you told me they were so dangerous. Now I'm taking half a pill every other day, and the itching is back again."

Interpreter: (Interprets previous statement into English)

Provider: (In English) "Wait a minute, wait a minute. You're just taking half a pill every other day? I've told you before, you can't go adjusting your own medication. This medicine has to be taken a certain way or it has serious potential side effects. You can't just lower the dose overnight. And if you ran out of the others, why didn't you call? Those pills aren't as toxic."

Interpreter: (Interprets previous statement into target language)

Patient: (In target language) "Oh...It's just that you kind of scared me when you told me that the pills could make my bones brittle. It doesn't seem right to be taking so many different pills."

Interpreter: (Interprets previous statement into English)

Provider: (In English) "I hear you. So, let us do this: start taking one whole pill every other day. And I'm going to give you another prescription for the other pills as well. If we can't get a handle on this in another month, I'll take the case to grand rounds. But no more fooling around with your medicines, OK?"

Interpreter: (Interprets previous statement into target language)

Interpreting Exercise #6

This scenario is for three people. Switch roles so that each person will have had a chance to play the interpreter.

The patient is a 47-year-old woman being seen in primary care for acute shoulder pain.

Provider: (In English) "Tell me, how long has your shoulder been hurting like this? Didn't one of our residents see you about this same problem last summer?"

Interpreter: (Interprets previous statement into target language)

Patient: (In target language) "Yes. You know, I've had this pain for a long time, but lately it's getting worse. It hurts to lift my arm, it hurts to move it. I'm sick and tired of hurting all the time."

Interpreter: (Interprets previous statement into English)

Provider: (In English) "I see you've already tried anti-inflammatories and hot soaks. I think I'm going to order some tests to see if we're not looking at something more serious here than strained muscles. I'd like to get some X-rays and some blood tests. Didn't you mention that your father suffered from rheumatoid arthritis?"

Interpreter: (Interprets previous statement into target language)

Patient: (In target language) "Well, he always said he had it, but who knows? Do you think I could have that?"

Interpreter: (Interprets previous statement into English)

Provider: (In English) "I don't really know. Let's get those tests and then discuss it. Here's a referral to radiology and a lab slip. How about if I see you back in 2 weeks?"

Interpreter: (Interprets previous statement into target language)

Clarifying

Interpreting Exercise #7

This scenario is for two people. There is a provider and an interpreter. Both group members may or may not speak the same target language. Only the provider should have his/her book open.

Instructions for a Flexible Sigmoidoscopy

Provider: (In English) "Your doctor has requested that you have a Flexible Sigmoidoscopy, which is a procedure that lets the doctor see the inside of the rectum and the sigmoid colon."

Interpreter: (Interprets previous statement into target language)

Provider: (In English) "To prepare for this procedure you need to do a number of things, all of which are very important."

Interpreter: (Interprets previous statement into target language)

Provider: (In English) "First of all, discontinue the following medications: iron, seven days before the procedure; aspirin 10 days before the procedure; and arthritis medications like Motrin or Advil two days before the procedure."

Interpreter: (Interprets previous statement into target language)

Provider: (In English) "You should **not** suspend any of the following: prednisone, heart medications, lung medications or diabetes medications. You may take Tylenol if you need it."

Interpreter: (Interprets previous statement into target language)

Provider: (In English) "The night before the procedure, drink one whole bottle of magnesium citrate."

Interpreter: (Interprets previous statement into target language)

Provider: (In English) "On the day of the procedure, don't eat anything for two hours before the exam, except maybe for a little water."

Interpreter: (Interprets previous statement into target language
[Continued on next page]

Interpreting Exercise #7 continued
(Instructions for a Flexible Sigmoidoscopy)

Provider: (In English) "Take two Fleets enemas, one two hours before the appointment, and the other just one hour before the appointment."

Interpreter: (Interprets previous statement into target language)

Provider: (In English) "Report to the Special Procedures Unit at least 15 minutes before the scheduled appointment."

Interpreter: (Interprets previous statement into target language)

Provider: (In English) "Don't forget, someone will have to drive you home, because the doctor will probably administer a sedative."

Interpreter: (Interprets previous statement into target language)

Interpreting Exercise #8

This scenario is for two people. There is a provider and an interpreter. Both group members may or may not speak the same target language. Only the provider should have his/her book open.

Preparation for a Barium Enema

Provider: (In English) "Your doctor has requested that you have a Barium Enema, which is a type of X-ray that will allow her to see if there are any problems in your colon."

Interpreter: (Interprets previous statement into target language)

Provider: (In English) "You need to prepare carefully for this procedure, because, if you don't, we will have to reschedule you."

Interpreter: (Interprets previous statement into target language)

Provider: (In English) "So, one day before the procedure, eat a clear liquid diet all day. That means things like apple juice, broth, plain jello, black coffee and tea without the cream. Also, drink five eight-ounce glasses of water."

Interpreter: (Interprets previous statement into target language)

Provider: (In English) "At 7:00 p.m., take 10 ounces of magnesium citrate, and at 10:00 p.m., take three tablets of Bisacodyl, without crushing the tablets, with a glass of water."

Interpreter: (Interprets previous statement into target language)

Provider: (In English) "On the day of the procedure, suspend all food and water for two hours before the appointment time. Also, insert one Bisacodyl suppository into the rectum and retain it for at least 15 minutes."

Interpreter: (Interprets previous statement into target language)

Provider: (In English) "Do not forget to take all your prescription medications, although if you take anything for diabetes, you'd better talk to your doctor first."

[Interpreter: (Interprets previous statement into target language)

Provider: (In English) "Please come to the Special Procedures Unit at least 15 minutes before your appointment time. Be aware that the medications they give you may cause some cramping afterward."

Interpreter: (Interprets previous statement into target language)

Lesson 6

MANAGING THE FLOW OF THE SESSION

GOAL

Develop techniques for facilitating a successful interpreting session and strategies for handling difficult interpreting circumstances.

KNOWLEDGE OUTCOMES

- Identify specific kinds of information to include in pre-sessions with the patient and provider

- Identify three types of interpreter positions and describe the benefits and risks of each

- Identify six guidelines for facilitating the flow of the conversation

Vocabulary

Pre-session

Position

> **Brainstorm**
>
> Imagine trying to interpret a conversation between two people who have never worked with an interpreter before. They look at the interpreter instead of each other, talk in long sentences without pausing.
>
> Why do you think this might be a problem?
> What are some strategies you might use as an interpreter to help manage the flow of the conversation?

Introduction

Although the patient and provider should always be in control of the medical interview, the interpreter is the best person to facilitate the flow of communication. Certain steps can enable that process and help the patient and provider focus on each other rather than on the interpreter.

Many patients and providers have limited experience with interpreters. It is important to teach both the patient and provider how to work successfully with an interpreter. This lesson will focus on skills and strategies that that can be done at the beginning and throughout an interpreting session that will help the interpreter facilitate the conversation effectively.

> **Vocabulary**
>
> **Pre-session:** a brief conversation with the patient or provider before an interpreted encounter, to establish expectations and guidelines about the interpreter's role

Pre-sessions

Trust among the three members of the interpreted interview is of utmost importance. Therefore, before the session starts, it is important for you to establish the beginnings of a trusting relationship. A **pre-session** is the time to introduce the role of the interpreter and to ask any questions before the interpreting begins.

A pre-session not only helps build trust, but also provides the interpreter with an opportunity to establish themselves as a professional, explain how the interpretation will work, and judge the linguistic level of the patient. Exactly what is included in a pre-session will depend on how much time is available and whether or not the interpreter has worked with the particular patient or provider before.

Pre-Session with the Patient

Ideally, the pre-session might sound like this:

*Hello. My name is **(your name)**. I'm the **(target language)** interpreter and I work for **(name of agency/organization)**.*

There are few important things to know that will help me interpret for you today:

- *Everything that you say today will be confidential, so please speak freely.*
- *I will interpret everything that you say, exactly as you say it. I will do the same for the doctor.*
- *Please speak directly to the doctor.*
- *Please pause frequently so that I can interpret what you say accurately.*
- *When I raise my hand, please pause so that I can interpret.*
- *I may need to take notes during the session, but if I do so, I will destroy them at the end of the session."*

Although including all of this information in the pre-session is ideal, in reality, you may not have time to convey it all. If you have less time, you might say something like this:

"Hello, my name is (your name), and I will be your (language) interpreter today. I will interpret everything you say and keep it confidential. Please speak directly to the doctor and pause frequently so that I can interpret."

The exact words and phrases that you use to conduct your pre-session may be slightly different. However, you should aim to include as much of the information as possible in the time you have available.

Pre-Session with the Provider

Pre-sessions with providers almost always take place as the provider enters the exam room to start the medical interview. Most providers do not expect it. There are many important pieces of information to communicate during the pre-session with the provider. The pre-session might sound like this:

"Hello. My name is (your name). I'm the (target language) interpreter and I work for (name of agency/organization). There are few important things to know that will help me interpret for you today:

- *I will interpret everything you say, exactly as you say it. I will do the same for the patient.*
- *Please speak directly to the patient.*
- *Please pause frequently so that I can interpret what you say accurately.*
- *When I raise my hand, please pause so that I can interpret.*
- *Is there anything special I need to know about this session?*

Again, you may not have time to cover all of this information with the provider. A shortened pre-session might sound like this:

"Hello, my name is (name), and I will be your (language) interpreter today. I will interpret everything you say. Please speak directly to the patient and pause frequently so that I can interpret."

Additional Pre-Session Guidelines

If you work with the same patient or provider repeatedly, you do not have to go through the entire pre-session every time. A simple greeting is enough.

In addition to these guidelines, remember the following:

- patient pre-sessions usually take place in the waiting room or in the exam room before the provider arrives
- a polite chat will help build trust and allow you to note a patient's accent, regional vocabulary, and level of speech
- if you arrive after the doctor has already started, the pre-session should still be conducted, but briefly

A patient may tell you all the details of their medical problem whether you want them to or not. Unfortunately, sometimes these patients will also then expect you to repeat it for the doctor ("Oh, just tell her what I told you in the waiting room.") This would not be appropriate; it is very important for patients to tell their own stories, because they often include details they omitted the first time around.

If possible, try to avoid putting yourself in a situation where you are alone with the patient without the doctor present. If a patient begins to tell her medical history, an interpreter can simply emphasize "how important it will be to tell that to the doctor." The best way to avoid this is to simply excuse yourself for 'a moment' and leave the room.

What Not To Cover in a Pre-Session

Topics that should **not** be included in a pre-session:

- a history of the patient's problem;
- topics that might be controversial, such as politics, religion, or morality.

The interpreter must always strive to be impartial, and discussing such topics generally do not help the interpreter be impartial. Guidelines for maintaining impartiality can be found in both the IMIA and NCIHC codes of ethics:

- The IMIA Standards state that the interpreter "refrains from asking personal probing questions outside the scope of interpreting tasks." (IMIA, IMIA)
- The NCIHC Standards state that "the interpreter does not allow personal judgments or cultural values to influence objectivity." (NCIHC, NCHIC)

Interpreter Positioning

The **position** of the interpreter can influence how the patient and the provider relate to each other. Does the interpreter sit or stand? Does she/he look at the patient or the provider when speaking? There are many decisions that an interpreter must make when they first step into a room. The ultimate goal of an interpreter is to facilitate and support the communication between the patient and provider.

Interpreter Position #1

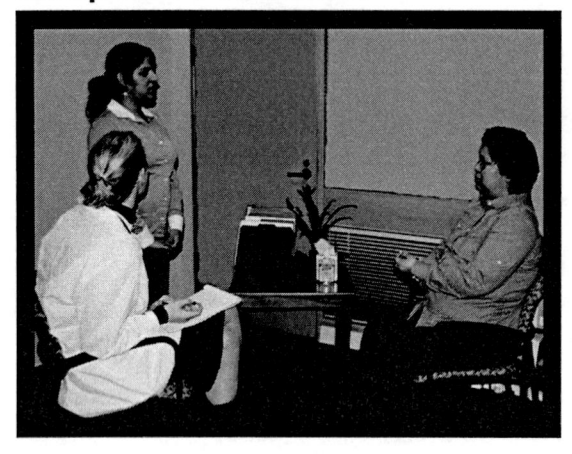

Interpreter position #1: The interpreter stands or sits beside the provider, facing the patient.

Benefits:
- the patient can easily see the interpreter and the provider
- the patient is more likely to talk to the provider

Risks:
- if the interpreter is on the same 'side' as the provider, it may set up a power dynamic and may intimidate the patient
- The interpreter may get in the way of the provider (National Council on Interpreting in Health Care)
- The patient may start speaking directly to the interpreter, as the position #1 photo shows

Vocabulary

Position: where the interpreter places themselves in the triadic encounter

Interpreter Position #2

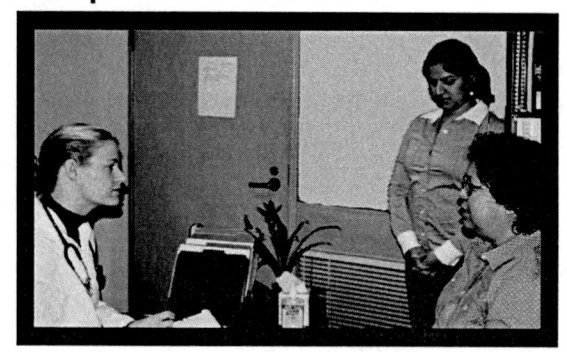

Interpreter position #2: The interpreter stands or sits beside the patient at a 45° angle to the patient.

Benefits:
- the patient is encouraged to speak directly to the provider
- the patient may have the sense that they are being supported by the interpreter beside them

Risks:
- the provider may start speaking directly to the interpreter, and not the patient
- the patient may feel that, because of the support of the interpreter, it is okay for them to confide in the interpreter, and not speak directly to the provider (National Council on Interpreting in Health Care)
- the patient may turn to look at the interpreter if they are more comfortable looking at the speaker's lips

Interpreter Position #3

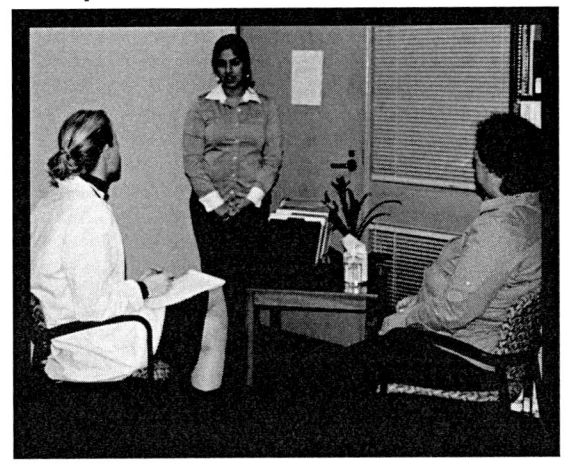

Interpreter position #3: The interpreter stands or sits between patient and provider, forming a triangle.

Benefits:
- in a triangle, each person can see the other two people equally well

Risks:
- the patient and provider will tend to speak to the interpreter instead of each other
- the interpreter can become the focus of attention
- this position does not support direct communication between the patient and the provider

The Ideal Interpreter Position

Each of the interpreter positions described above have their benefits and disadvantages. The ideal position is Interpreter Position #2, where the interpreter is beside the patient and at a 45° angle to the patient.

The interpreter should be positioned in a way that facilitates and encourages the patient-provider communication. The interpreter should be unobtrusive, and eye contact between the patient and the provider should be encouraged. It may not always be possible for the interpreter to be in this ideal position, so it is important to be aware of the benefits and drawbacks of the other possible positions.

It may seem that Interpreter Position #1 (where the interpreter stands or sits beside the provider and in front of the patient) encourages direct communication between the patient and the provider, similar to the way that Interpreter Position #2 does. However, this position also contributes to a potentially disruptive and intimidating power dynamic.

In Western biomedicine, there is typically an imbalance of power, where the provider has more power and control in a medical setting. An interpreter can exercise the same dominance and power as the provider if they are not careful. However, by being a trained professional and an advocate when necessary, an interpreter can help to equalize the power balance.

By choosing to sit or stand beside the patient, (Interpreter Position #2), the interpreter not only encourages direct patient-provider communication but also contributes to a more equal power balance between the patient and the provider.

When the Ideal Position Is Not Possible

There are some situations when the interpreter will not be able to position themselves next to the patient. In these situations, remember that the goal of the interpreter is to facilitate communication between patient and provider without being disruptive. With this in mind, the interpreter should position themselves accordingly.

During physical exams, the best option is for the interpreter to stand behind a curtain. Sometimes there is no curtain, but the interpreter needs to be present. In these cases, one option is to stand at the head of the exam table, where you can speak easily to the patient and doctor but cannot see under the sheets. Another option is for the interpreter to remain in the room, but face the wall, so that she can hear what is being said but not see.

The same logic is applied for positioning in surgery or during other procedures: you should be out of the provider's way, close to the patient's head to aid communication, but not so close so as to be intrusive.

There are many situations where the ideal position for the interpreter may not be clear. For instance, there may be many non-English speaking family members present. Or, you may work in a teaching hospital, where there are other doctors and medical students in the room. There may not be any room to sit or stand beside the patient.

Each situation will be different, and the interpreter will have to make a decision about which position will help them to best facilitate the conversation, encourage direct communication between the patient and the provider, and contribute to a more equal power balance between the patient and the provider.

Eye Contact

Not only is the position of the interpreter important, but where the interpreter looks is also important. In many cultures, people are expected to look at the person to whom they are talking. The listener's eye contact tells the speaker that he is being listened to.

Sometimes, you can be effective in getting a provider to talk to the patient by looking at the patient, not the provider, while the provider speaks. Similarly, by looking at the provider while the patient speaks, the interpreter can direct the patient's attention. By looking down and avoiding eye contact altogether, the interpreter can "remove" herself/himself and discourage others from speaking to the interpreter directly.

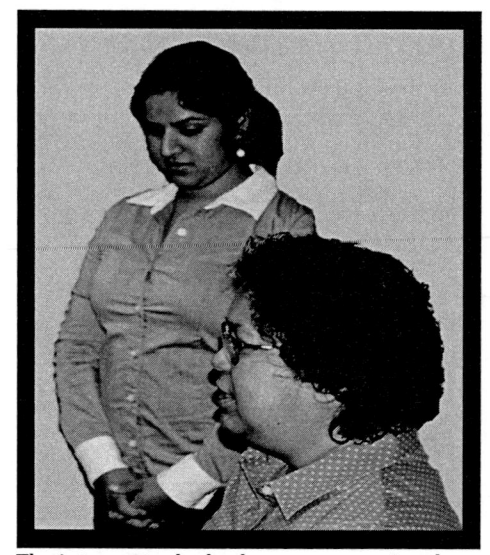

The interpreter looks down, encouraging the patient to look at the provider.

Looking at someone directly in the eye may be considered disrespectful in some cultures. With that in mind, remember that regardless of the culture of the patient and the provider, the ultimate goal of the interpreter is to facilitate the communication and understanding between the patient and provider. The techniques and strategies we have discussed here are simply guidelines. You must make decisions that will allow you to most effectively facilitate the conversation.

Handling Difficult Interpreting Circumstances

There will inevitably be challenging situations that arise while interpreting, despite the interpreter's best efforts to lay the groundwork for a successful encounter. It is not your responsibility to handle medical concerns, but it is your responsibility to resolve situations that arise from communication problems or differences in culture.

Although it is important to strive for the ideal interpreted encounter, the interpreter must be prepared for unexpected difficulties that may arise. Sometimes problems occur because providers or patients are not used to working with an interpreter. It is important for the interpreter to remain flexible and have tools and guidelines for when things do not go as expected. For instance:

Family members' input: You should interpret everything that is said during the interpreted session by anyone involved, including family members. If a family member starts to consult with the patient during a medical interview, begin a simultaneous interpretation for the provider if you are comfortable with simultaneous interpreting. If everyone is talking at once, you may intervene and ask each person to take turns speaking. This will allow you to interpret more effectively.

Discussions between residents and attending physicians: The only partial exception to the rule of "interpret everything" relates to the educational discussions that go on between residents and attending physicians at teaching hospitals. If, during a medical interview, the attending begins to discuss technical aspects of the case with the resident, it is usually difficult, if not impossible, to interpret everything, simply because the vocabulary is so technical. Many interpreters deal with this situation by telling the patient that the senior doctor is teaching the student doctor about the case using very technical words.

The patient refuses the services of the interpreter: Patients refuse interpreters for many reasons. They may feel their English is good and does not require interpretation. They may prefer to have a family member interpret. They may feel some rejection of the interpreter because of racial, political or religious biases. In these cases, it is important for you to know the institution's policy on the issue. Some clinics may allow you to leave if the patient declines the service and signs a waiver, while others leave the decision up to the doctor.

Many hospitals will explain or allow you to explain that the interpreter is also there for the doctor and the hospital's benefit to make certain that the interpretation is accurate.

The provider feels that they speak enough of the target language to "get along": In this situation, the interpreter can remain present in the room while the provider speaks to the patient in the target language, staying alert to any errors. The interpreter can intervene as needed to make corrections or clarifications.

When these situations arise, the interpreter should follow the guidelines laid out in this lesson and remember to use the Code of Ethics as a guide. In addition to the practice provided in this training, medical interpreters need a support network that will allow them to discuss these situations and decide how best to respond to them.

Summary

Conducting pre-sessions develops trust, and interpreter positioning facilitates the patient-provider relationship. These steps lay the groundwork for a successful interpreting session.

During the interpreted encounter, the interpreter can use positioning, eye contact, and intervening as needed in order to facilitate the flow of communication. When difficult situations arise, the interpreter should remember to use the strategies outlined in this lesson and use the Code of Ethics as a resource to guide their response.

Skill Development

Interpreting in Difficult Situations

How would you handle the following challenging interpreting situations? Brainstorm strategies and ideas about how to facilitate effective communication in each of these situations.

Remember: Refer to the Code of Ethics as needed to determine the best course of action. There may be more than one good way to handle difficult situations.

- The provider wants to practice his language skills and doesn't feel the need to have an interpreter.

- The speaker talks without pausing for the interpreter to interpret.

- When the interpreter arrives, the provider has already started.

- When the provider arrives, he/she is in a hurry and is not interested in a pre-session.

- Many family members are present in the room and talking at the same time.

- The attending physician is discussing the case with residents in front of the patient.

- The nurse starts to chat with the interpreter in front of the patient.

- The patient refuses interpreter services.

- The patient enters the hospital in an emergency situation.

- The patient's family member insists on interpreting for the patient.

Skill Development

Role-play: Pre-session

This exercise can be done in pairs or groups of three, with an interpreter, a patient, and/or a provider. The interpreter can practice introducing themselves to the patient and/or provider in the appropriate target language. Remember to include the following points in your pre-session as appropriate:

- Interpreter name
- Agency
- Interpret everything said
- Confidentiality
- Note-taking if applicable

Role-play: Managing speakers who don't pause

This exercise can be done in pairs or groups of three, with an interpreter, a patient, and/or a provider. The patient or provider should speak without pausing, so that the interpreter can practice effective intervention to manage the flow of the conversation. Participants can make up dialogue, or use the following scripts to get started:

"It appears you have a bacterial infection. I am going to prescribe an antibiotic to fight the bacteria that are causing your symptoms. It's very important that you take this medicine exactly as prescribed, and that you take all of the medicine in your prescription, even if you feel better before you finish the prescription. Even if you feel better, it's possible that you might still have an infection, and if you stop taking the medicine too early, your symptoms could come back. You can get the prescription filled at your pharmacy; just let the nurse know where you would like to pick up the medication so that we can call it in. You'll want to take the medication with some food, or else it might upset your stomach. You'll take the medicine twice per day, once in the morning, and once at night. You should feel better within a day or two, but remember to take the entire course of antibiotics to ensure that the treatment is effective. Be sure to make a follow-up appointment before you leave with the front desk. I'd like to see you back here in two weeks. If you aren't feeling better within a few days, you should come back sooner."

Skill Development

Role-play: Managing speakers who don't pause, continued

The following script can be used for the patient. Remember to speak without pausing, so that the interpreter can practice intervening.

"Doctor, I'm very worried about my daughter. I have been using the ear drops you gave me last time I came in, but she doesn't seem to be getting better. She cries and cries, and I can't seem to do anything to help her. She keeps touching her ears and crying, and she hardly sleeps. Her fever went down, but then this morning, it was back up to 102, and that's when I decided to bring her in to see you again. It just doesn't seem like she's getting better. My sister's son had an ear infection that got out of control, and now he has partial hearing loss! I don't want that to happen to my daughter. That would just be terrible; she's so young. I'm so worried, and she won't sleep at all. I'm up all night with her. She's always been so healthy; I just can't understand why she's not getting better. I'm doing everything you told me to do, but it doesn't seem like anything is working. I can't take her to daycare until she's all better, so I've been missing work. Money is already tight as it is, and I can't afford to miss any more work. I just feel so bad for my little girl! I wish there was something I could do to help her. What else can we do?"

Lesson 7

MEMORY DEVELOPMENT

GOAL

Develop techniques to help increase short-term memory and accurate recall.

KNOWLEDGE OUTCOMES

- Identify techniques to improve short-term memory

Vocabulary

Chunking

Long-term memory

Shadowing

Short-term memory

Very short-term memory

Visualization

> **Brainstorm**
>
> Why do you think it is important for an interpreter to develop their memory?
>
> What techniques have you used when you needed to remember words or concepts in the past? Think about taking tests, memorizing a password, or remembering an unfamiliar address while you look for a building.

Introduction

Memory is an essential tool for an interpreter. Improving memory skills, like learning new vocabulary, must be done continually, little by little. This lesson describes techniques to help improve general memory, number retention and note-taking skills.

Types of Memory

For an interpreter, a good memory is an absolute necessity. In interpreting, we use three different types of memory.

Very short-term memory allows you to hold an exact string of numbers in your head for 5-7 seconds. After that amount of time, those numbers will be forgotten.

Short-term memory helps you recall concepts or ideas for a short period of time. Working to improve short term memory will provide the most immediate results for a medical interpreter. **Short term memory is the focus of this lesson.**

Long-term memory is what you have learned in the past that stays with you over time. Long-term memory can be improved by studying something over a long period of time. For example, long term memory is used to remember vocabulary words that you need to recall regularly.

Techniques for Improving Short-Term Memory

Some techniques that can be used during the process of medical interpreting are:

- concentrating
- visualizing
- repeating key phrases
- counting points
- writing down numbers
- chunking
- word association

Concentrating

Concentrating is perhaps the most basic and important memory development technique. You cannot retain what you have heard accurately unless you are focused on what is said. You may need to clear your mind of any thoughts unrelated to what you are hearing. Silence your own mental voice so that you can hear the voice of the person for whom you are interpreting.

Visualization

When listening to a speaker, visualize the series of events being recounted. Playing

Memory Development

back this "video" of events can help you remember the series of events.

Visualization might look something like this:

Patient: (In target language) "I usually go to bed at 11:00 p.m. Then I usually wake up in pain around 4:00 a.m. and toss and turn and try to get comfortable. Sometimes I put my feet up on pillows, and then I usually doze off until I wake up for work.

Interpreter: (While patient is speaking, visualize the series of events)

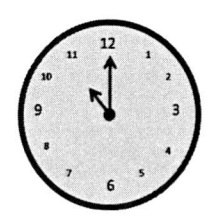

"I usually **go to bed** at 11:00 PM."

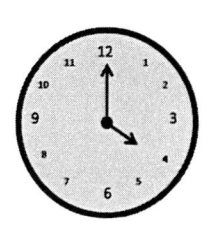

"Then I usually **wake up in pain** around 4:00 a.m., **toss and turn** and **try to get comfortable**.

Sometimes I put my **feet up on pillows**, and then I usually **doze off** until **I wake up for work**."

Repeating Key Phrases

Repeat key phrases in your mind and repeat those key phrases until you have an opportunity to interpret. By repeating the key phrases as you listen, you create a pathway in your brain that makes it easier to "find" those key words again. Be sure to still interpret everything that is said.

In the following paragraph, the bold words are those the interpreter might want to repeat in their head while listening:

"Well, doctor, I **don't know** how it started, really. I mean, **one day** I was **fine**, then the **next day**, I **woke up** so **weak** and **nauseated**. **Suddenly**, I started **vomiting**, maybe **four or five times** I vomited."

Counting Key Points

When a speaker is listing a number of items, you can count off the items in your head.

For example, the nurse asks:
"Have you or has anyone in your family suffered from a serious disease, such as diabetes, cancer, heart disease or glaucoma?"

It may help to count off the diseases when you get to the list:

- [diabetes] one
- [cancer] two
- [heart disease] three
- [glaucoma] four

Now, when you get to this list, you know that you have four diseases to name.

Writing Down Numbers

You can write down numbers as they are said so that you can look at them as you interpret. It can also help to picture the number in your mind.

© 2014 Cross Cultural Health Care Program

Chunking

When you hear large amounts of material to be interpreted, you can find patterns in the information and arrange it into groups or "chunks" in your mind to make it easier to remember.

For example, the provider might ask the patient, "Have you had any symptoms such as dizziness, shortness of breath, heart palpitations, numbness in your hands or feet, confusion, or memory loss?"

You might find it easier to remember each symptom if you associate each one with an area of the body. You might think:

- [Head]: dizziness, confusion, memory loss
- [Chest]: heart palpitations, shortness of breath
- [Extremities]: numbness in hands and feet

Chunking can be helpful when trying to remember long strings of numbers.

For instance, it would be hard to remember **3849872547** as one long string.

However, chunking this number into phone number format makes it easier to remember: **384 – 987 - 2547.**

Word Association

Word association involves linking a word with a concept or another word that you are more familiar with. If you have established word associations with key interpreting terms prior to an interpreting session, the word associations will help you remember during a session.

Imagine that you have associated the word "otorhinologist" with the word 'rhino.' When you think of a rhino, you think of an animal with a big nose, and this reminds you that an otorhinologist is an ear and nose doctor. Now, when the provider mentions that the patient needs to see an otorhinologist, you immediately associate the word with a 'rhino' and this will help you remember until you have an opportunity to interpret.

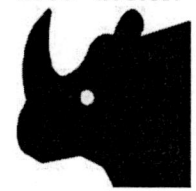

Shadowing

Shadowing is a strategy that can be used to help develop short-term memory when you are not in an interpreting session. Shadowing involves listening to a section of spoken words, then repeating back what was said in the same language.

You can do this exercise with a friend, by having them tell a story or read text to you aloud. Then you can repeat the story back and have your friend check your recall. If you do not have a partner to practice with, you can use a recording of material being read aloud. For example, your local library will most likely have a large collection of books on tape. Start the tape and let it run for a sentence. Stop the tape and repeat the sentence. Then let the tape run for two sentences. Stop the tape and repeat the sentences. When you start to miss words, go back and listen again.

Taking Notes

Some interpreters like to take notes to help them remember key phrases, numbers, dates, etc. This is a technique used extensively in court interpreting, but less in medical interpreting.

It is important to note that to some people, the sight of the interpreter taking notes during an interview can be very distressing if it brings back memories of surveillance and repression in their country of origin. Others may simply be uncomfortable about privacy issues if an interpreter is taking notes.

If you want to take notes, consider the following guidelines:

- Ask the patient's permission first.
- In your pre-session, mention that you may take notes, but that those notes will be destroyed after the session.
- Take notes discretely and in a small notebook, rather than in an obtrusive way that makes the note-taking obvious.
- Dispose of your notes in such a way that confidentiality is maintained, even if your notes would not make sense to anyone else.

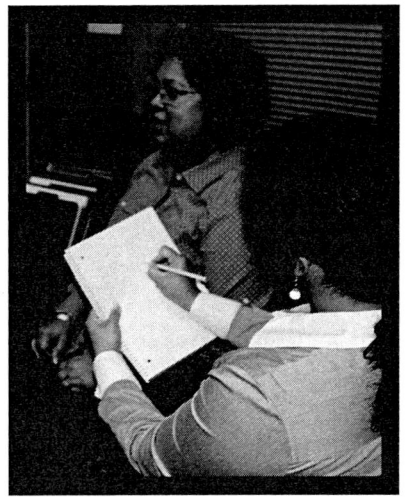

The way the interpreter is taking notes here may be distracting and disruptive.

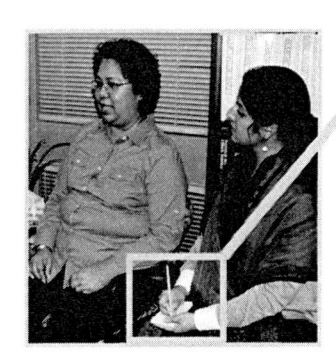

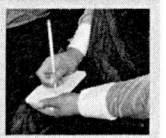

Note the size of the notepad, where the interpreter is holding the notepad, and how the interpreter's note-taking is discreet and unobtrusive.

Developing Symbols and Shorthand for Note-Taking

Many interpreters who take notes develop their own kind of shorthand based on symbols that have meaning only to them. This allows the interpreter to let the speaker continue for a longer time without interrupting the flow of the message. Each interpreter usually develops their own style of note taking. The purpose of shorthand note-taking is not to write down every word a speaker says, but to jog the interpreter's memory of what was said.

Note-taking is a skill that requires quite a bit of practice. You should not make up the symbol patterns on the spot. Instead, develop a personal shorthand for the kind of things that come up frequently in medical interpreting. This shorthand must become largely automatic, so that taking notes does not get in the way of actually listening to what was said. The best way to develop this skill is, not surprisingly, to practice, practice, and practice!

Summary

Interpreters use different types of memory when interpreting. They use very short-term memory to remember strings of numbers and words for a very short time. They use short-term memory to remember what a speaker said until they can interpret. They use long-term memory to remember vocabulary words in both languages.

It is important for interpreters to develop all three types of memory in order to interpret effectively. The best way to do this is to employ multiple memory development techniques and practice regularly. The following skill development exercises will provide tools for interpreters to develop their memory capacity.

Skill Development

Shadowing activity

You can do this exercise with a friend or with recorded material. Each person should have a partner. Each partner will take turns telling one story of a happy childhood memory. Once each partner has shared, everyone will come back together in one large group. Each person will then exercise their short term memory, use the strategy of shadowing, and retell the story that their partner had told them in as much detail as possible.

Shadowing Scenario Instructions (next page)

This exercise requires two people working as partners. There are two scenarios, so each person has a chance to be both the reader and the repeater.

Instructions for the Repeater:

The repeater will practice the technique of shadowing - repeating what is said in the same language (in English). When comfortable, the repeater can also practice interpreting the scenarios into their target language.

Instructions for the Reader:

The reader is the only one with their book open. The reader will first read only the first set of sentences and wait for the repeater to repeat. Then the reader will read the first set of sentences and the second set of sentences, and wait for the repeater to repeat both. Then the reader will read the first, second and third set of sentences, and so on. The reader will not correct or prompt the repeater at any time. If the repeater cannot continue repeating the latest set, the reader will start again from the beginning and again add the next set of sentences.

Skill Development

Shadowing scenario #1

1st Set of Sentences: Hello, my name is Adelaida.

2nd Set of Sentences: I've had heartburn for a long time. Lately, I feel it is getting worse.

3rd Set of Sentences: I used to get heartburn after I ate pepperoni pizza. Now I have it when I eat spicy food, too. I have a lot of trouble sleeping when I have heartburn.

4th Set of Sentences: I take Mylanta Maximum Strength for my heartburn, and I drink lots of water. I even tried drinking almost a liter of club soda because my sister-in-law said it would help!

5th Set of Sentences: I have gone to three doctors about this problem. The first one just gave me over the counter medicine, but that didn't help. The second one did an x-ray and gave me a prescription, but the heartburn still occurs. Now I am seeing a specialist called a gastroenterologist. I wonder what she will do.

6th Set of Sentences: One of the tests they did was an endoscopy. They put a tube into my mouth, through the esophagus and into my stomach. I was sedated where I could follow the doctor's instructions but not feel any discomfort. The doctor told me that the tube she inserted had a camera that projected a picture of my insides on a TV monitor. This allowed her to see if anything was wrong in my digestive tract.

7th Set of Sentences: Today I have an appointment with the gastroenterologist at Group Health Outpatient Clinic in Burien. To get to the hospital by 2:00, I have to leave home at 12:45. I take a bus to downtown where I change. If I'm lucky, I can catch my next bus at 1:30. That way I will get to the clinic on time. Last time I went I was late, and the doctor couldn't see me. This time I will be on time!

Skill Development

Shadowing scenario #2

1st Set of Sentences: This is John, my baby.

2nd Set of Sentences: Yesterday, I took my baby for a checkup. We went to see Dr. Tran.

3rd Set of Sentences: Dr. Tran is a specialist for children. He's a pediatrician. It was the first time we had seen him.

4th Set of Sentences: First, Dr. Tran examined John. Then he asked me a lot of questions about how John was doing. He asked about how he eats, how he sleeps and how he wets himself. He asked me about what things he can do, like smile.

5th Set of Sentences: Dr. Tran said John was doing just fine. But then he got out a big needle! Why did he want to stick my baby if he was doing fine? It turns out he wanted to give John a vaccination. Vaccinations help babies stay well.

6th Set of Sentences: Dr. Tran actually gave John two vaccinations. One was for diphtheria, tetanus, and whooping cough. The other was just three drops of a liquid. That one was to protect John against polio. He didn't seem to mind the drops. But he sure screamed when Dr. Tran gave him the injection!

7th Set of Sentences: It's hard for me to get John to the doctor. I have so much to do. I get my children ready for school in the morning. The bus picks one up at 7:30 and the other at 8:00. Then I have to take John to my mother-in-law's house and get to work by 9:00. I often don't get home until 7:00 at night. Still, I liked Dr. Tran and I think it is important for John to stay healthy.

Lesson 8

SIGHT TRANSLATION

GOAL

Develop skills and strategies to accurately sight translate patient education material.

KNOWLEDGE OUTCOMES

- Identify appropriate and inappropriate requests for sight translation

- Understand and apply the guidelines of sight translation

- Understand how to respond to inappropriate sight translation requests

---

Vocabulary

Non-vital documents

Sight translation

Vital documents

> **Brainstorm**
>
> What types of materials do you think you might be asked to sight translate in a medical setting?
> Think about written documents you may have received at a doctor's office or hospital.
> What would you do if you couldn't read or understand these documents?

Introduction

In lesson 3, we discussed four modes of interpreting: consecutive interpreting, sight translation, simultaneous interpreting, and summarization. The most commonly used mode is consecutive interpreting. The second most common mode is sight translation. It is important to understand the term "sight translation" in the context of interpreting and translating.

Any document written in English that English-speaking patients could read for themselves needs to be translated or sight translated for limited English speaking patients. Ideally, the best practice is to create professionally translated documents *before* they are needed in a patient-provider interaction. However, this is not always the reality; medical interpreters are often asked to provide written and sight translations.

> **Interpretation and Translation**
>
> **Interpretation** is the oral rendition of a spoken communication from one language into another. This is the primary role of a medical interpreter.
> **Translation** is the rendition of written text in one language into a comparable written text in another language. In medical settings, translation of documents should be done by professional translators, for legal purposes.
> **Sight Translation** is the oral rendition of a text written in one language into another language. Medical interpreters are often asked to provide this service spontaneously when they are in their primary role as a medical interpreter.

Recognizing Appropriate Sight Translation Requests

Documents to be sight translated generally fall under three categories:

- documents that must be translated by a professional translator and should not be sight translated by the interpreter
- documents that can be sight translated by an interpreter, but only in the presence of a provider
- documents that can be sight translated by an interpreter without the provider present

An interpreter should not be put in the position of having to answer technical questions or choose what part of the information should be summarized or omitted. However, the reality is that, as a medical interpreter, you may still be asked to sight translate documents, even though it may not be in the scope of your work. It is important to know what kinds of requests for sight translation fall within the scope of medical interpreting so that you can respond appropriately.

Types of Documents to Be Sight Translated

Vital documents that provide general information about how an institution functions (HIPAA, Patient Bill of Rights) must be translated into an institution's commonly used languages. They should not be sight translated by an interpreter.

Vital legal documents (financial agreements, consent forms, advance directives) may be professionally translated or interpreted in the presence of a provider, but may not be sight translated without the provider present. If the interpreter is not comfortable interpreting complicated legal language, she can ask the provider to summarize and interpret their summary.

Vital documents with specific instructions about a patient's condition (patient education materials, brochures, flyers) may be professionally translated or sight translated in the presence of the provider. They should not be translated without the provider present, in case the patient has questions.

Vital documents that contain specific instructions for patient care (prescriptions, instructions for procedures, discharge instructions, technical instructions) may also be professionally translated or sight translated only in the presence of the provider.

Non-vital documents (registration forms, financial aid forms, accident report forms for workman's compensation, work releases, questionnaires and surveys, appointment reminder cards) may be sight translated without the provider present, as long as the interpreter is comfortable with the information, and the agency or hospital policy allows this.

Types of Documents to Be Sight Translated

Vital documents that provide general information about how an institution functions (HIPAA, Patient Bill of Rights) must be translated into an institution's commonly used languages.

Vital legal documents (financial agreements, consent forms, advance directives) may be professionally translated or interpreted in the presence of a provider.

Vital documents with specific instructions about patient's care or condition (patient education materials, brochures, flyers, prescriptions, instructions for procedures, discharge instructions,) may be professionally translated or sight translated in the presence of the provider.

Non-vital documents (registration forms, financial aid forms, accident report forms for workman's compensation, work releases, questionnaires and surveys, appointment reminder cards) may be sight translated without the provider present.

Vital and Non-Vital Documents

Determining whether a document is considered "vital" or "non-vital" for the purposes of sight translation depends on the document's original purpose. A vital document is any document that would be provided to an English proficient patient to inform them of their rights or provide essential information related to their health and well-being.

In determining whether a document is vital or not, some questions that need to be answered include (Department of Health and Human Services):
- What is the importance of the program/process/service it represents?
- What is the consequence for the limited English proficient (LEP) person if the information is not provided accurately or in a timely manner?

According to the U.S. Department of Health and Human Services, the following are some examples of vital and non-vital written documents:

Vital written documents may include:
- consent and complaint forms
- intake forms with the potential for important consequences
- written notices of eligibility criteria, rights, denial, loss, or decreases in benefits or services, actions affecting parental custody or child support, and hearings
- notices advising LEP persons of free language assistance
- applications to participate in a federally funded organization's program or activity or to receive benefits or services from the federally funded organization

Non-vital documents may include:
- hospital menus
- third party documents, forms, or pamphlets distributed as a public service
- large documents such as enrollment handbooks (although vital information contained in large documents may need to be translated)
- general information about a program intended for informational purposes only

Sight translation guidelines

If you have determined that you have received an appropriate sight translation request, follow these guidelines:

Read the document all the way through so that you understand what it says before starting to translate.

Ask for clarification of any words or concepts that you do not understand.

Translate at a steady, moderate pace. If you read a few lines very quickly and then leave long pauses before continuing, it is difficult for the patient to understand and remember what you have read.

Translate exactly what is written. Add nothing; omit nothing; change nothing.

Provide only an oral sight translation of the written document. As an interpreter, you should not provide written translation, unless you are also a qualified professional translator.

Inappropriate Sight Translation Requests

If you have determined you have received an inappropriate sight translation request, intervene and politely decline to sight translate the document. Explain that since you are a medical interpreter and not a professional translator, you cannot translate the document.

If it is appropriate for you to sight translate the document with the provider present, politely ask the provider to remain in the room while you sight translate the written document. Remind the provider that you will be sight translating all of the information exactly as it is written. Also, remind the provider that their presence will allow the patient to ask the provider any questions that might arise.

If you have determined that the document involves language of a very high register (for example a legal document) that you are not familiar with, politely decline to sight translate the document. You can also ask the provider to provide a summary of the information (or pick out key points) contained in the document, which you will then interpret for the patient. This option gives the provider the appropriate responsibility of editing and summarizing.

Summary

Ideally, all documents that would be provided to an English-proficient patient would be translated into an LEP patient's preferred language by a professional translator. However, in reality, an interpreter will often be asked to sight translate documents.

Providers may not know what documents an interpreter can appropriately sight translate. Therefore, interpreters should be familiar with sight translation guidelines. Interpreters should not attempt to sight translate a document that is beyond their skill level. If the interpreter is concerned that they will not be able to provide an accurate sight translation, they should decline the request.

Skill Development

Sight Translation Practice Exercise #1

An Appropriate Sight Translation

A patient has come to the clinic for a non-critical work related injury. Prior to the start of the examination, the provider asks the interpreter to sight translate the workman's compensation form that is required before seeing the patient.

The interpreter determines that it is appropriate to sight translate the Workman's Compensation Form.

(The interpreter can practice translating the document **Workman's Compensation Form** included in Appendix A).

Sight Translation Practice Exercise #2

An Appropriate Sight Translation with the Provider Present

Provider: (In English) Mrs. Khan, your son has the flu. I would like you to have this informational brochure about the flu. It will explain how to recognize if someone else in your family gets the flu and how to prevent the flu from spreading in your house and out into your community.

Interpreter: (Interprets previous statement into target language):

The interpreter recognizes that this informational brochure about the flu needs to be sight translated in the presence of the provider, so that the patient can ask questions. Since the provider has made no indication of leaving, the interpreter can begin the sight translation.

(The interpreter can practice translating the document **Preventing the Spread of Influenza** in Appendix B).

Skill Development

Sight Translation Practice Exercise #3

An Inappropriate Sight Translation Request

Provider: (In English) Mr. Trung, you will need to have a Flexible Sigmoidoscopy, which is a procedure that lets the doctor see the inside of the rectum and the sigmoid colon.

I don't have this brochure in Vietnamese, but the interpreter will be able to translate it for you. I have to go for my next appointment, but I will see you tomorrow morning for the procedure.

The interpreter recognizes that instructions for a procedure should be sight translated only in the presence of the provider. Since the provider has indicated she will be leaving, the interpreter needs to intervene and respond appropriately. Review the guidelines in this lesson for help on how to respond.

See Appendix C: Instructions for a Flexible Sigmoidoscopy

Appendix A: Workers Compensation Form

Please send this form to the Claims office. By law, employers must keep accurate records of all work-related injuries and illness. Employers must report all claims to the Claims office. This report must be filed for all injuries that result in the loss of more than five regular workdays. This information is confidential.

Date of report		
Employer's Name		
Employer's Mailing Address	Nature of Business or service	
Name of workers' compensation carrier	Policy #	
Employee's full name	Social Security #	Employee's address
Circle One: Male or Female	Circle One: Single, Married	Number of Dependents
Employee's average weekly wage	Job Title or Occupation	Date Hired
Time employee began work: AM/PM	Date and time of accident	Last day employee worked
If the employee died as a result of the accident, give the date of death	Did the accident occur on the employer's premises?	
Address of accident	What was the employee doing when the accident occurred	
How did the accident occur?	What was the injury or illness? List the part of the body affected and explain	
What object or substance, if any, directly harmed the employee?	Name and address of physician/health care professional.	
If treatment was given away from the worksite, list the name and address of the place it was given	Was the employee treated in an emergency room?	
Was the employee hospitalized overnight as an inpatient?	Report prepared by Title/Phone Number	

Appendix B: Seattle and King County Public Health: Preventing the Spread of Influenza

Office of the Director
405 Fifth Avenue, Suite 1300
Seattle, WA 98032
206-296-4600 Fax 206-296-0166
TTY Relay: 711
www.kingcounty.gov/health

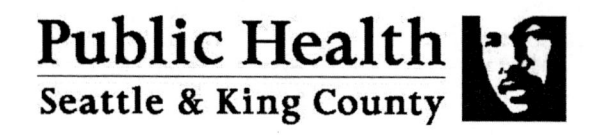

Public Health
Seattle & King County

Preventing the Spread of Influenza

Most patients with pandemic influenza will be able to remain at home during the course of their illness and can be cared for by others who live in the household. This information is intended to help you recognize the symptoms of influenza and care for ill persons in the home, both during a typical influenza season and during an influenza pandemic.

At the outset of an influenza pandemic, a vaccine for the *pandemic* flu virus will not be available for several months. However, it's still a good idea to get a *seasonal* flu vaccine to protect from seasonal flu viruses (see Influenza Vaccine Information Sheet).

Know the Symptoms of Influenza, which may include:

- Sudden onset of illness
- Fever higher than 100.4° F (38° C)
- Muscle aches
- Chills
- Feeling of weakness and/or exhaustion
- Cough
- Headache
- Diarrhea, vomiting, abdominal pain (occur more commonly in children)
- Sore throat

Prevent the Spread of Illness in the Home

Because influenza can spread easily from person to person, anyone living in or visiting a home where someone has influenza can become infected. For this reason, it is important to take steps to prevent the spread of influenza to others in the home.

What Caregivers Can Do
- Physically separate influenza patients from other people as much as possible. When practical, the ill person should stay in a separate room where others do not enter.

Other people living in the home should limit contact with the ill person as much as possible.
- Designate one person in the household as the main caregiver for the ill person. Ideally, this caregiver should be healthy and not have medical conditions that would put him or her at risk for severe influenza disease. Medical conditions that are considered "high risk" include the following:
    - Pregnancy
    - Chronic lung disease, including asthma, emphysema, cystic fibrosis, chronic bronchitis, bronchiectasis and tuberculosis (TB)
    - Diabetes
    - Heart problems
    - Kidney disease
    - Disease or treatment that suppresses the immune system
    - Age over 65.
- Watch for influenza symptoms in other household members.
- If possible, contact your health care provider if you have questions about caring for the ill person. However, it may be difficult to contact your usual healthcare provider during a severe influenza pandemic. Public Health–Seattle & King County's pandemic flu website (listed below) will provide frequent updates, including how to get medical advice. If special telephone hotlines are used, these numbers will also be on the website and announced through the media.
- Wearing surgical masks (with ties) or procedure masks (with ear loops) may be useful in decreasing spread of influenza when worn by the patient and/or caregiver during close contact (within 3 feet). If masks are worn, to be useful they must be worn at all times when in close contact with the patient. The wearing of gloves and gowns is not recommended for household members providing care in their own home.

What Everyone in the Household Can Do

- Wash hands with soap and water or, if soap and water are not available, use an alcohol-based hand cleanser (like Purell® or a store-brand) after each contact with an influenza patient or with objects in the area where the patient is located. Cleaning your hands is the single best preventive measure for everyone in the household.
- Don't touch your eyes, nose, or mouth without first washing your hands for 20 seconds. Wash hands before and after using the bathroom.
- Wash soiled dishes and eating utensils either in a dishwasher or by hand with soap. It's not necessary to separate eating utensils used by a patient with influenza.
- Laundry can be washed in a standard washing machine with warm or cold water and detergent. It is not necessary to separate soiled linen and laundry used by a patient with influenza from other household laundry. Do not grasp the laundry close to your body or face, in order to avoid contamination. Wash hands with soap and water after handling soiled laundry.

- Place tissues used by the ill patient in a bag and throw them away with other household waste. Consider placing a bag at the bedside for this purpose.
- Clean counters, surfaces and other areas in the home regularly using everyday cleaning products.

Prevent the Spread of Illness in the Community

- Stay at home if you are sick. Ill persons should not leave the home until they have recovered because they can spread the infection to others. In a typical influenza season, persons with influenza should avoid contact with others for about 5 days after onset of the illness. During an influenza pandemic, public health authorities will provide information on how long persons with influenza should remain at home.
- If the ill person must leave home (such as for medical care), he or she should wear a surgical or procedure mask, if available, and should be sure to do the following:
    - Cover the mouth and nose when coughing and sneezing, using tissues or the crook of the elbow instead of the hands.
    - Use tissues to contain mucous and watery discharge from the mouth and nose.
    - Dispose of tissues in the nearest waste bin after use or carry a small plastic bag (like a zip-lock bag) for used tissues.
    - Wash hands with soap and water or use an alcohol-based hand cleanser after covering your mouth for a cough or sneeze, after wiping or blowing your nose, and after handling contaminated objects and materials, including tissues.
- During an influenza pandemic, only people who are essential for patient care or support should enter a home where someone is ill with pandemic influenza unless they have already had influenza.
- If other persons must enter the home, they should avoid close contact with the patient and use the infection control precautions recommended on this sheet.

This guidance is based on current information from the U.S. Department of Health & Human Services Pandemic Influenza Plan and is subject to change. Up-to-date guidance will be available from your healthcare provider and at these websites:

Public Health – Seattle & King County: www.metrokc.gov/health/pandemicflu **Official U.S. Government pandemic flu website:** www.pandemicflu.gov/plan/tab3.html

For more information on "How to Care for Someone with Influenza":
www.metrokc.gov/health/pandemicflu/prepare/care.htm

Appendix C: Instructions for a Flexible Sigmoidoscopy

Your doctor has requested that you have a Flexible Sigmoidoscopy, which is a procedure that lets the doctor see the inside of the rectum and the sigmoid colon.

To prepare for this procedure you need to do a number of things, all of which are very important.

First of all, discontinue the following medications: iron, seven days before the procedure; aspirin 10 days before the procedure; and arthritis medications like Motrin or Advil two days before the procedure.

You should **not** suspend any of the following: prednisone, heart medications, lung medications or diabetes medications. You may take Tylenol if you need it.

The night before the procedure, drink one whole bottle of magnesium citrate.

On the day of the procedure, don't eat anything for two hours before the exam, except maybe for a little water.

Take two Fleets enemas, one two hours before the appointment, and the other just one hour before the appointment.

Report to the Special Procedures Unit at least 15 minutes before hour scheduled appointment.

Don't forget, someone will have to drive you home, because the doctor will probably administer a sedative.

Section 2

Culture and its Impact on Interpreting

Lesson 9

INTRODUCTION TO CULTURE

GOAL

Introduce the concept of culture and its impact on medical interpreting.

KNOWLEDGE OUTCOMES

- Define culture in general terms
- Understand the importance of culture in the medical interpreting process

Vocabulary
Acculturation
Active culture
Assimilation
Bicultural
Bilingual
Cultural lens
Culture

Brainstorm

What does the word "culture" mean to you?
What comes to mind when you think of your own culture?

Introduction

Culture is not only an important and significant part of our personal and professional lives, but is also a crucial element in communication and health care. To become culturally competent means we must educate ourselves about the needs of the communities we serve, as well as our own culture.

However, by studying specific cultural information about a given community, there is a risk of further adding to the stereotypes about members of that community. Our purpose in discussing this information is to describe the general cultural frameworks within which each individual develops in a unique way. These cultural frameworks will differ on the basis of ethnicity, national origin, race, religion, class, sexual orientation, gender, and age.

As we recognize these basic cultural frameworks, it is equally important to point out that there are many differences between individuals who come from the same community. To be culturally competent, we need to learn specific information about a community, as well as simultaneously treat each person as a unique individual who is not necessarily representative of his or her whole group.

In addition, we must gain an understanding of our own culture and how it affects the way we perceive the world and others. This delicate balance may not be easy to learn, but we must do so in order to work successfully in diverse environments.

What is Culture?

"Culture" is a complex word, which, because it has been used in so many different ways, has come to mean many things. When many people think of culture, they think of the aspects of their lives that are both components of culture and influenced by culture. These may include things like food, dress, holidays, art, music, language, etc. But culture impacts our lives in even more profound ways. It determines how we perceive our world on the most fundamental level, how we assign meaning to what we see, and how we respond to it.

One way of saying it is that **culture** is a shared set of belief systems, values, practices, and assumptions which determine how we interact with and interpret the world.

Our personal worldview is the product of many **cultural lenses**. Each lens represents a different influence that shapes how we understand and interpret the world around us. Every new or repeated experience adds another lens or dimension to our worldview. These lenses affect our thoughts, values, opinions and actions.

> **Vocabulary**
>
> **Active culture:** a person's unique outlook, shaped by their individual life experiences
>
> **Culture:** a shared set of belief systems, values, practices and assumptions which determine how we interact with and interpret the world
>
> **Cultural lens:** the values, beliefs, assumptions, and practices through which we see and understand the world around us

Why Consider Culture?

Language differences are not the only barrier separating an English-speaking provider from a non-English-speaking patient. Imagine a provider and a patient with different views on how the world works, what is important in life, what causes an illness or how to treat an illness. These different views are heavily influenced by each person's culture and can potentially cause misunderstanding between the patient and provider.

People tend to be unaware of their cultural influences and assume that others share the same basic views. As a result, people from different cultures often find themselves confused by the behavior of others who work from a different set of understandings. The patient and the provider may not even be aware that they have different views.

An action or message in one context may have a completely different meaning in another context. In a medical setting, the clarification of these cultural norms may be crucial to understanding. This clarification of cultural norms is the job of the interpreter when acting in the role of a culture broker.

Active Culture

While most people identify with at least one culture, even people from the same culture may be very different from each other. People from the same cultural group frequently have different values, different beliefs and different customs. How can we be the same, and yet so different?

The key is in our **active culture**. While we may share a general culture with other people, each of us has grown up with a special set of experiences and influences that have formed us as unique individuals. This unique outlook resulting from individual experiences is known as active culture.

Each person's 'active culture' changes and grows constantly. This makes culture a dynamic entity that is open to new influences every day. Because every person's active culture is different, every encounter with another person, even with someone from our own culture, is a cross cultural encounter.

Factors That Influence Active Culture

A person's active culture reflects the influences of many factors. Some of these factors include:

- history (the moment in history into which a person is born, leading to unique political and economic experiences)
- place (the place in which a person is born - urban/rural, country, climate - and lives throughout their lives)
- influence of family and friends
- primary language
- formal and informal education
- religion
- key people who have influenced a person's thinking (including sources like the Internet and mass media)
- the presence, or non-presence, of a disability
- economic experiences
- traumatic or significant life events

Consider the following example: two Vietnamese women may share many common aspects of Vietnamese culture. However, a younger woman, who grew up in a well-to-do family that immigrated to the U.S. at the end of the Vietnam War may carry significantly different values and beliefs than an older woman who came to the U.S. as a refugee after living under Communist rule for many years. Some of the factors that influence active culture can be so strong that these differences might be found even in two Vietnamese women who belong to the same family.

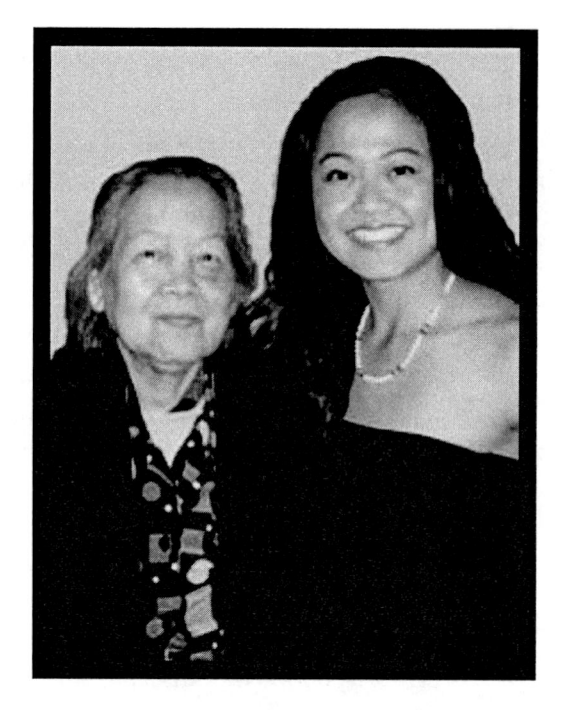

Acculturation and Assimilation

Acculturation, **assimilation**, and social class are three often-overlooked factors that greatly influence active culture. In addition to creating barriers between patients and providers, differences between interpreters and patients in these areas can potentially cause distrust and may even become barriers to the provision of quality interpretation.

> ### Vocabulary
>
> **Acculturation:** the process of adapting to a new culture without losing one's original culture
>
> **Assimilation:** to fully become part of a different society, country, or culture other than the original
>
> **Bilingual:** speaking two languages
>
> **Bicultural:** identifying with two cultures

Acculturation is the process of adapting to a new culture, without losing one's original culture. A person begins to blend together two cultures and identifies with aspects of both of them. As a person acculturates (integrates and adapts), old cultural values, language, belief systems, religion, and traditions are integrated with the new. Becoming **bilingual** and **bicultural** may be part of this process.

Acculturation is a dynamic process which moves along a continuum. **Assimilation** is the extreme end of the process of acculturation. When a person assimilates, the new culture is completely incorporated. New cultural values, practices, and beliefs may be adopted. This may happen when the old values are in conflict with the new ones.

Summary

Culture is a shared set of belief systems, values, practices and assumptions which determine how we interact with and interpret the world. Our personal worldview or personal culture is the product of many cultural lenses. Each lens represents a different influence that shapes how we understand and interpret the world around us.

Skill Development

Acknowledging your own active culture

What communities are you a part of? (You may define community as a cultural community, a religious community, a community based on age group, activity or something else entirely).

What people or experiences in your life have helped to form an idea of what community you belong to?

Think about times when you have experienced cultural differences in communication at home or at work. How did these cultural differences play out?

Lesson 10

CULTURAL BUMPS

GOAL

Understand the factors that affect communication in cross-cultural situations.

KNOWLEDGE OUTCOMES

- Define "cultural bump"
- Apply the concept of cultural relativity to resolving communication issues

Vocabulary
Cultural bump
Cultural competence
Cultural relativity
Generalization
Stereotype

Introduction

Understanding one's own culture and how it affects interactions is the first step in becoming culturally competent. Without this awareness, it is unlikely that an interpreter will be able to be an effective culture broker.

An interpreter may need to act as a culture broker when different cultures in the encounter between patient and provider result in miscommunication or misunderstanding. In order to do this, the interpreter must understand the concept of cultural bumps and how to handle them when they arise.

Cultural Bumps

When people expect one type of behavior, and cross-cultural interactions result in something different, this is known as a **cultural bump**. To navigate cultural bumps and overcome the barriers associated with them, medical interpreters must develop **cultural competence**.

Cultural competence is the ability to function effectively in the context of cultural differences (Cross). In any interaction, one person's actions or communication is determined by that person's active culture. We must be able to understand another person's actions as they themselves would view it within their cultural framework.

People from different cultures might interpret the situation in the case study above in different ways and give Mr. Albert different advice about what is appropriate behavior. They might say:

- Mr. Mohammed is prejudiced against people of other races and is unwilling to accept anything Mr. Albert has touched.
- Mr. Mohammed regards the left hand as unclean and cannot knowingly swallow something he considers contaminated.
- Mr. Mohammed is a fatalist and believes that nothing can be done to cure his ulcer.

Cultural Bump Case Study

An Egyptian Muslim, Hussein Mohammed, comes to the gastrointestinal clinic and, after examination, is diagnosed as having a duodenal ulcer. The nurse tells Mr. Mohammed how to get to the hospital pharmacy for a free prescription.

Mr. Mohamed goes to the pharmacy and is given the free medicine by Tom Albert, a left-handed African American, who carefully reviews the dosage instructions with him. Mr. Mohammed is seen throwing away the bottle after he leaves the hospital grounds.
(Gropper, Culture and the Clinical Encounter: An Intercultural Sensitizer for the Health Professions)

How do you explain Mr. Mohammed's behavior?

Why does Mr. Mohammed throw the medicine away?

What do Mr. Mohammed's actions mean?

How should Mr. Albert respond?

- Mr. Mohammed does not like taking charity, and he feels that accepting free medication from the pharmacy would disgrace him.

Culture tells us how to interpret what we see. Mr. Mohammed's action isn't inherently rude. It is interpreted as being rude by someone from a culture in which throwing away free medication is considered rude and wasteful, regardless of the source. Another person from a different culture will interpret this event in a completely different way.

> **Vocabulary**
>
> **Cultural bump:** when different expectations based on different cultural contexts result in misunderstandings
>
> **Cultural competence:** the ability to function effectively in the context of cultural differences
>
> **Cultural relativity:** the idea that behavior must be evaluated and understood within the cultural context where it occurred

Cultural Relativity

Understanding and accepting cultural differences allows for the concept of **cultural relativity**: any behavior must be judged first *in relation* to the culture in which it occurs. Often, people's behavior can seem very strange until you put it into the context of their own culture; then suddenly it seems perfectly reasonable.

Mr. Albert may be thinking, due to his culture, that Mr. Mohammed is very rude for throwing away free medicine, until he finds out that Mr. Mohammed, because of his culture, believes that anything given with the left hand is contaminated because the left hand is used for toilet functions, while the right hand is used for eating and touching people. For Mr. Albert and Mr. Mohammed, being able to judge each other's behavior within its own cultural context may be the key to a successful relationship.

Stereotypes and Generalizations

The concept of cultural relativity helps us understand that people from different cultures may see a situation from completely different perspectives. In order to understand how someone from a different culture might see something, it can be useful to make **generalizations** about certain cultural groups with which you are familiar. Often, these generalizations are useful to promote general understanding between the patient and the provider.

However, generalizations are also the starting point for **stereotypes**. Stereotypes are dangerous, because, as we have discussed, each member of a cultural group has a unique individual culture. The generalizations that may apply to the group as a whole may not apply to the specific individual.

A medical interpreter must be able to recognize the difference between using generalizations as a useful tool to anticipate cultural misunderstandings and stereotypes as a tool for making inaccurate and harmful assumptions. Generalizations are useful if they help anticipate possible barriers and challenges. Generalizations are not useful if they lead to stereotypes that are incorrect and further increase misunderstanding.

> **Vocabulary**
>
> **Generalization**: a general statement or assumption based on past experience or general knowledge
>
> **Stereotype**: an oversimplified image or idea of a person, culture, or concept

Consider the following example: In general, family is valued very highly in Hispanic/Latino cultures. Many Hispanic patients may want to consult with family before deciding on a major health intervention. If a patient is hesitating to proceed with the doctor's recommendations, it may be because they need to consult with family members first. If the interpreter communicates this possible explanation to the provider, it may facilitate culturally competent health care. The provider may be able to find a way to allow the patient to consult with the family first. As long as the interpreter remembers that this may not be true for every individual patient of Hispanic/Latino culture, this can be a successful use of a generalization.

There is a delicate balance to be reached between being aware of cultural generalities and being aware of potential individual differences. People who speak the same language are not necessarily from the same culture, and even people who are from the same culture may have very different beliefs and values. Interpreters must be ready to recognize and respect individual differences and avoid the tendency to form or reinforce cultural stereotypes.

Summary

People tend to be unaware of their culture and assume that others share the same basic views. As a result, people from different cultures often find themselves confused by the behavior of others who work from a different basic set of understandings. In a medical setting, the clarification of these cultural norms may be crucial to understanding.

Critical Incidents

Use the examples in this section to develop your awareness of other cultures. Be aware of how the examples might differ from your own personal beliefs and worldview. Try to see each incident in a culturally relative context, understanding how the behavior in each example is perfectly logical within the context of that culture. Try to determine the key piece of information that will help the characters in these situations resolve their misunderstandings.

Critical Incident #1: Laundry Starch

Ruth Clay, a twenty-eight year old African American female with two children who is paraplegic, craved Argo laundry starch while she was hospitalized following an auto accident. Since she had few visitors, she asked the staff to bring her the starch so she could eat it. The staff, who thought this craving was 'crazy,' told her they did not have any. Eventually, Ruth became very depressed during her long hospitalization. (Galanti)

What should the staff do?
Why would Ruth be craving laundry starch?

Critical Incident #2: Whose baby?

A four o'clock appointment had been scheduled for Antonio Reyes, a one-month-old Mexican American. When four o'clock arrives, the nurse, Ms. Chin, recognizes Sra. Maria Lopez sitting in the reception area and holding a little baby.

Ms. Chin goes over to greet Sra. Lopez and look at the baby, presumably a new arrival since the last prenatal visit. Sra. Lopez says she has brought her son for his first well-baby visit. Ms. Chin knows that no baby with a last name of Lopez had been scheduled for today. (Gropper, Culture and the Clinical Encounter. An Intercultural Sensitizer for the Health Professions)

What should Ms. Chin do?

Critical Incidents

Critical Incident #3: The Rejected Drink

Kiyoko Miramoto, a twenty-six year old Japanese woman in her third trimester of her pregnancy arrived at the clinic on an unusually warm day. She looked dangerously pale and was trembling. When the nurse, Ms. Sommerville, who knew Mrs. Miramoto quite well, commented on her appearance, Mrs. Miramoto told her she had waited in the sun for almost an hour before a bus - without air-conditioning - arrived. "I am sorry I am late," she added quietly. "Oh," said Mrs. Sommerville, "don't worry about being late. We are running a little behind schedule ourselves today. Do sit down, please, and relax. May I get you a cold drink?"

Mrs. Miramoto sat down but said she did not want anything to drink. A few minutes later when the nurse passed by, she noticed that Mrs. Miramoto was still pale and trembling and looked like she was going to faint.

What, if anything, should Ms. Sommerville do? (Gropper, Culture and the Clinical Encounter. An Intercultural Sensitizer for the Health Professions)

Critical Incident #4: Paying the Hospital Bill

Marie Louise and Jean-Claude Poitier, who are political refugees from Haiti, take their eight-year-old son to a private family physician for acute earache. After the doctor examines the boy, he instructs the family to see the nurse in the reception area. The nurse reviews the doctor's instructions and extends a bill for services and a prescription to Mrs. Poitier, who accepts the prescription but tries to return the bill to the nurse. (Gropper, Culture and the Clinical Encounter. An Intercultural Sensitizer for the Health Professions)

Why might Mrs. Poitier behave this way?

Critical Incidents

Critical Incident #5: The Bar of Soap

Sandra Miller, a young Rom (Gypsy) woman, is in the hospital recovering from a major surgery. This morning she asked Martha Beck, the nurse assigned to her room, for a washcloth, towel and a bar of soap so that she could wash up. Ordinarily, Ms. Beck would have complied with her wishes without giving it a second thought, but just yesterday the staff had been scolded for wasteful practices that were increasing hospital costs. So today, the nurse feels she must remind Ms. Miller that she had been given personal bath supplies when she was first assigned to a bed.

Ms. Miller very apologetically said she had misplaced the washcloth, towel and soap and could not find them. She even offered to pay for another set. Ms. Beck smiled and said that it was not necessary to do that. She then went to the supply room, got the requested items, and gave them to Ms. Miller.

The next morning when performing her duties in Ms. Miller's room, Ms. Beck noticed that Ms. Miller had two bars of soap, two washcloths and two bath towels. (Gropper, Culture and the Clinical Encounter. An Intercultural Sensitizer for the Health Professions)

What should Ms. Beck do?

Why would Ms. Miller go to such lengths to get a supply of bath items?

Critical Incidents

Critical Incident #6: Bruises

The Nguyen family had been bubbling with excitement and pleasure the last time they had visited the clinic. They were to be reunited with Mr. Nguyen's parents, an event for which they had prayed for months. "What an unusual and marvelously loving family," commented Margo Smith to her fellow nurse, Lang Duong, herself a Vietnamese American.

"Actually, Margo," laughed Lang, "they are not particularly remarkable. Almost any Vietnamese family would be just as delighted. Family is about the most important consideration in our lives, you know."

Two months later, Margo stopped Lang at lunchtime. "We need to talk," said Margo, frowning. "The Nguyen family brought in the baby today. She had an acute respiratory infection and a serious cough and fever. The ARI is not the problem, though. What bothers me is that I saw many bruises on her chest and back. When I asked Mrs. Nguyen about them, she said the grandfather had been responsible for them. But she got embarrassed and changed the subject when I asked for more details. And I thought they were such a loving family. Now what should I do about this child abuse? Is the grandfather senile? Where should I refer the family?" (Gropper, Culture and the Clinical Encounter. An Intercultural Sensitizer for the Health Professions)

What could Ms. Lang Duong advise?

Critical Incidents

Critical Incident #7: The Weapon

Raj Singh, a seventy-two year old Sikh from India had been admitted to a hospital after a heart attack. He was scheduled for a heart catheterization to determine the extent of blockage in his coronary arteries. The procedure involved running a catheter up the femoral artery located in the groin. The doctor has previously fully explained the procedure to him in detail.

Susan, his nurse, entered Mr. Singh's room and explained that she had to shave his groin to prevent infection from the catheterization. As she pulled the razor from her pocket, she was suddenly confronted with the sight of metal flashing in front of her. Mr. Singh had a short sword in his hand and was waving it at her as he spoke excitedly in his native tongue. Susan got the message. She would not shave his groin.

She put away 'her weapon' and he did the same. Susan, thinking the problem was that she was a woman, said she would get a male orderly to shave him. Mr. Singh's eyes lit up again as he angrily yelled, "No shaving of hair by anyone!" (Galanti)

What should Susan do?
Why did Mr. Singh react this way?

Critical Incident #8: Car Seat for the Baby

Nancy Grimes, a social worker, talked to Ayesha Faud, a 23-year-old Syrian Muslim, about her impending delivery. "Have you gotten a car seat for the baby yet?" she asked. The young woman replied that she had not. Further conversation revealed that other baby equipment, such as a crib, changing table and stroller, had not been purchased, or even ordered. No arrangements had been made to borrow any of these items either.

Since Mrs. Faud seemed very embarrassed and unhappy, Ms. Grimes volunteered the information that some of the local merchants had established a fund to help clinic patients obtain needed items for their babies and offered to help Mrs. Faud submit an application. However, Mrs. Faud refused, firmly insisting, "All will be supplied when the time comes, Allah willing." (Gropper, Culture and the Clinical Encounter. An Intercultural Sensitizer for the Health Professions)

Should Ms. Grimes drop the subject, or should she pursue the matter further?

Lesson 11

THE CULTURE OF BIOMEDICINE

GOAL

Gain a basic overview of the culture of Western biomedicine.

KNOWLEDGE OUTCOMES

- Understand how Western biomedical culture may influence a provider's problem-solving strategies

- Understand how cultural bumps may occur between Western biomedical culture and a patient's culture

Vocabulary
Diagnosis
Diagnostic questions
Informed consent
Medical interview
Symptom
Symptom descriptor

> A successful interpreter must take culture into account. There are at least five different cultures that influence the health care setting:
> - the culture of biomedicine
> - the provider's culture
> - the culture of the health care institution
> - the patient's culture
> - the interpreter's culture
>
> **Brainstorm**
> What does "the culture of biomedicine" mean to you?
> What about the provider's culture?
> How do you think the culture of biomedicine is related to the provider's culture?

Introduction

When the patient comes to a doctor with a problem, they most likely already have some idea of what is wrong and what should be done about it. Both the patient and the provider are there to solve a problem. However, the way in which the provider seeks to solve the problem may be different from the way the patient might solve the problem.

This difference is primarily due to the influence of the culture of biomedicine and the culture of the provider. The culture of biomedicine affects how the provider goes about solving the questions: What is wrong with the patient? What should be done about it?

Steps in Problem-Solving

Problem solving, whether in a medical setting or in our everyday lives, usually follows a sequence of four steps:

Step 1: Collect information.
Step 2: Decide what is wrong.
Step 3: Make a plan to solve the problem.
Step 4: Follow through with the plan and evaluate the outcome.

Consider the following example of the problem solving steps applied to an everyday situation:

PROBLEM:
Your baby is crying, and you are wondering, "What is wrong? What should I do?"

1. **Collect information:** You pick up the baby, check with your spouse to see when she last ate, check to see if she's too hot or too cold, and check her diaper.
2. **Decide what is wrong**: Based on the information you gathered, you decide that she is hungry.
3. **Make a plan to solve the problem:** You decide to feed her.

4. **Follow through with the plan and evaluate the outcome:** You pick her up and begin to feed her. Does she stop crying? Does she seem content? If not, you go back to collecting more information to see what is wrong.

Medical problem-solving is done the same way. The same four steps are used by the provider and the patient. What is important to recognize is that when a provider applies these problem solving steps to the medical problem, the culture of the provider, of biomedicine, and of the health care institution influence how these four steps are carried out. When a patient uses these four problem solving steps, it may look different, because it is usually not influenced by the culture of biomedicine, but by the culture of the patient.

The Provider's Approach To Problem-Solving

Step 1: Collecting information

Just as in everyday problem solving, the first step that a provider takes when solving problems is to collect information. The provider uses a variety of sources to collect information. Some of the sources include:

- laboratory tests (X-rays, blood tests, etc.)
- physical examinations (taking temperature, measuring blood pressure, etc.)
- medical histories

Medical interviews, or histories, are one of the most important tools that a provider

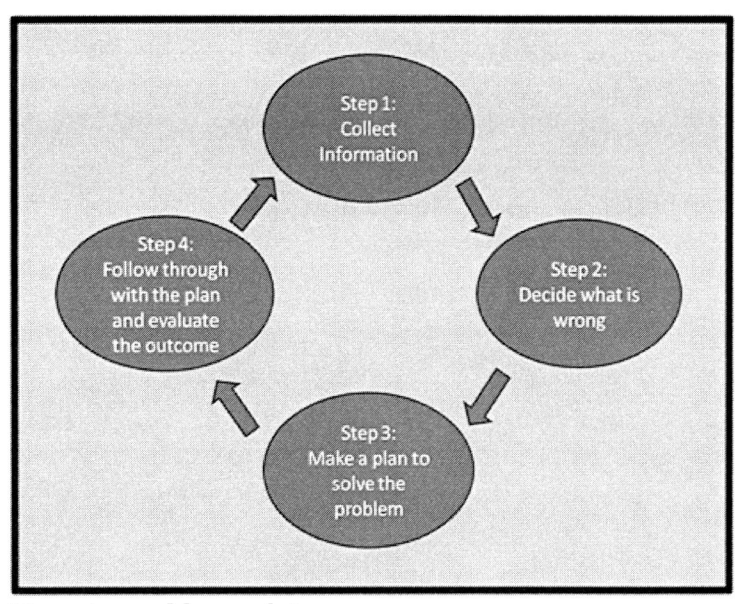

Steps in problem solving

has for collecting information. The provider takes the medical interview by talking to and listening to the patient. The medical history includes the patient's and their families' questions, concerns or complaints. Providers listen for the patient's chief complaint and the history of the present illness.

During the problem-solving process, the provider is heavily influenced by what patients have to say during the medical interview. Providers often make decisions about what to ask next and which exams or laboratory tests are needed based on the patient's circumstance and health history.

Providers often jump back and forth between these four problem-solving steps. For example, a patient may say something during a follow-up session that initiates another problem-solving session.

The purpose of collecting information through tools like laboratory tests, physical exams and medical histories is to make a decision about what is wrong with the patient, the next step in problem solving.

Step 2: Deciding what is wrong

In a medical setting, deciding what is wrong involves making a problem list or statement and then making a **diagnosis.**

The goal of the medical history is to create a problem statement or list of problems. By collecting as much relevant information as possible, the provider strives to accurately describe the problem the patient is facing. The problem statement is a list of the issues that need attention. Each patient's problem list is unique to that individual.

A medical diagnosis is when the nature or cause of the patient's condition is determined. The problem statement itself may or may not contain a diagnosis. It will contain the chief complaint of the patient ("chest pain," "difficulty breathing," etc.). The more accurate a problem list/statement is, the easier it is to make an accurate diagnosis. Once the provider has what they believe is the correct diagnosis, the provider can go on to the

> **Vocabulary**
>
> **Diagnosis**: the identification of the nature of an illness or other medical problem
>
> **Medical interview**: a series of questions that a provider asks to understand a patient's medical history

The Medical Interview

The medical interview is the provider's most important source of information. The purpose of the medical interview is to gather information to aid in the process of problem solving. It can be done in a variety of settings, each of which has a slightly different focus. Some situations require a complete history, such as when:

- a new patient or a patient with unknown or undiagnosed problems is being admitted to a hospital
- a new patient is being referred to a specialist for a special evaluation such as long term care for chronic illnesses
- a new patient is beginning treatment in an outpatient setting

Other situations require a more specific and focused medical history. This might occur during a brief clinic visit or in an emergency room situation.

When specialists see patients multiple times, they often repeat questions that have already been recorded, because new or different details often emerge when patients repeat their stories. This is important to know because patients (or interpreters) are often puzzled by the need to start over and re-describe events.

In each situation it may be difficult to determine the ultimate purpose of the provider's questions. Therefore, it is imperative that the interpreter accurately interpret what the patient is saying.

Diagnostic Questions

Diagnostic Questions usually fall into two categories:
- questions about the body and body systems
- questions about life history and other events

Questions about the body and body systems might include questions about the different body systems:
- circulatory system
- digestive system
- endocrine glands system
- musculoskeletal system
- nervous system
- respiratory system
- skin system
- urinary system
- female reproductive system
- male reproductive system

Questions about life history and other events are important because they may often be connected to the symptoms and chief complaints that the patient has. Topics that might be covered in these types of diagnostic questions include:
- history of present problems
- past medical history
- allergies
- habits such as the use of tobacco, alcohol, or drugs
- travel
- immunizations
- family history
- social history
- current medications
- health maintenance – previous evaluations and preventative exams

next step of making a treatment plan. The problem statement can be any one of the following: a symptom or set of symptoms, a diagnosis, an abnormal laboratory test or physical finding, or a statement of psychosocial issues.

The problem list may change once a clear diagnosis is determined. For example, "chest pain" may turn into "rib fracture" because a rib fracture was determined to be the cause of the chest pain, *or* "chest pain" may turn into "pleurisy" because it was determined that the pleura around the lungs was inflamed, causing the chest pain.

Depending on the problem statement, certain next steps and treatment plans can follow. For example, the provider may only be able to identify problems or characteristics related to the patient's:

- general medical problems
- social problems - family problems, recent widowhood, etc.
- psychiatric problems
- demographic - age, gender, ethnicity

Sometimes, the provider is only able to identify physical problems that need to be investigated further such as:

- edema (swelling)
- lymphadenopathy (enlarged lymph nodes)
- chest pain/pressure in the chest
- high blood sugar
- urinary frequency

The provider may need to go back to collect more information, but now is more informed about which tests to do and which questions to ask.

Other times, the provider may have enough information and be able to identify the specific cause of the problem, such as:

- pneumonia with chest pain due to pleurisy
- diabetes
- rib fracture
- depression

In this situation, the provider already has a diagnosis and can begin to formulate a plan for treatment.

When collecting information (step 1) the provider is attempting to make a medical diagnosis (step 2). Both steps often happen simultaneously. While collecting information and attempting to make the problem list, the provider may already have many ideas about what the diagnosis might be. The ideas about potential diagnoses help the provider know which questions to ask. The provider will test out different ideas by asking for more information about each of the symptoms the patient reveals.

A **symptom** is something that the patient experiences that is different from normal and indicates the presence of a particular disease. The different questions a provider can ask about the symptoms are known as symptom descriptors. The provider uses **symptom descriptors** to help refine the problem list and make it as specific as possible.

> **Vocabulary**
> **Symptom**: a physical, mental, or emotional feature that indicates the presence of disease
>
> **Symptom descriptor**: words used to describe what the patient is experiencing
>
> **Diagnostic questions**: questions a provider asks to gain information about a patient's condition

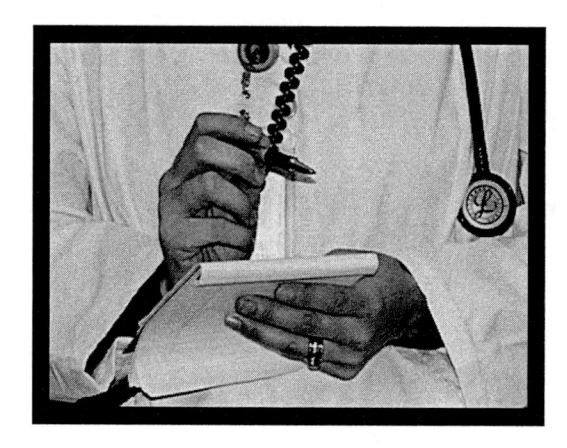

If the patient has complained of "chest pain," the chest pain is most likely the symptom of a particular disease. The provider will then go through a list of symptom descriptors and try to determine more specific information about the symptom. The provider might ask about the following symptom descriptors:

Onset: How did it start? Did it start slowly, gradually, abruptly?

Duration: How long does it last? Does it reoccur, is it constant, intermittent?

Location: Where is it? Where did it start?

Precipitant: What makes it start? Has it happened before?

Radiation: Where does it (the pain) go?

Relieved by: What makes it better? What makes it start or stop?

Quality: What does it feel like? Is it sudden, gradual, sharp, dull?

Patients often have more than one answer to any one of these questions. A careful history takes time, but it leads to a more accurate problem list/statement and a more accurate diagnosis. This then leads a provider to make a more effective treatment plan (step 3).

As a provider collects information, she/he is usually already thinking about what is wrong (step 2 in the problem solving process). Skilled providers may consider 15 to 20 diagnoses until a diagnosis is firmly established. At any one time during an interview, providers may have 5 or 6 possibilities in mind.

As the patient responds to each question, the provider uses the information to direct the next question. By asking specific questions, the provider is eventually able to eliminate the possibilities one by one until a definite diagnosis can be reached. These are called **diagnostic questions.**

Step 3: Figuring out what to do and making a plan.

When providers have made a decision about what is wrong with the patient, they move on to the next step: creating a plan for action.

When making this plan, they generally think about four things:

- the end goal
- collection of more data (more tests)
- treatment
- patient education

Providers ask themselves what their goal is in treating the patient. Their goal may not necessarily be to make the patient well. In some cases, there may be no way to make the patient well. In these cases, the goal may be to control pain, or to keep the illness from spreading.

Setting an appropriate goal is an important first step in deciding what to do. After that, doctors may want to collect more information (perhaps by doing more tests), treat the patient's problem, and educate the patient about his part in treatment. Education may also include how to avoid getting sick again, how to manage a chronic problem, or how to avoid spreading the sickness to others.

Step 4: Follow through with the plan and evaluate the outcome.

The final step in the problem solving process includes following through with the plan and evaluating if the outcome was satisfactory. After some period of time, the doctor will want to know how the patient is doing. Is the patient getting better? Is the problem under control? Has the problem reoccurred? In effect, the doctor will want to be able to see if the goal is being met. If not, the process of problem solving starts over again.

Conversation between patient and provider	What the provider is thinking
Provider: Hello Mrs. Chen. How are you doing today? How are the children? **Mrs. Chen:** Oh yes, the twins are doing just fine. They are now sleeping through the night. **Provider:** That's great to hear. Now, please tell me why you are here?	The provider has seen Mrs. Chen before and knows that she is a new mother. He is asking about the children to find out some information about her family history to see if there is any cause for concern there. The provider is trying to determine the chief complaint, an important part of the medical interview.
Mrs. Chen: I'm having chest pain.	As soon as the patient says this, the provider begins thinking of a possible diagnosis. He begins to think that it might be one of the following: • lung problems • heart problems • gastrointestinal tract problems • a pulled muscle
Provider: Can you describe what the pain feels like? **Mrs. Chen:** The pain feels like a pressure in my chest. **Provider:** Can you describe to me exactly where in your chest it hurts?	The provider will need more information about the symptom of chest pain that has been described. He begins to ask a series of symptom descriptor questions.

The Culture of Biomedicine

Conversation between patient and provider	What the provider is thinking
Mrs. Chen: I'm not sure. Sometimes I feel like it is up near my shoulders. Sometimes it feels like it is right below my ribs. **Provider:** Does the pressure occur when climbing stairs? **Mrs. Chen:** No. **Provider:** Does the pressure occur when you are resting? **Mrs. Chen:** No.	The provider now thinks that the cause of the chest pain may be a heart problem. He has a tentative diagnosis of angina. He begins a series of questions that are related to the heart. These are questions about Mrs. Chen's body systems. From what the provider knows about the cardiovascular system, he knows that heart problems will typically show a pattern of pain linked to exertion.
Provider: Does anyone in your family have a history of heart disease? **Mrs. Chen:** No, not that I know of. **Provider:** Does anyone in your family have high blood pressure? **Mrs. Chen:** No, not that I know of.	At this point, the provider is less certain of his tentative diagnosis of angina. He decides to ask a few more diagnostic questions about Ms. Chen's family medical history.
Provider: Have you been experiencing any nausea or vomiting lately? **Mrs. Chen:** Yes, actually I have. I've been quite nauseous lately. **Provider:** Mrs. Chen, I'd like to do an ultrasound and ask you a few more questions.	Now the provider thinks that perhaps it is not related to a heart problem. So, he moves on to another possible diagnosis and another line of questioning. He knows that problems related to the heart often look/feel similar to problems related to the gastrointestinal system so he begins to ask questions about the gastrointestinal system. These are more diagnostic questions about Mrs. Chen's body systems. The provider thinks that the cause of the chest pain is gallstones as a result of the information Mrs. Chen has provided him. Before he discusses a final diagnosis and treatment plan with Mrs. Chen, he will need to conduct a lab test.

© 2014 Cross Cultural Health Care Program

Informed Consent

Informed consent is a part of the culture of biomedicine with which interpreters must be familiar. In order to do any procedure on a patient, providers in the U.S. are required to get "informed consent." With informed consent, the patient knows what is going to be done, what the risks are in doing it, what the alternatives are, and gives the provider permission to go ahead.

> **Vocabulary**
>
> **Informed consent**: the process of making sure a patient knows what is going to be done and ensuring the patient gives the provider permission to perform a procedure or treatment

The concept of informed consent may seem very strange to some patients unfamiliar with the culture of biomedicine. In many cultures, a patient expects to trust the doctor to do what is best and does not expect to have to give permission at every step along the way. For these patients, the process of informed consent can weaken their trust in the provider. For some, talking about informed consent and the potential risks of a procedure could cause complications.

Informed consent is a complicated issue that challenges many professionals in the medical field. If a patient seems concerned or confused about the concept of informed consent, an interpreter can explain why a patient may be confused and let the provider decide what to do. Some institutions have a limited consent form, which the patient signs to say that he does not want to know the details of what is going to be done.

> **The Importance of Informed Consent**
>
> A patient who spoke English well, but did not read well, visited her gynecologist for her annual women's health exam. After a lengthy discussion, her doctor left her with multiple forms to sign. The patient trusted her doctor to do what was right for her. After signing the forms, she underwent the procedures recommended by her doctor.
>
> Two weeks later, the patient entered the clinic for a follow up appointment. The nurse greeted her and said, "How are you feeling after your hysterectomy?" The patient's jaw dropped. She did not have any idea that the procedure she had undergone two weeks before was a hysterectomy. She did not know that she had agreed to a procedure that would prevent her from having children. (American Medical Association)

The Patient's Approach to Problem Solving

Providers in western biomedicine try to fit a patient's symptoms into a recognizable pattern that can be labeled, and therefore treated. Just knowing that someone has "chest pain" does not tell the doctor how to treat it. Once the provider has decided the patient has "angina," there are recognized approaches to further diagnosis and treatment.

Unfortunately, this can sometimes lead physicians to ignore patients' ideas about what is wrong with them. Patients and providers use the same four steps towards problem solving. However, the patient is typically not influenced by the culture of biomedicine when engaging in the problem solving process. The patient typically relies on different sources of information. This means that the provider and the patient may come to different conclusions of what is wrong and how it should be treated. If this happens, the patient-provider relationship can deteriorate.

When a patient is problem solving and collecting information about what is wrong, she/he may collect information from the following:

- prior life experiences
- recent events in his/his life
- an analysis of what is happening to her/him right now, during the illness
- information gained from her/his cultural processes

A patient is not limited to these sources of information. He/she may use the information from the biomedicine problem solving procedure as well. Note that this list is different from the provider's primary sources of information.

Power and Bias in the Culture of Biomedicine

The previous section explained the importance of incorporating both the provider and the patient's methods of problem solving. A challenge in incorporating both modes of problem solving is the perceived imbalance of power, in which most of the power seems to be in the hands of the provider and those familiar with the culture of biomedicine.

What does the dominance of the provider culture look like?

- the provider has been asked to help, diagnose, counsel, treat, and often to certify the patient as "sick" in a socially approved fashion
- through the use of the medical interview, the provider organizes the discussion between patient and provider according to their knowledge of biomedical problems
- the provider takes the patient's responses and fits them into recognizable, manageable patterns through the use of diagnostic questions
- the provider determines which part of what the patient says will be regarded as significant, independent of the patient's views
- the provider describes both the diagnostic and therapeutic actions to be taken based on the provider's method of problem solving
- The health care providing facility determines the payment criteria. They decide when and how the bill is to be written and which services are on the bill.

While certain aspects may be changing, this sense of power on the part of the providers in the biomedical culture can easily lead to bias. Providers may have a sense of correctness, authority and superiority. By overlooking the patient's culture and views, the medical process is overwhelmingly biased toward that of biomedicine and the provider's culture.

> **Case Study - Domestic Violence Case and Power Imbalance**
>
> A 28-year-old Vietnamese woman came to the clinic after a number of brief emergency room visits for breathlessness and chest pain. Her complaints had been attributed to hyperventilation. Her history revealed an abusive husband, violence, and fright preceding the hospital visits. She had a long history of unwillingness to deal with her marital circumstances and rejected advice as well as referrals for help.
>
> The physician checked three items at the end of the patient's visit: chest pain, family problems, and breathlessness. The billing clerk listed family problems first, and the insurance company refused to pay the bill for the visit. A resubmission of the bill under the problem labels "breathlessness" and "chest pain" was quickly paid.
>
> The physician, independent of the patient, decided that 'chest pains,' 'family problems' and 'breathlessness' was the proper diagnosis for this woman's medical concerns. The billing clerk decided, again without the input of the patient, that 'family problems' should be listed first on the bill. The insurance provider made a decision *not* to pay the bill when 'family problems' was listed as the first diagnosis.

Hearing What the Patient Has to Say

In patient care settings, the provider and the patient are often both simultaneously engaging in problem solving processes. It is necessary to reach an accommodation between them. The patient's views must be taken into account and incorporated.

Patients may have special knowledge or views about the cause, necessary therapies, or specific family and community problems. These issues often play a role in a patient's understanding about illness and how the patient chooses to seek help and therapy. A skilled medical provider may be able to incorporate both their style of problem solving and their patient's style of problem solving into one coherent and effective solution.

Preserving the Patient's Language

Because each descriptor may lead to a different diagnostic direction, it is important to preserve the language the patient uses to describe a symptom. If the patient says, "The pain is like a pressure," and the interpreter misinterprets it to say, "The pain is like burning in my chest," that alone may cause the provider to shift his ideas about a final diagnosis.

If the provider asks the patient, "Do you have chest pain?" a patient may say "It's not pain, it's discomfort...an uncomfortable sensation ...distress." The patient may go on to describe the quality and the character of the discomfort: "It's...sharp...dull... crushing...tight...like something sitting on me...burning...like something that cuts off my breath." Each of these characterizations is important for the interpreter to convey to the provider.

It is important to hear about a patient's concern in the patient's own words. Interpreting words, phrases, and expressions related to the subjective experience of pain is a challenging subject matter for medical interpreters.

Understanding what influences both the provider's and the patient's approaches to problem solving can help you understand how to facilitate communication.

Different Approaches to Problem Solving

The provider's approach to problem-solving is:

- influenced by biomedical culture and provider's culture
- based on data, facts, science
- influenced by what is learned in medical school (body systems, anatomy, physiology)
- informed by developments in the field of medicine
- influenced by having the most power to make decisions

The patient's approach to problem-solving is:
- influenced by their active culture
- based on cultural beliefs
- influenced by life experiences (family problems, emotions, environment)
- informed by ideas about 'sicknesses' and what is happening to "me"
- may be influenced by thinking she has little or no power

Consider the example of a patient complaining of 'chest pain.' See the examples on the following pages to see different ways of problem solving. The first example shows how this problem might be resolved when the provider's and the patient's problem solving strategies occur simultaneously but independently of each other. The second example shows the more ideal setting, in which the problem is resolved by incorporating both the patient's and provider's methods of problem solving.

Problem Solving: <u>Not</u> Hearing What the Patient Has to Say

SCENARIO:
A 75-year-old Mexican woman comes into the clinic with chest pain.
She has just left her life-long home in Michoacan to come live with her youngest daughter.
She has left her other grown children and grandchildren behind.

Patient Problem Solving	Provider Problem Solving
↓	↓
1. Collects information through: • cultural beliefs • life experiences • thinking about "what is happening to me right now"	**1. Collects information** through • medical history • laboratory tests • physical exams
↓	↓
2. Decides what is wrong The patient thinks her chest pain might be due to • *nostalgia* (debilitating longing), or • *susto* (fright), or • witchcraft She decides that the cause of her chest pain is witchcraft.	**2. Decides what is wrong** The doctor thinks her chest pain might be due to • heart problems, or • pulmonary problems, or • GI problems, or • musculoskeletal problems The doctor decides that the cause of her chest pain is angina, a heart problem.
↓	↓
3. Figures out what to do She decides to see a *curandero,* a traditional healer, to help solve the problem of being a victim of witchcraft.	**3. Figures out what to do** Doctor prescribes her pills to help with the angina.

↘ ↙

4. Patient follows through with decision and evaluates
She does not believe that the pills will address her concern and so throws them in the garbage and continues to see only the *curandero,* completely disregarding the doctor's problem solving. Her chest pain may or may not get better.

The Culture of Biomedicine

Problem Solving: Hearing What the Patient Has to Say

SCENARIO:
A 75-year-old Mexican woman comes into the clinic with chest pain. She has just left her life-long home in Michoacan to come live with her youngest daughter. She has left her other grown children and grandchildren behind.

Patient Problem Solving   Provider Problem Solving

1. Collects information
through:
- cultural beliefs
- life experiences
- thinking about "what is happening to me right now"

Information is shared between patient and provider

1. Collects information
through
- medical history
- lab tests
- physical exams

2. Decides what is wrong
The patient thinks her chest pain might be due to
- *nostalgia* (debilitating longing), or
- *susto* (fright), or
- witchcraft.

She tells the provider that she believes the cause of her chest pain is that she is the victim of witchcraft

Based on the methods of problem solving they are familiar with, the patient and provider come to different conclusions about what the nature of the problem is.

2. Decides what is wrong
The provider thinks her chest pain might be due to
- heart problems, or
- pulmonary problems, or
- GI problems, or
- musculoskeletal problems

The provider tells the patient that he thinks the cause of her chest pain is angina, a heart problem.

3. Figures out what to do
Together the patient and provider decide what to do. They decide that the patient will see a *curandero*, a traditional healer, to help solve the problem of being a victim of witchcraft as well as take the pills the doctor has prescribed for the angina.

4. Patient follows through with decision and evaluates
She sees the *curandero* and takes the pills.
Both the patient and provider methods of problem solving are utilized.
Her chest pain may or may not get better.

Interpreting Within the Culture of Biomedicine

Interpreters are involved in every step that requires patient-provider communication. And, in every step, they must be conscious of the different cultures that are involved. The following are five guidelines for interpreting within the context of the biomedicine culture.

1. Interpret everything that is said, as faithfully and as accurately to the meaning as possible. The interpreter needs to interpret everything the patient and provider say, even if it seems irrelevant.

2. Interpret the "small talk." Providers who know a patient well will occasionally make inquiries about past events that they have discussed with the patient, or they may socialize with the patient by asking about family, job or recent events. This often plays an integral part in the building of a patient-provider relationship. Interpreters need to interpret this small talk as well.

3. Communicate all patient ideas about why they think they are ill. When patients describe to doctors why they think they are ill, they may use specific, culture-bound terms to talk about their illness and their concerns. By communicating these terms, interpreters can play a key role in helping both the patient and the provider understand each other's points of view.

4. Communicate clearly with the provider and the patient. Communication is the most important tool used for evaluation in health care. The interpreter's role is very important here. Key decisions are often based on the quality and character of what patients have to say. The interpreter's ability to faithfully portray the patient's views, emotions and language is the critical link in the process.

5. Interpret with an awareness of your own biases. The interpreter can exercise the same power and dominance as the provider, with the same negative results. As the only member of the group who understands everyone, the interpreter has a great deal of power to influence the course of the interaction. Interpreters must be careful to not let their personal biases influence their interpretation. These issues will be discussed further in the lessons on culture brokering and advocacy.

Summary

As a bridge between patient and provider, the interpreter must be familiar with the cultural influences that affect communication between patient and provider. By understanding the culture of the provider and that of biomedicine, the interpreter can more effectively identify cultural bumps and facilitate understanding.

Skill Development

Role-play: Medical interview

This role-play, taken from the sample medical interview earlier in this chapter, can be performed like the previous interpreting practice exercises, with a patient, a provider, and an interpreter. As you interpret, think about what informs the provider's questions and the patient's answers.

Provider: Hello Mrs. Chen. How are you doing today? How are the children?

Mrs. Chen: Oh yes, the twins are doing just fine. They are now sleeping through the night.

Provider: That's great to hear. Now, please tell me why you are here?

Mrs. Chen: I'm having chest pain.

Provider: Can you describe what the pain felt like?

Mrs. Chen: The pain felt like a pressure in my chest.

Provider: Can you describe to me exactly where in your chest it hurts?

Mrs. Chen: I'm not sure. Sometimes I feel like it is up near my shoulders. Sometimes it feels like it is right below my ribs.

Provider: Does the pressure occur when climbing stairs?

Mrs. Chen: No.

Provider: Does the pressure occur when you are resting?

Mrs. Chen: No.

Provider: Does anyone in your family have a history of heart disease?

Mrs. Chen: No, not that I know of.

Medical interview role-play, continued

Provider: Does anyone in your family have high blood pressure?

Mrs. Chen: No, not that I know of.

Provider: Have you been experiencing any nausea or vomiting lately?

Mrs. Chen: Yes, actually I have. I've been quite nauseous lately.

Provider: Mrs. Chen, I'd like to do an ultrasound and ask you a few more questions.

Skill Development

Pain descriptors activity

PART A: Find equivalents for these English pain terms in your own non-English target language.

Ache
Burning pain
Cramps
Dull pain
Pain that comes and goes
Annoying pain
Constant pain
Crushing pain
Gnawing pain
Numbing pain
Pins and needles

Shifting pain
Sickening pain
Spasms
Stinging pain
Throbbing pain
Sharp pain
Shooting pain
Soreness
Stabbing pain
Tenderness
Tingling

PART B: List specific terms used in your non-English target language to describe pain and then find the English equivalent.

Skill Development

Understanding the pain scale

Pain management is an important aspect of health care. Many hospitals' patient bill of rights includes a patient's right to timely, effective pain management.

In order to provide pain management, a provider might ask a patient to rate their pain on a scale of 1-10.

Many patients may not be familiar with the concept of rating their pain on a scale of 1-10.

It is important to make sure you, as the interpreter, clearly understand what the provider is asking when telling the patient to rate their pain on a scale.

The provider may be asking the patient to rate their pain from 1-10, with 1 being no pain at all, to 10 being the worst possible pain they can imagine.

Since the patient and the provider might have different cultural beliefs about pain and how to handle it, it is essential that the interpreter understand what both the patient and provider mean when rating pain.

Lesson 12

THE CULTURE BROKER ROLE

GOAL

Develop the skills of the culture broker role so that, when faced with a cultural bump, the interpreter will be able to facilitate mutual understanding.

KNOWLEDGE OUTCOMES

- Understand content-based cultural barriers vs. process-based cultural barriers

- Understand the steps of the culture broker role

Vocabulary
Content-based cultural bump
Process-based cultural bump

Introduction

In the previous lessons, we discussed some of the cultural factors that may inform the worldview, behavior, and decision-making process of the patient and the provider. When these cultural factors result in conflicting expectations and misunderstandings, it is the interpreter's job to step in as the culture broker to facilitate understanding. This section will help develop awareness of the nature of these misunderstandings and introduce the skills necessary to be an effective culture broker and resolve the misunderstandings.

Types of Cultural Bumps

Cultural bumps occur when people expect one type of behavior, and cross-cultural interactions result in something different. Interpreters might encounter two types of cultural bumps. One type is found in the *content* of the communication and the other in the *process*.

Content-based cultural bumps are related to what is said or done in an interaction. Content-based bumps occur when a person says or does something that has different meaning within his or her cultural context than in the cultural context of the listener.

For example, an oncologist asks an advanced cancer patient who wants to return home to rural Peru if she will have access to adequate medical care there. She says "yes." However, "adequate medical care" may mean different things to the patient and the provider. The patient may be envisioning a public clinic with minimal stocks of medicine. The physician is more likely to be envisioning a full-service hospital with hospice care. These assumptions could result in misunderstandings that could negatively affect the patient's health.

Process-based cultural bumps are related to *how* things are said or done. Process-based bumps occur when the way something is done or said has a meaning which is different between the cultures.

An example of a process-based bump is when a provider comes into the room with her head buried in a chart or laptop and begins to talk to the patient without even greeting her. The provider may be short on time. To save time, the provider may want to get right to the patient's concerns. The patient, however, may believe the provider's lack of greeting indicates a lack of courtesy and respect.

> **Vocabulary**
>
> **Content-based cultural bump**: when what is said or done has a different meaning to each of the people involved in an interaction
>
> **Process-based cultural bump**: when the way things are done has a different meaning to each of the people involved in an interaction

Guidelines for the Culture Broker Role

The first step in the culture broker role is to be aware that a cultural misunderstanding may be occurring. Often some key information is enough to alert the provider to ask more questions. Therefore, the interpreter should intervene in a transparent way. Then, the interpreter should let the patient know in general terms what he/she is going to do. Then, the interpreter can offer the key information to the provider. The goal is to get back to conduit interpreting as fast as possible.

The culture broker role can be understood as a five-step process:

1. The interpreter is alert to potential cultural barriers to understanding.

2. The interpreter explains to the patient what she wants to tell the provider, or vice versa.

3. The interpreter briefly tells the provider or patient the appropriate information, stating it as something that is generally true in the culture. She avoids stereotyping.

4. The interpreter lets the doctor decide what to do with this information.

5. The interpreter goes back to conduit interpreting as quickly as possible.

When acting as a culture broker, the interpreter should:

- be respectful in what is said, and how it is said
- make no assumptions
- avoid creating or reinforcing stereotypes

The Five Steps of Culture Brokering

1. Be alert to potential cultural bumps, whether process-based or content-based.

2. Explain to the patient or provider what you want to tell the other.

3. Briefly provide the appropriate cultural context, avoiding stereotypes.

4. Let the provider decide what to do with the information provided.

5. Return to conduit interpreting as quickly as possible.

We can apply these guidelines to the content-based cultural bump example of the cancer patient discussed earlier.

Doctor: Mrs. Chungara, I know you want to go home, but I'm concerned about your medical needs at this point. Will you have access to adequate health care there?
Patient: Oh yes, there's a hospital in my town.
Doctor: Well, in that case, maybe there's no problem.

STEP 1: The interpreter is alert to potential cultural barriers to understanding

The interpreter knows that the patient is from a small town in rural Peru. She is familiar with Peru's health care system and the level of care often available to rural dwellers. She is also aware of the type of care needed for an end-stage cancer patient. She suspects a misunderstanding, judges that it could have serious results. The interpreter decides to intervene.

STEP 2: The interpreter explains to the patient what she wants to tell the doctor.

Interpreter: (To the patient) This is the interpreter speaking. I'd like to mention to the doctor a little information about the health care system in Peru.
Patient: Oh. That would be all right.

STEP 3: The interpreter briefly tells the doctor the appropriate information, stating it as something that is generally true in the culture. She avoids stereotyping.

Interpreter: (To the doctor) This is the interpreter speaking. I would like to inform you that in many parts of Peru, people use the word "hospital" to refer to any health care facility. Mrs. Chungara is from a rural area of the country. It would be unusual if there was an inpatient hospital there.

> **Remember**
>
> Be respectful.
>
> Make no assumptions.
>
> Be transparent.

STEP 4: The interpreter lets the doctor decide what to do with this information.

Doctor: Hmm, that would be a concern. Mrs. Chungara, tell me exactly what you mean by "hospital." Would they have an oncologist there? Could they hospitalize you if necessary? Would there be a pharmacy where you could get a prescription for pain killers?

Patient: Well, not really. I guess it's not a hospital really, but there's a nurse there most days who could give an injection. And there's a pharmacy in town where you can buy anything. You don't need a prescription.

STEP 5: The interpreter goes back to conduit interpreting as quickly as possible. Having clarified the cultural misunderstanding, the interpreter can return to the less invasive conduit role.

We can also apply these guidelines to cultural barriers that are caused by a patient misunderstanding of the biomedical culture. In this situation, the interpreter may need to provide a key piece of information to the patient. The same guidelines for culture brokering still apply regardless of who is being misunderstood.

Some examples of when the patient may require a piece of key information include:

- a patient being seen by a resident insists on being seen by a "real doctor"
- a patient feels that only having 15 minutes with her primary care provider is a sign of discrimination

- a patient doesn't understand why the provider is focused on looking at the computer instead of looking at the patient when the patient is trying to describe the problem

Sometimes it helps to let patients know about the norms of the health care facility. The same guidelines for culture brokering apply. Make sure communication is transparent, give appropriate information in a general way, and go back to conduit interpreting as quickly as possible.

Summary

It is important for interpreters to be aware of potential misunderstandings based on cultural differences. When these arise, the interpreter can intervene and clarify the misunderstanding, using the five steps of culture brokering. By using these five steps effectively, the interpreter can go back to their primary Conduit role as quickly as possible.

Skill Development

Now that you are familiar with three of the roles of the interpreter – conduit, clarifier, and culture broker, you can write your own role-plays demonstrating these three roles.

Incorporate the skills you have learned so far, including pre-sessions, managing the flow of the session, interpreting in the first person, and handling cultural bumps.

You can create your own skits based on real life or hypothetical experiences. If you use real-life experiences, be sure not to include any information that could identify real patients.

If you need help getting started, consider the following ideas:

- You are interpreting for a patient at a routine doctor visit. The nurse asks what type of medications the patient takes, and the patient shows the nurse some medications that a friend sent her from her home country. The nurse is confused about how the patient got the medication without a prescription.

- You are interpreting for a patient, who has gone to the emergency room for a non-urgent matter, such as a mild but persistent cold. The triage nurse is clearly annoyed that the patient is using the emergency room for a non-urgent matter.

- You are interpreting for a patient in a small clinic, who is there for a physical for their job. The patient also brought in their two small children and asks if they can be seen during the same appointment.

- You are interpreting for a patient in a mental health setting, who is talking very quickly and won't pause for you to interpret.

- You are interpreting over the phone and cannot see the patient's body language, and you are having trouble hearing well.

Section 3

Navigating the Health Care System

Lesson 13
THE UNITED STATES HEALTH CARE SYSTEM

GOAL

Gain a basic overview of the United States health care system.

KNOWLEDGE OUTCOMES

- Understand some of the factors that shape the United States health care system

- List different types of providers, facilities, and settings that interpreters may encounter

- Understand when professional interpreters or bilingual staff are required by federal law

---

Vocabulary

Allopathic medicine

Alternative or complementary medicine

Attending physician

Copay

Deductible

Dental student

Fellow

Medical student

Resident

Teaching hospital

> **Brainstorm**
>
> Have you had experiences in the United States health care system?
> Have you had experiences in health care systems outside of the United States?
> What differences or similarities did you notice?

Introduction

Health care in the United States is a complex system that has been evolving since the country was first formed. There is an increasing list of new and different health care professionals offering services. Additionally, a vast array of insurance options limit where, when, how much, by whom, and for what a patient can be seen. Even for people who speak English fluently, this system can be very confusing.

As an interpreter, it is not your job to know everything about the health care system, to act as a social worker, or to refer patients to providers or coverage options. However, it is important that you have an overview of how the health care system works in the United States. It is important for interpreters to be familiar with different types of providers and facilities that they may encounter while working as an interpreter. Interpreters need to understand how to talk about different types of providers and procedures in their source and target languages.

In addition, the advocate role deals with systemic barriers that patients may encounter when navigating an unfamiliar health care system. Interpreters working in the United States should have a basic understanding of the United States health care system in order to advocate successfully when necessary.

Health care providers in the U.S.

Types of health care providers and the title they are given in the U.S. may differ from those in other countries. Each of these professionals has a different role to play.

A "doctor" may be anyone from a first year **resident** just out of medical school to a specialist with 18 years of post-high school education. A doctor could practice **allopathic medicine** or **alternative or complementary medicine.** In addition to doctors, there are a variety of other providers that a patient might see during the course of their treatment.

> **Vocabulary**
>
> **Allopathic medicine:** mainstream medical care in the United States; the use of drugs and surgery to combat disease
>
> **Alternative/complementary medicine:** health care practices that are not considered part of mainstream medical treatment; may include acupuncture, herbal remedies, homeopathy, etc.
>
> **Resident:** a person who has received a medical degree and is practicing medicine, usually under supervision

Medical Education and Residency

Doctors and dentists are required to complete many years of schooling and supervised practice before they can practice on their own. Patients may be seen in teaching hospitals, where medical students practice under the supervision of **attending physicians**.

In a **teaching hospital** or clinic, the patient may be seen by medical students or physicians at various stages of their education and training. Medical students should introduce themselves as such. Be aware that residents and fellows *are* doctors who are involved in advanced studies under the senior physician's direct supervision. Patients should also know that they have a right to be seen by the attending physician.

Vocabulary

Attending physician: doctors who have finished their education and training and have the primary responsibility for patients

Dental student: a person studying to become a dentist

Fellow: a medical doctor who is pursuing additional training in a specialty field

Medical student: a person studying to become a doctor

Teaching hospital: a hospital where medical students see patients under the supervision of attending physicians

Doctors and dentists follow a similar pathway through education and residency:

After 4 years of college:
Receive a Bachelor of Arts (BA) or a Bachelor of Science (BS) degree

↓

+4 years of medical or dental school
These students are called **medical students** or **dental students**.

↓

After medical or dental school
Students receive their MD, DO, DDS, or DMD degree and are known as and certified as doctors or dentists.

↓

Depending on their specialty, doctors go through 1-5 years of residency in a hospital, under the supervision of an attending physician. During this time, they are called residents.
Dentists may also go through 2-3 years of specialized study, but not all dentists are required to specialize.

↓

+ 3-7 years of specialization
Some residents go on to a fellowship, under the supervision of an attending physician. **Fellows** can operate as an attending physician in the area of their residency. Not all doctors are required to go on to fellowships.

↓

Attending physicians:
Have finished their residency and/or their fellowship and can supervise Residents and/or fellows. They have the primary responsibility for the patient.

Types of Health Care Providers in the United States	
Provider	**Scope of work and training**
Primary Care Provider (PCP)	A person that a patient may see first for general checkups and health problems. A primary care provider is not a specific type of doctor, but is generally the person designated as the patient's main, general health care provider.
Generalist	An MD or DO who specializes in internal medicine, family practice, or pediatrics, rather than a specific disease or body system.
Medical doctor (MD)	An MD evaluates and treats illness. An MD generally receives 12-20 years of training after high school. They may specialize in a certain type of medicine or may be a generalist.
Osteopath/Doctor of Osteopathy (DO)	A DO evaluates and treats illness just as an MD would, but with a "whole person" approach, including manipulative treatment of bones and muscles.
Physician assistant (PA)	A PA may provide health care services under the supervision of a physician, such as history-taking, physical examination, and diagnosis. Their education varies, but they generally hold a bachelor's degree, plus about 4 years of health related experience, in addition to a 2+ year PA program.
Registered nurse (RN)	A person who has graduated from a nursing program, passed a state board examination, and is licensed by the state. They work in all medical settings.
Nurse practitioner (NP)	A registered nurse with graduate training. They may serve as a primary care provider. An NP can prescribe medicines. They may work with or without doctor supervision, depending on state laws.
Advanced practice nurse	A person who has education and experience beyond basic training and licensure required of all RNs.

The United States Health Care System

Types of Health Care Providers, continued	
Provider	**Scope of work and training**
Clinical nurse specialist (CNS)	A CNS has specialized training in a field such as cardiac, psychiatric, or community health.
Certified Nurse Midwife (CNM)	An RN with specific training in women's health care, including prenatal care, labor and delivery, and postnatal care.
Certified registered nurse anesthetist	A person who has training in the field of anesthesia.
Licensed practical nurse (LPN)	An LPN works in all medical settings, but is less advanced than an RN. They do not have a degree in nursing, but have state licensure plus training.
Certified nursing assistant (CNA)	A CNA has training and certification, but not a nursing degree.
Dentistry	
Dentist (DDS/DMD)	A person who evaluates and treats tooth and/or gum problems.
Dental assistant	A person who assists dentists and performs some dental procedures according to state laws, which vary.
Dental hygienist	Someone who cleans teeth and may assist dentists with dental procedures.
Pharmacy	
Licensed pharmacist	Someone who holds a graduate degree from a college of pharmacy. They may prepare and process drug prescriptions from a health care provider.
Pharmacy technician	A person who dispenses medications in a pharmacy under the supervision of a pharmacist.
Specialists	
Anesthesiologist	A person who provides general anesthesia or a spinal block for surgeries and pain control.
Audiologist	A person who measures hearing.

© 2014 The Cross Cultural Health Care Program

Types of Health Care Providers, continued	
Provider	Scope of work and training
Cardiologist	Someone who specializes in heart disorders.
Dermatologist	Someone who specializes in skin disorders.
Endocrinologist	Someone who specializes in hormonal or metabolic disorders.
Gastroenterologist	Someone who specializes in digestive system disorders.
Hematologist	Someone who specializes in blood disorders.
Immunologist	Someone who specializes in immune disorders.
Obstetrician/Gynecologist (OB-GYN)	Someone who specializes in pregnancy and women's reproductive health.
Oncologist	Someone who specializes in cancer treatment.
Ophthalmologist	Someone who specializes in eye disorders.
Orthopedic surgeon	Someone who specializes in surgery of bones and connective tissue.
Otorhinolaryngologist	Someone who specializes in ear, nose, and throat disorders.
Radiologist	Someone who specializes in x-rays and related procedures.
Urologist	Someone who specializes in the male and female urinary system, as well as the male reproductive system.

Types of Health Care Providers, continued	
Provider	**Scope of work and training**
Mental health	
Psychiatrist	Someone who specializes in emotional or mental disorders. They may prescribe medicines, while a counselor, MSW, or psychologist may not.
Psychologist	Someone who treats mental health disorders but cannot prescribe medications.
Counselor (MSW/MA)	Someone who provides mental health counseling.
Social worker	Someone who helps patients access social services. They may have a degree in social work.
Other	
Dietician/Nutritionist	Someone who counsels patients on diet and nutrition.
Medical assistant	Someone who assists medical professionals and may perform tasks such as measuring vital signs, administering medications, and preparing medical instruments and supplies, among others.
Phlebotomist	A person who draws blood and may perform some tests.
Physical therapist (PT/MSPT)	A person who provides rehabilitative treatment for injuries, pain, and other issues.

Health Care Facilities in the U.S.

Today, health care in the United States is provided in many different settings and facilities. Some facilities have specialties. For example, they might only work with older people, or only with AIDS patients, or only with burn care, or only with mental health. The following are a few examples of different types of health care facilities. Although it is not a comprehensive list, you can get an idea of some of the different types of facilities where you might interpret.

- Clinics (public and private) provide primary and/or specialty care for outpatients
- Hospitals (public and private) often provide primary care and specialty care, but they also provide inpatient care and emergency care
- Home care services provide care for people in their own homes
- Hospice provides palliative care for people who doctors believe are terminal and will not survive past six months

- Long term care, like nursing homes, provide care for people who need medical care over a long period of time
- Respite care provides a break to family caregivers by taking an aged or disabled patient for a few days

Health Insurance and Coverage

Unlike many other countries, the United States does not have a universal health care system. In the United States today, there are numerous funding sources and health care providers at the national, state, and local level. There are public, private, and nonprofit hospitals, clinics, local health departments, and free clinics in the United States. This can make the system difficult to understand for United States-born citizens, immigrants, and refugees alike.

The cost of health care is very high in the United States. Many people cannot afford health care without insurance. Health insurance helps people pay for a portion of their health care costs. However, patients are also expected to pay for a portion of the care they receive. Often, health insurance plans have **deductibles** and **copays** for medical appointments, procedures, and prescriptions.

A significant number of people in the United States receive health insurance through their employer, but not all employees qualify for health insurance this way. There are government-sponsored health coverage programs as well, whose requirements and restrictions vary from state to state. Each state funds and regulates health care in different ways. As a result, each community may have different sources of medical care and funding. A person's ability to access care in different facilities is determined by the type of health care coverage they hold.

> **Vocabulary**
>
> **Deductible**: an amount of money that a person must pay before an insurance company will pay for a claim
>
> **Copay**: an amount of money that an insured person must pay, in addition to what their insurance pays

Health Care Laws and Regulation

One of the challenges in understanding health care payment options is that there are many government laws and organizations that dictate and oversee health care coverage, methods and payment options. Although providing an exhaustive explanation of all of the laws affecting health care in the United States is outside the scope of this text, there are a few laws which may affect interpreters more than others. These include:

- Title VI of the Civil Rights Act of 1964
- Culturally and Linguistically Appropriate Service (CLAS) Standards
- The Joint Commission
- The Affordable Care Act

Title VI of the Civil Rights Act of 1964

Title VI of the Civil Rights Act of 1964 states that "no person in the United States shall, on the ground of race, color, or national origin, be excluded from participation in, be denied the benefits of, or be subjected to discrimination under any program or activity receiving Federal financial assistance." Here, we will examine what each part of this statement means as it relates to interpreters.

"...on the grounds of...national origin..."
National origin refers to being from a particular country or part of the world. National origin also means belonging to or being associated with a particular ethnic or cultural group. For the purpose of this law, a person's preferred language falls under their national origin.

"...be denied the benefits of, or be subjected to discrimination..."
Discrimination refers to treating a person differently. This means that a person who does not speak English fluently should not have to pay more or have more difficulty accessing health care than a person who does speak English fluently. According to this law, health care facilities must provide a qualified interpreter to a patient free of charge.

"...under any program or activity receiving federal financial assistance."
This part of the law refers to organizations that receive money from the federal government. It is important to know that this law does not require all health care facilities to provide interpreters free of charge. A private clinic or doctor's office may not be required to provide interpreters for their patients, if the facility does not receive money from the federal government.

Title VI

Title VI of the Civil Rights Act of 1964 provides that "no person in the United States shall, on the ground of race, color, or national origin, be excluded from participation in, be denied the benefits of, or be subjected to discrimination under any program or activity receiving Federal financial assistance."

Title VI
- applies to all programs that receive federal funding
- is enforceable by law
- requires all programs and facilities that receive federal funding to provide appropriate language services, including professionally trained interpreters when needed

According to this law, ineffective methods of communication between providers and LEP patients would be a form of discrimination based on country of national origin. Effective methods of communication include the use of professionally trained interpreters. The use of family members or minors as interpreters can be a violation of Title VI if it is shown that the family member or minor that was interpreting was inadequate and compromised the delivery of effective health care services.

CLAS Standards

CLAS stands for "Culturally and Linguistically Appropriate Services." The CLAS Standards are produced by the Office of Minority Health, which is part of the national Department of Health and Human Services. These standards seek to ensure that everyone receives quality care that is respectful of their cultural beliefs and meets their language needs. This includes identifying patients' language preferences, translating important forms into commonly used languages, and using skilled and trained professional interpreters or bilingual staff with interpreter training.

The Joint Commission

The Joint Commission is a nonprofit organization that accredits hospital departments and programs. When a hospital is accredited, this means that that the Joint Commission has examined the way a hospital provides care and has determined that it meets national standards. With an accreditation from the Joint Commission a hospital is eligible for Medicaid and/or Medicare reimbursement.

The Joint Commission standards include a commitment to culturally and linguistically appropriate care. This means that all patients should receive care that is in a language that they can understand and respectful of their cultural beliefs. Interpreters are a significant part of providing appropriate care to LEP patients.

The Affordable Care Act (ACA)

On March 23, 2010, President Obama signed the Patient Protection and Affordable Care Act (ACA).

The intention of the ACA is to:

- help people maintain health coverage
- make private insurance more accessible
- bring down health care costs
- give individuals and families more control over their own health care

The ACA aims to do this by:
- providing a stronger safety net and making it more difficult for insurers to cancel or deny health insurance coverage
- investing in preventative services and providing preventative services without copays in many cases
- covering more services, including emergency care, mental health, maternity and newborn care, substance abuse treatment, and prescription drugs (Hodos)

Summary

It is not an interpreter's job to know everything about the United States health care system, nor to counsel patients about their rights. However, it is important that you have a basic understanding of some of the different factors that shape the system. You may end up working within a specialized field of medicine, such as oncology or pediatrics, in which case, you will learn more specifics about that particular area of medicine. You can use this lesson as a jumping-off point for further research and learning.

Skill Development

Identifying health care facilities and specialists in your community

What type of service or specialization do these providers offer? Can you provide examples of these types of providers in your community?

Nurse practitioner (NP)
Certified Nurse Midwife (CNM)
Dentist (DDS/DMD)
Licensed pharmacist
Dermatologist
Obstetrician/Gynecologist (OB-GYN)
Orthopedic surgeon
Psychiatrist
Dietician/Nutritionist
Generalist
Oncologist
Counselor
Urologist
Social worker
Anesthesiologist

Brainstorm examples of these health care facilities that are found in your community.

Doctor's offices
Community clinics
Free clinics
Urgent care clinics
Outpatient surgery center/surgicenter
Dentist's offices
Hospitals
Children's hospitals
Cancer/Oncology center
Nursing home
Assisted living
Inpatient mental health
Mental health clinic
Alternative medicine providers

Skill Development

Understanding the United States health care system

Consider your own experiences in the United States health care system.

Use these questions to engage with your fellow interpreters in a discussion about health care systems.

What is your experience with the U.S. health care system?

Do you have health care coverage? If so, what type?

Have you had different kinds of health care coverage in the past?

What is your experience with health care in other countries?

In your experience, how would you compare and contrast the U.S. health care coverage to that found in other countries?

How is your experience with the U.S. health care system similar or different to other interpreters in this course?

What other kinds of health care coverage/payment options/facilities have you heard of or encountered?

Lesson 14

DEFINING THE ADVOCATE ROLE

GOAL

Develop a definition of the advocate role, understand arguments for and against advocacy, and develop the ability to advocate effectively.

KNOWLEDGE OUTCOMES

- Define advocacy

- Understand arguments for and against advocacy

- Identify situations when advocacy is not appropriate

- Identify guidelines for how to advocate effectively

- Practice applying professional judgment to situations that require a decision about advocacy

Vocabulary
Advocacy

> **Brainstorm**
>
> Have you ever had to advocate for yourself in a situation where you did not feel your needs were being met? How did you do so? What was the outcome?
>
> Has anyone tried to advocate on your behalf? How did you feel about this? What was the outcome?

Introduction

Advocacy is the most controversial of the interpreter roles because traditionally, the interpreter is seen as being "neutral." The interpreter is not supposed to influence the outcome of the interpreted interview. However, there are some situations where it may be appropriate for an interpreter to speak up on behalf of a patient. When the interpreter becomes concerned about the quality of care the patient is receiving, it may be appropriate for the interpreter to advocate.

In conference, court, and business interpreting, the interpreter is restricted to interpreting exactly what is said. In medical interpreting, an interpreter should have no voice in which treatment options a patient chooses or whether the patient follows through with a diagnosis and treatment plan. Some people believe that medical interpreters should not act as advocates at all. However, others feel that there are many reasons that advocacy *should* be a part of the medical interpreting process. As a result, there is a debate about the role of advocacy in the health care setting.

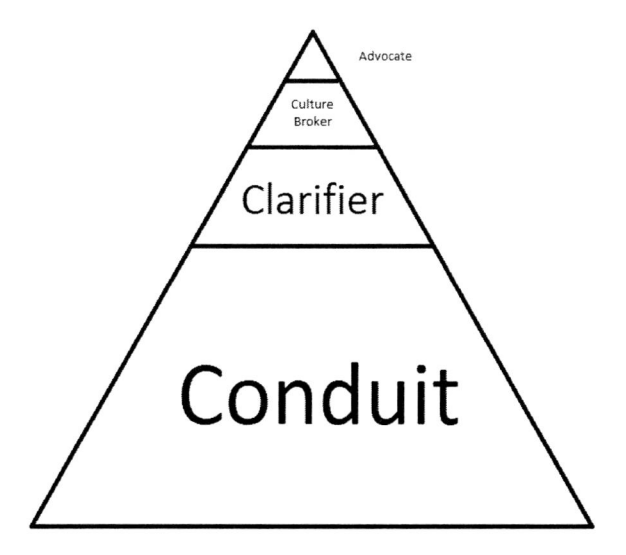

> **Vocabulary**
>
> **Advocacy**: supporting or acting in favor of a person or idea

Distinguishing between the four interpreter roles

Advocacy is any action taken on behalf of the patient that does not deal with the message that one person is trying to communicate to another. Normally, advocacy takes place outside of the interpreting session with the provider. Think of the roles of the interpreter:

In the conduit role, the interpreter is focused solely on interpreting the message.

In the clarifier role, the interpreter is asking for clarification or checking to see if the patient understood. The interpreter is still focused on the message.

In a culture broker role, the interpreter may be pointing out a cultural difference that is causing a misunderstanding. The interpreter is still focused on clarifying a cultural misunderstanding and not on taking any actions outside of the interpreted encounter.

It is only when the interpreter acts on behalf of the patient outside of the communication between patient and provider does the interpreter step into the role of advocate. For example, the interpreter might decide to inform the patient of her right to see the patient advocate or protest when a patient is turned away from a clinic even though she has a valid appointment card. These acts are not focused on the communication at all, but on the quality of service that the patient is receiving.

Who do we advocate for?

Why is advocacy defined as an action taken only on behalf of the patient? Can an interpreter advocate for a provider or the health care system?

Advocacy is usually undertaken to help equalize an imbalance in power. The provider or health care institution usually has the most power in an interpreted encounter. The interpreter also has power because she speaks the language of the dominant culture and is more likely to be familiar with the dominant culture.

In advocacy, a person with power (the interpreter), adds his/her voice to that of a person with less power (the patient). An interpreter does this in order to achieve a desired response from a person with more power (usually the provider or health care institution).

In a health care setting, those who represent the health care institution, especially the doctors, already hold power, because they control access to the care that the patient needs. They don't need interpreters to advocate for them. The patient, however, may need an advocate.

Unfortunately, LEP patients in the U.S. health care system are often marginalized in many ways. Systems are regularly set up to accommodate only English speakers. Some examples include:

- interpreters may be available for clinic visits, but there is often no system to help an LEP patient who calls to make an appointment, ask about medications, or consult with a nurse
- written materials and letters about policy and procedural changes are routinely written only in English

- traditional values held by patients may be ignored or belittled
- patients who are unfamiliar with American society and the health care system often are unaware of their rights and responsibilities
- many immigrants and refugees come from cultures where it is inappropriate to directly challenge people in authority

English speakers often have difficulty navigating the health care system. For LEP patients unfamiliar with how the system is supposed to work, the challenges are even greater.

Debating the Role of the Advocate

Those who argue for advocacy typically feel that it is the humanitarian thing to do. Their support of advocacy is usually based on:

- compassion and empathy for the patient
- feeling that helping a person without power is the right thing to do
- wanting to ensure that the patient receives the best possible treatment
- having concern for other's welfare

Those who argue against the role of advocacy in medical interpreting suggest reasons based on guidelines established for professional behavior. Those who are against it generally argue that advocacy:

- compromises the interpreter's neutrality and can undermines the provider's trust in the interpreter
- cause interpreters to be seen as bothersome people who are constantly demanding more or better care for their LEP patients than an English-speaking patient would receive
- patronizes patients who are perfectly capable of standing up for themselves
- can create patient dependency, not only on interpreters in general, but on certain interpreters in particular
- is not an interpreter's job, and there are already people in the health care system whose job it is to resolve patient problems, i.e., patient advocates and social workers

How can this issue be resolved? Advocacy must be clearly defined. Guidelines should be established to help interpreters know when they are advocating appropriately and when they are invading the patient - provider relationship. Interpreters need to have the skills necessary to advocate well so as to increase trust rather than undermine it.

Both the National Council on Interpreting in Health Care (NCIHC) and the International Medical Interpreters Association (IMIA) have issued Standards of Practice that address advocacy. The NCIHC Standards of Practice suggest that an interpreter may take on the role of the advocate if they must "speak out to protect an individual from harm" or "to correct mistreatment or abuse" (NCIHC, National Standards of Practice for Interpreters in Health Care).

The IMIA Standards of Practice suggest that the interpreter has a duty to "deal with discrimination". These standards also suggest that an interpreter use effective strategies when "the interpreter feels strongly that either party's behavior is affecting access to or quality of service, or compromising either party's dignity" (IMIA, Medical Interpreting Standards of Practice).

When to Advocate in a Medical Setting

Knowing when and how to advocate can be challenging. Different institutions have different policies about who can and should advocate. Doctors, nurses, receptionists and other support staff may advocate from time to time when they perceive a need, even if it is not technically a part of their job. Whether an institution considers this to be part of an interpreter's job will depend on many internal factors. It is important to be aware of the internal policies of the institution(s) where you interpret.

Assuming that an institution wants to provide quality services to every patient, you can justify advocating if you perceive that a patient is not getting quality care. Medical interpreters provide their services through a variety of contractual arrangements. The institution you work for and the type of contract you have with them will often define when and how you can appropriately advocate for a patient. The more an interpreter is a part of the health care facility, the more she may be able to advocate effectively.

An interpreter who is unsure about the scope of advocacy that is appropriate should consider the norms of the health care institution in which he/she works. She/he must also consider how knowledgeable she/he is about the particular institution and the relationship she/he has with the employees and administrators there. Advocacy, in the end, is the choice of the individual interpreter, and there is no easy answer to the question of when to advocate.

Whichever contractual arrangement applies, the most important thing to remember is that different health care facilities have different policies about how an interpreter can advocate. You must know the institution's guidelines and respect them when interpreting in that facility.

An interpreter with good interpersonal skills and a clear understanding of when and how to advocate appropriately can be effective, and welcome, in any institution. Although it may vary greatly between each institution and each interpreter, the following are some guidelines about how the type of contract relates to the scope of advocacy allowed.

Staff Interpreters are employed at a health care facility as a dedicated interpreter for that facility. Staff interpreters:

- may have a broader scope for advocacy than other types of contracts
- usually have clear guidelines set for the scope of advocacy
- have the benefit of knowing their specific health care system well
- may have the opportunity to build trusting relationships with providers and patients by working with them repeatedly

Freelance/contract interpreters are contracted independently by a hospital or clinic. Contract interpreters:

- have the freedom to reject or accept appointments
- are usually paid only for the time they interpret
- may be less familiar with policies and procedures unique to each facility, because they are often contracting to a variety of facilities, leading to challenges in advocacy

- may find it more difficult to develop relationships with patients and providers when working at a variety of facilities
- may have less time available to advocate if they have to leave for another appointment at a different facility

Agency Interpreters are hired by interpreter agencies. Agency interpreters:

- are usually contracted by an agency, not by a hospital
- may have advocacy guidelines set by their agency
- rarely interpret in the same facility all the time and therefore may face challenges in being an advocate, similar to the role of a freelance/independent interpreter
- are removed from the health care facility's procedures and opportunities to build relationships; therefore, the scope for advocacy is often quite limited for agency interpreters

Remote interpreters interpret over the phone or video. Remote interpreters:

- often do not work in the same building, city, or even the same country as the person for whom they are interpreting
- will likely find it very difficult or impossible to advocate, as their contact with the patient usually ends when they disconnect the phone or video interpreting session

When Advocacy Is Not Appropriate

Although the appropriateness of advocacy generally depends on the institution and the individual interpreter, there are times when advocacy is not appropriate.

Some situations where advocacy would not be appropriate include:

- there does not appear to be a misunderstanding or oversight
- the patient does not want to continue with advocacy
- the patient needs a service not provided for anybody in the clinic in question
- advocacy would involve breaking confidentiality
- the advocacy is primarily for the benefit of the interpreter, not the patient

Remember, advocacy is action that an interpreter takes and, as such, the interpreter can decide whether or not to go ahead. If the patient takes the initiative to complain or insist on a particular action, you must accompany him or her to interpret, whether you think it's a good idea or not.

Summary

Advocacy is the most controversial of the four interpreter roles. Despite this controversy, it is possible for an interpreter to advocate effectively, without undermining the patient's autonomy, or the patient-provider relationship.

In order to advocate effectively, an interpreter should understand arguments for and against advocacy, so that they can determine appropriate actions. Interpreters need to understand when it is not appropriate to advocate, as well as how to do so effectively. In the next lesson, we will discuss developing communication skills to support effective advocacy.

Skill Development

Debating the Advocate Role

There are two sides to the debate about advocacy in medical interpreting: those who support advocacy, and those who do not.

With your group members, brainstorm arguments for the position your instructor asks you to defend.

Applying professional judgment

Consider the following scenario:

A Spanish speaking husband and wife have come to the provider to find out how to prevent further pregnancies. Upon seeing the interpreter, the husband angrily says "I've been living in this country for 7 years, I don't need an interpreter!" According to hospital policy, you remain in the room but do not actively participate in the conversation.

While listening, you observe that the husband seems to understand English, but is speaking for the wife and answering all of the provider's questions on her behalf.

When the provider explains the birth control pill method, the husband is interested and agrees to this course of action. As the couple gets ready to leave, you realize the husband may believe that he is supposed to take the birth control pills (and not his wife).

Is advocacy appropriate in this situation?
If so, why is advocacy appropriate?
If appropriate, what would this advocacy look like?

Brainstorm examples of situations when an interpreter may be in a position to advocate for a patient. Determine whether advocacy would be appropriate in each situation.

Remember, the 'answers' may not be as simple as "Yes, advocate" or "No, do not advocate." This is a challenging exercise that requires you to utilize your professional judgment and recognize that there might not be just one 'right answer.'

Lesson 15

Effective Advocacy

Goal

Develop communication skills to support effective advocacy.

Knowledge Outcomes

- Understand guidelines for appropriate and effective advocacy
- Develop effective communication skills
- Identify communication styles

Vocabulary

Aggressive

Passive

Passive-aggressive

Assertive

Effective Advocacy

Introduction

Now that we have discussed when it is appropriate to advocate, it is important to understand how to advocate, if you determine it is appropriate to do so. Advocacy requires sensitivity and good communication skills. By developing your communication skills, you can help ensure that your message comes across clearly. People are often more receptive and willing to help when they are approached in a clear and respectful way.

In this lesson, we will discuss general guidelines for advocacy. We will also cover strategies to help you communicate effectively within the US health care system.

How to Advocate Effectively

The following are some guidelines to help you advocate in a professional and non-threatening manner. These guidelines may not fit every situation. With experience, interpreters will be able to adapt these guidelines to fit their personal style of communication. Knowing when and how to advocate is an art that requires mature professional judgment. Interpreters who are conscious about what they do will develop that judgment and become effective advocates.

Identify the problem. Clearly identify the problem in your own mind. Ask enough questions of the patient or provider to determine if there really is a problem.

Explain the problem to the patient. Ask the patient if he or she would like you to pursue the question further. If the patient says no, do not continue. If the patient says yes, continue.

Use resources that are already available. Using the mechanisms already in place in the institution, choose the most appropriate person to whom to bring your concern. Make sure you are talking with the person who can resolve the problem. If the person you are talking to is not being helpful, politely ask to speak to that person's supervisor.

Introduce yourself and the patient to the person whose help you need. Clearly explain the problem. Sometimes, simply explaining the problem is enough. Enlist that person's help in solving the problem instead of blaming that person.

Ask questions. Ask questions to discover what options are available to resolve the problem, instead of telling the person what needs to be done.

Advocacy Guidelines

- Identify the problem
- Explain the problem to the patient
- Use resources that are already available
- Introduce yourself and the patient to the person whose help you need
- Ask questions
- Use non-threatening language
- Use non-threatening body language
- Represent your patient
- Know where to go for help

Effective Advocacy

Avoid:
- blaming
- raising your voice
- threats
- sarcasm
- contradicting
- interrupting

Use non-threatening language. Use statements like:

"I am concerned about...."
"Would it be possible..."
"What do you think about...?"
"What do you usually do when..."

Use non-threatening body language. When approaching someone for help, greet them in a friendly, non-confrontational way.
- focus your full attention on the person, keeping your eyes on his/her face
- avoid crossing your arms in front of you or standing with your hands on your hips

Represent your patient. Always make sure the patient knows what you are doing and is in agreement. Represent your patient's circumstances and wishes faithfully.

Know where to go for help. The interpreter services office of the institution where you are interpreting should support you. When a situation gets too difficult, or if you are unsure how to proceed, ask the interpreter services supervisor to help you. If there is no interpreter services office, call your agency or the person who assigned you to the job.

Effective Communication

When advocating for a patient, it is important that you present your message in a way that will be as well-received as possible. If you come across as rude and overbearing or unsure of yourself, people may be less responsive. It may be helpful for you to think of communication styles in four categories: aggressive, passive, passive-aggressive, and assertive.

Aggressive: A person who is communicating aggressively uses any means possible to achieve the goal of winning. This includes such things as putting others down or hurting and humiliating them. This behavior can sometimes get the aggressor what he or she wants, but at the expense of other people. Being the target of an aggressive communicator makes most people feel defensive and angry.

Communicating aggressively may be useful in certain circumstances. It may be tempting to communicate aggressively when you perceive injustice that upsets you, and you want to correct it. In fact, it

---

Vocabulary

Aggressive: ready to attack or confront

Assertive: confident and self-assured; expressing needs clearly with respect for self and others

Passive: allowing what happens or what others do without resisting or responding

Passive aggressive: indirectly resisting without directly stating one's needs or feelings

---

© 2014 Cross Cultural Health Care Program

may get you what you want the first time. However, clinic staff and providers will remember you, and the next time you need help, you may discover that people are unwilling to help you.

Passive: A person who communicates passively does not express preferences, allowing others to make decisions.

This communication style may be appropriate for certain people under certain circumstances; but for an interpreter trying to advocate for a patient's needs, this communication style will probably not help resolve the problem.

Passive-aggressive: The passive-aggressive communicator generally attempts to get his or her needs met through deception and manipulation. The key to recognizing passive-aggressive communication is that the words say that everything is all right, but the way the words are said communicates the opposite.

This communication style is common, especially among people who do not feel they have the right to request what they really need. As an interpreter, this communication style will simply leave you and the clinic staff confused and frustrated. It is unlikely to help you resolve problems or advocate successfully.

Assertive: Assertive behaviors are verbal and non-verbal responses which enable one to act in one's own best interests, to stand up for oneself, to express one's opinions, feelings, needs, and wants without violating another person in the

> ### Assertive Communication
>
> Here are some tips about responding assertively when trying to resolve a problem or advocate for a patient.
>
> - Start by thinking: "My concern is important and deserves to be addressed," and, "The person I'm talking to is also important and deserves my respect."
> - When you describe your concern, provide specific information about the immediate situation. Avoid general comments about everything you feel is wrong.
> - Be clear about what you want in order to fix a situation instead of simply complaining about it.
> - Focus on changes the listener is able to make, rather than ones that are out of the listener's control.
> - Consider the value of the information to the listener, rather than how much you want to say.
> - Try to share ideas and information rather than suggest specific solutions
> - Use "I" statements instead of "you" statements. For example, instead of complaining "You're always running late!" try saying "I'm worried about how late it is getting."

process. Although assertive behavior does not guarantee you will get what you want, it makes it much more likely. The message you send when you communicate assertively is "Let's work together so that both of us get our needs met."

In the dominant professional biomedical culture, this communication style will likely be the most useful in resolving problems faced by medical interpreters. Assertive communication will enable the interpreter to build strong and lasting relationships with the patients and providers they work with.

Effective Listening

An essential part of effective communication is not only getting your message across but listening carefully to what the other person has to say. It is important to listen well, even if you disagree with what the other person is saying. Here's how to ensure you are listening effectively (and that others can tell you are listening):

- face the speaker when they are talking, lean forward, and nod your head when appropriate
- make an effort not to become interested in something else
- don't interrupt, but ask questions if you don't understand
- maintain good eye contact if appropriate
- verify and validate what you are hearing by summarizing what is being said, even if you don't agree

Summary

Advocacy is a sensitive topic that needs to be approached with sensitivity and care. Effective communication can produce better results when advocating. You may not have effective communication skills overnight, especially if this is a new concept for you. However, these are skills that can be learned and developed with time.

Start by being aware of your usual communication styles and notice how people react. You may want to try practicing assertive communication skills. This way, you may feel more comfortable when you need to advocate.

Skill Development

Identifying Communication Styles

It is important for you to be able to recognize communication styles and respond to situations in an assertive manner. Read each of the scenarios below, and decide if the communication style is aggressive, passive, passive-aggressive, or assertive. If the communication style used is not assertive, figure out how to convey the same message using an assertive communication style.

Situation #1: At a meeting, someone interrupts you when you're speaking.
Your response: "Excuse me, I would like to finish my statement."

Situation #2: A patient tells you she will bring you a gift of fruit at the next visit.
Your response: You roll your eyes and say, "That is nice, but I'm just doing my job!"

Situation #3: An acquaintance has asked to borrow your car for the evening.
Your response: "I don't know... Well, I suppose so. You can borrow it, but I warn you that I've been having trouble with the brakes."

Situation #4: Your supervisor has just reprimanded you for your work.
Your response: "I think some of your criticisms are true, but I would have liked you to be less personal in telling me my shortcomings."

Situation #5: A provider asks you to state what you just interpreted for the patient.
Your response: "Why? Don't you believe I said the right thing? If you can speak the language, then you should talk to the patient yourself."

Situation #6: A nurse asks you if you can take a patient to the pharmacy.
Your response: "Sure I can. Just give me five minutes to answer a page and I'll be ready."

Situation #7: Another interpreter with a busy schedule asks if you can take an appointment that was just added to their schedule.
Your response: "Well, I guess so, but don't take advantage just because my schedule is open!"

Identifying Communication Styles Continued

Situation #8: You overhear a nurse loudly making anti-immigrant comments.

Your response: Who do you think you are? You'd better shut up and apologize!

Situation #9: A doctor is annoyed that you won't sight translate a vital document while the doctor is not in the room.

Your response: I understand you have a busy schedule. However, I will not be able to answer any questions the patient has about this document, which is why I cannot sight translate this document alone with the patient.

Situation #10: You are done with an interpreting appointment, and the receptionist asks if you can stay to help him make a quick phone call to an LEP patient. You have another appointment starting soon, and you need to leave now in order to be on time.

Your response: What do you people think? I can't be everywhere at once!

Situation #11: A patient asks you to help him understand a utility bill that has nothing to do with his treatment in the hospital. You have another appointment starting soon and haven't eaten lunch yet.

Your response: Um, well, okay, I can help you do that.

Situation 12: The nurse asks you to babysit a patient's children during the patient's physical examination.

Your response: I cannot do that, as it is not within the scope of my job as an interpreter.

© 2014 The Cross Cultural Health Care Program

Section 4

Professional Development

Lesson 16

PROFESSIONAL CONDUCT AND SELF-CARE

GOAL

Develop professional conduct, professional judgment, and self-care strategies for interpreters.

KNOWLEDGE OUTCOMES

- Identify professional and non-professional conduct, as well as conduct that may be considered professional in some situations, but not others

- Develop strategies for self-care during and outside of interpreting sessions

Vocabulary
In-service self-care
Professional
Professional within limits
Self-care outside of service
Self-care
Unprofessional

> **Brainstorm**
>
> What does the term "professional conduct" mean to you?
> What actions do you take in order to appear professional?

Introduction

All professions have limits and guidelines for behavior. For medical interpreters, sometimes the boundaries are fairly clear, and sometimes they are a question of professional judgment. Such professional judgment can only be developed with time and experience. This lesson is designed to help review and clarify what behaviors constitute professional conduct and what behaviors do not.

Self-care is part of professional conduct. Self-care includes drawing boundaries to prevent an interpreter's work from spilling over into their personal life when it is not appropriate. Interpreters need to take good care of themselves in order to avoid burnout and maintain a professional demeanor.

Identifying Professional Conduct

One of the greatest challenges for an interpreter is to decide how to respond to the many different demands and situations which may arise during their interpreting work. Acting as a professional does not always seem natural; interpreters must always be conscious of their professional boundaries.

As an interpreter, there are certain behaviors that are considered to be **professional** and appropriate. Additionally, some behaviors may always be considered to be **unprofessional** or inappropriate for an interpreter. However, not every situation is clearly "right" or "wrong". Certain behavior may be considered to be **professional within limits**: the same behavior could be considered appropriate or inappropriate, depending on the situation.

Consider the following examples:

You ask the radiology technician to clarify a word you don't understand.

Since an interpreter needs to be able to interpret the meaning of the message at all times, this behavior is professional.

You give your telephone number to the doctor and offer to call the patient to report lab results.

> **Vocabulary**
>
> **Professional**: following accepted standards of behavior
>
> **Professional within limits**: acceptable in some situations, but not others
>
> **Unprofessional**: not following accepted standards of behavior
>
> **Self-care**: actions and attitudes which contribute to your well-being

This behavior can be professional within limits. If you and the doctor have arranged beforehand that receiving the lab results via phone through an interpreter and is important to the health of the patient, then this behavior can be professional. If the doctor is asking you to do this because it is more convenient than using other established means of giving the lab results (like a remote interpreting service), then this behavior is unprofessional.

An appointment is taking longer than usual, so you tell the provider you need to leave the interpreting session because you will be late for your next appointment in a clinic across town.

Leaving an interpreting session in the middle because of another appointment is unprofessional, even if the session went on longer than expected. A better course of action would be to ask the provider to give you a few minutes to make a phone call to your agency, if you have one, to arrange for a substitute for your next appointment or to come and replace you at your current appointment.

You interpret for a patient whom you know outside of the hospital. Later, when you are not at work, a mutual friend asks what happened to the patient, and wants to know how they are doing.

Interpreting for people you know may put you in an awkward position, but it may be difficult to avoid, especially if you work in a small community. You must not break patient confidentiality by sharing information that you discovered in an interpreted encounter. This would violate HIPAA, as well as compromise your professional integrity and reputation with the health care institution, the patient, and the patient's community.

Maintaining a Professional Appearance

Be sure to dress professionally and according to the norms and dress code of the facility where you work. Some facilities may have required uniforms for interpreters; if not, be sure your clothes are neat, clean, and professional. Most facilities will require anyone providing services to wear an identification badge. Ensure that you are familiar with the dress code for your institution and be sure to follow it.

Avoid talking or texting on your cell phone. If you use any electronic tools while interpreting, such as a glossary on a tablet or smartphone, it is important to advise the patient and provider beforehand, so they do not think you are engaging in unprofessional behavior while using your device.

Besides maintaining your appearance as a professional, it is also important to keep in mind your personal comfort. Interpreters may work long hours and may end up walking a significant amount to different appointments or standing for the duration of an encounter. Wearing comfortable, professional-looking clothing will ensure that neither you nor those for whom you are interpreting are distracted by your appearance or physical comfort level.

Self-care

Many of us are drawn to interpreting because we want to help people. It may seem that by taking care of yourself, you are being "selfish" or not helping a patient as much as you could. It is important to remember that, as a person providing a service, it is essential that you take care of yourself to avoid burnout and to be able to provide the highest level of service possible. When you take care of yourself, it is easier to think clearly, listen carefully, interpret well, and maintain a professional demeanor.

Self-care may include:

- utilizing techniques to reduce stress both during and after an interpreted encounter
- being sure to eat properly and stay hydrated while working
- wearing comfortable shoes and clothing while working
- setting appropriate boundaries

Stress Factors

The medical interpreting profession is often a stressful one, due to the pressures involved in interpreting, as well as the difficulties inherent in working in a health care setting. The conflicts that arise from different expectations held by the provider, the patient, the health care facility and the interpreting profession can lead to high levels of stress. The following are just some examples of stressful situations that occur in medical interpreting.

Logistical stresses can include:

- being asked at the last minute to interpret for more patients, providers, and clinics than originally scheduled
- having to stay later than planned when appointments run late or continue longer than expected
- worrying about being late for your next appointment
- being unable to locate resources for patients and/or not having the time to help them

Stresses due to the relationship between interpreter and patient may include:

- dealing with patients who are emotionally upset or aggressive
- handling unreasonable role expectations from the patient
- interpreting for patients who are lying and/or giving you information, but withholding it from the provider
- trying to communicate with patients who don't listen
- patients refusing interpreters based on gender, culture, and political or religious affiliation
- having to communicate bad news to the patient
- being subjected to racial and sexual harassment from the patient
- reliving past personal trauma through hearing the patient's experiences

Stresses due to the relationship between interpreter and provider/health institution may include:

- dealing with providers who don't listen
- being subjected to cultural stereotypes from the provider
- being subjected to racial or sexual harassment
- dealing with a provider's lack of understanding about the appropriate role of the interpreter
- handling unreasonable expectations of skill level from providers
- interpreting for providers who omit important information when talking to the patient

Secondary and Shared Trauma

It is not uncommon for interpreters to work with patients who have shared or similar experiences that were traumatic in nature. This may be especially true when interpreting for refugees or in mental health settings. An interpreter may find that their own emotions about their personal trauma can be awakened by hearing about and interpreting the patient's experience.

Additionally, it is possible for interpreters to experience secondary trauma. Secondary trauma can occur when you become traumatized by listening to and empathizing with others' traumatic experiences.

As an interpreter, it is important that you be aware of the existence of shared or secondary trauma and how it may affect you. If you feel like you are being affected by exposure to trauma in your workplace, you should seek help from a counselor or someone who can listen and support you.

> **Vocabulary**
>
> **In-service self-care**: actions and attitudes you take to support your health and wellbeing while working
>
> **Self-care outside of service**: actions and attitudes you take outside of work to support your health and well-being

In-Service Self-Care

Interpreters can practice self-care strategies during, as well as outside of, the interpreted encounter. Strategies that can be utilized while interpreting are called **in-service self-care strategies**.

The following are examples of in-service self-care strategies:

- involve the patient and provider in a pre-session interview, no matter how short, so they understand your role as an interpreter
- set boundaries with the patient as needed
- explain the process of interpreting to the patient and the provider in order to manage expectations
- treat everyone with professional courtesy and expect the same in return
- stay calm in all situations
- do not give your personal phone number to clients
- separate your emotions from the client's, and remember that being empathetic does not mean you are responsible for fixing the patient's problems

- recognize when your emotions are interfering with your work
- withdraw from a session if you believe that your personal feelings may get in the way of providing adequate interpretation
- be aware of your limitations and refuse an assignment that is beyond your area of expertise or that is too close to unresolved personal experiences
- learn to say "no" in a way that does not undermine the trust of the provider or the patient
- take care of your physical comfort and well-being by eating at regular intervals, staying hydrated, and wearing comfortable shoes and clothing

> **Remember...**
> ...you cannot help others unless you take care of yourself both physically and emotionally.
> ...do not feel you have abandoned a patient if you are unable to assist due to linguistic, professional, time or other limitations.
> ...acknowledge and value your contributions as a professional and as an individual.
> ...maintain your sense of humor in the serious business of helping people.

Self-care outside of service

Some self-care strategies can be done outside of the interpreted session and these are called **outside of service self-care strategies.**

The following are examples of outside of service self-care strategies:

- If a situation is bothering you, discuss it with appropriate people, but remember to avoid revealing any confidential information.
- Do not discuss service activities with a patient outside of the service environment.
- Work with a professional counselor to resolve trauma, including secondary trauma that may be the result of interpreting for traumatized patients.
- Join a professional organization to update skills and connect with colleagues in the field.
- Engage in regular exercise.
- Find time for fun activities that are not related to professional duties.
- Set priorities for yourself and take time out for your personal life.
- Prepare healthy snacks/meals to take with you during long interpreting appointments.
- Ask about the nature of the appointment and what precautions will be taken to protect your health if needed. For instance, if you are interpreting for a patient with an infectious disease.

Summary

Behaving professionally involves abiding by rules, norms, and regulations, as well as setting appropriate boundaries. Certain behavior is considered professional and appropriate at all times, while some conduct is appropriate only in certain situations. Other conduct is never appropriate. It is important to understand when and how it is appropriate to take certain actions.

Self-care is part of professional conduct. By practicing self-care, it is easier for interpreters to maintain a professional demeanor. Self-care helps an interpreter avoid getting "burned out" and maintain appropriate, effective relationships with patients, providers and colleagues.

Skill Development

Examine the following situations and discuss with your fellow students, or brainstorm on your own, what would be an appropriate, professional response:

A patient with a serious health condition is very distressed and says that they have no friends or family in this country to help them. They ask for your personal number in case they need help or have a medical emergency when you are not there to interpret.

You are scheduled with back-to-back appointments. A provider asks you to stay after one appointment ends to make a follow-up phone call to a patient you interpreted for in the past. If you do so, you will be late to your next appointment.

A patient is talking about a very traumatic experience, and you find yourself becoming very emotionally upset, to the point that you don't think you can interpret effectively.

You work in a small community, and you have another job outside of your work as an interpreter. You interpret for one of your coworkers, who was injured in an accident. When you go to work at your other job, you discover that the patient/coworker did not let the job know they would not be into work. Their boss is very upset, and you feel like you should let the boss know why your coworker is not at work.

You work from home as a telephone interpreter. In the middle of an interpreted phone call, someone starts knocking at your door.

Your hospital requires you to wear a certain uniform, but wearing the uniform conflicts with your cultural beliefs about appropriate dress.

What other situations have you experienced where you had to make a judgment about what would be professional behavior?

Lesson 17
TELEPHONIC AND VIDEO REMOTE INTERPRETING

GOAL

Understand factors related to telephonic and video remote interpreting in health care settings.

KNOWLEDGE OUTCOMES

- Understand what telephonic and video remote interpreting are and where these types of interpreting take place

- Identify challenges and benefits unique to remote interpreting

- Understand how to work effectively as a remote interpreter

Vocabulary

Remote interpreting

Telephonic interpreting

Video remote interpreting (VRI)

> **BRAINSTORM:**
>
> What do you think are some of the challenges faced by interpreters who interpret over the phone or video and not in person?
>
> What do you think might be some benefits of interpreting over the phone or video, rather than in person?

Introduction

Video remote and telephonic interpreting are becoming increasingly common. While many interpreters prefer to interpret in person (Locatis, Williamson and Gould-Kabler), this is not always possible. Many interpreters will do at least some telephonic or video remote interpreting, even if they are employed on-site at a hospital.

Although the same general code of ethics and standards of practice apply to remote interpreters as in-person interpreters, there are some unique factors affecting remote interpreting. Therefore, it is important for interpreters to understand these unique factors and be able to work effectively with these modes.

Telephonic Interpreting

Just as in in-person interpreting, a telephonic interpreter interprets between two people who do not speak a common language. The difference is that the interpreter is not in the room with the people for whom they are interpreting but connected via telephone.

Some health care facilities have special telephone interpreting equipment, which often looks like a corded telephone with two handsets; one for the patient and one for the provider. The interpreter may be in a call center on or off the health care facility grounds, or they may work from a home office.

Video Remote Interpreting

Video remote interpreting uses devices such as web cameras, videophones, or tablets to provide either sign language or spoken interpretation. As in telephonic interpreting, many facilities that use video remote interpreters have special equipment with a video screen that allows the interpreter to see the patient and provider, and vice versa.

Video remote interpreters may work from home offices or in call centers. One benefit of video remote interpreting is that is allows the interpreter to see the patient and the provider. The patient and provider can also see the interpreter.

> **Vocabulary**
>
> **Remote interpreting:** interpreting that takes place in a different location than the people who require interpretation
>
> **Telephonic interpreting:** remote interpretation where the interpreter hears the patient and provider and interprets over the telephone
>
> **Video remote interpreting:** remote interpreting where the interpreter hears and sees the patient and provider, and vice versa, over video

Remote Interpreting Settings

Remote interpreters may work in several settings:
- a call center or office within a health care facility
- a call center outside of a health care facility, usually for an interpreting agency
- a home office

Many health care facilities employ interpreters on-site, but still have them do a significant portion of their work over the phone or video. This cuts down on the time an interpreter spends waiting for the patient or the provider. Rather than having the patient, provider, or interpreter wait when not all of them are present, the provider can simply call and use interpretation services over the phone when they are needed.

Some facilities that use on-site telephonic or video interpreters may use in-person interpreters only for specific situations, such as very sensitive appointments. For instance, in-person interpreters may be used for mental health or assault cases or communicating bad news to a patient or their family.

Other health care facilities may contract an outside interpreting agency to provide remote interpreting services. The agency generally has call routing software or operators who connect the caller to an interpreter in the desired language. The agency may have a call center where interpreters work. The interpreters will likely interpret for a variety of clients, not just one health care facility. Some language agencies contract remote interpreters to work from home offices.

There are some remote interpreting agencies that specialize in health care, but many have clients in varied sectors. Interpreters who work for these agencies will likely interpret not only for health care, but for other settings ranging from tourism to customer service.

Advantages of Remote Interpreting

Although patients, providers, and interpreters generally report higher levels of satisfaction with in-person interpreters than remote interpreters (Craig Locatis), there are some advantages to remote interpreting.

Patient privacy: Patients may feel a greater sense of privacy when speaking through a telephonic interpreter. Since the patient cannot see the interpreter, they may be less concerned with the interpreter knowing confidential information about them, especially if the interpreter is part of a small community.

Emphasis on the patient-provider relationship: Since the interpreter is not in the room, the patient and provider may be more likely to look directly at each other when speaking. The interpreter is emphasized as a medium for communication, rather than being on the patient's side or the provider's side. It may be easier for an interpreter to maintain professional distance from the patient's situation when they are not present in the room.

Less waiting and travel time: Remote interpreting eliminates the time an interpreter spends traveling to and from appointments and waiting for patients or providers who may be running late. Because they don't have to spend time traveling and waiting, the interpreter will likely spend more time interpreting when working remotely.

Easier for the interpreter to access resources: It may be easier for a remote interpreter to discretely use electronic glossaries and other resources when they are not in the room with the patient and provider.

Easier to obtain less common languages: With remote interpreting, a health care facility can access less common languages for which interpreters may not be readily available.

Challenges of Remote Interpreting

Less personal connection: When the interpreter is not present in the room, the interpreter may feel distant and disconnected from the patient-provider interaction. Additionally, while some patients may appreciate the extra privacy afforded by telephonic interpreters, others may not feel comfortable discussing sensitive topics over the phone or video.

Concerns about confidentiality: On the flip side of confidentiality, there may be concerns with the security of the phone or video connection being intercepted or overheard. Most language agencies require that interpreters who work from home have a dedicated line that is only used for interpreting. This reduces the chance that someone could listen in. Interpreters who work from home must take precautions to ensure that the phone or internet connection they are using is secure.

Technological difficulties: Telephonic or video equipment may present technical challenges. Whether you work from home or in a call center, it is important to be familiar and comfortable with the equipment you are using. Be sure to take the time to learn how to use the equipment properly and ask for guidance or technical support if needed.

Background noise: Especially when working from home, background noise can interfere in the interpretation. Interpreters who work from home must take special care to ensure that background noise, such as children or pets, do not interfere in the interpreted session. Interpreters also may have difficulty hearing the patient or provider if there is background noise on either end. Using a good quality headset with a mouthpiece can help ensure good sound quality.

May be difficult to manage the flow of the session: Without using visual cues, telephonic interpreters may have more difficulty managing the flow of the session, especially when interpreting for people who talk on and on without pausing. If possible, remote interpreters should conduct a pre-session where they remind the patient and the provider to pause frequently.

Inability to see non-verbal cues: Although remote interpreters can pick up on a speaker's tone, inflection, and volume, telephonic interpreters are unable to see visual cues that may add meaning to the conversation. They must rely entirely on what is said and how it is said in order to interpret the meaning. This is less of a concern for video remote interpreters.

Less down time for the interpreter: Since remote interpreters don't have to travel to appointments and can be called only when needed, they may be likely to get back-to-back calls without a break in between. Remote interpreters need to ensure that they are engaging in appropriate self-care by taking breaks when necessary in order to avoid fatigue from back-to-back calls.

Often unable to advocate: When working remotely, the interpreter generally does not have contact with the patient after the interpreted encounter ends. As a result, advocacy may be extremely challenging or impossible. Remote interpreters should familiarize themselves with their agency's or organization's policies and procedures regarding advocacy and consult their supervisor if needed.

Tips for Remote Interpreters

Tips for Remote Interpreting

Develop consecutive interpreting skills. Remote interpreting, like other health care interpreting is conducted almost exclusively in consecutive mode.

Understand your needs and limitations. Be sure to take breaks as needed to avoid fatigue and burnout. Realistically assess whether you are able to set up an appropriate home office space if needed.

Include a pre-session. Remind the patient and provider to pause frequently and that you cannot see any gestures or visual cues if you are interpreting over the phone.

Be aware of policies and procedures. Whether you work for a language agency or directly for a hospital, there may be specific procedures that a remote interpreter will need to follow.

Memory development for consecutive interpreting: Remote interpreting for spoken language, especially telephonic interpreting, is almost exclusively done in the consecutive mode (Kelly). Simultaneous interpreting would likely be quite confusing if done over the phone, and sight translation is effectively impossible.

Just like in-person interpreters, remote interpreters should develop their consecutive interpreting skills, as they will be using this mode almost exclusively. Additionally, since remote interpreters may find it more difficult to control the flow of the interpreted session, they may be asked to interpret longer chunks of information, which requires increased memory capacity. Remote interpreters may be able to take notes less obtrusively than in-person interpreters, but they must be sure to destroy all notes at the end of the session.

Understand your needs and limitations: Since remote interpreters are likely to spend more time interpreting than waiting between appointments, they may become more easily fatigued. Interpreters must possess enough self-awareness to know when fatigue is affecting the quality of their interpretation and be sure to take breaks when needed.

Working from home: If you plan to work from home, you should honestly assess whether your home environment is realistic for interpreting. Are you able to have a line dedicated solely to interpreting? Many language agencies that employ interpreters who work from home require that they use a land line, rather than a cell phone or internet-based phone. Do you have a quiet, secure area where you can work and not be distracted by children, pets, other family members, or noises inside or outside of the house? Are you able to set up a comfortable workstation? These are all important considerations to keep in mind (Kelly).

Be aware of policies and procedures: Whether you work as a contractor or employee of a hospital or agency, be sure that you know their policies. There will likely be procedures in place for dealing with dropped calls and other issues that arise. Additionally, make sure you are prepared if the provider places you on hold with the patient or leaves the room briefly without disconnecting the call. Since the interpreter can't leave the room as they would with in-person interpreting, you will need to come up with another way of dealing with this situation. The interpreter may want to mute their phone to discourage the patient from having a side conversation with the interpreter. The interpreter may also need to politely inform the patient that they are not permitted to have conversations without the provider present, if the patient tries to do so.

Include a pre-session: If you work for an agency, they may have a scripted pre-session that you are required to use. Ideally, a remote pre-session should emphasize the need for the speaker to speak in short sentences and pause frequently. Additionally, a telephonic interpreter may want to remind the patient and provider that they cannot see visual cues or gestures.

Summary

Realistically, most interpreters will spend at least part of their time interpreting over the phone or video. While the same code of ethics and practices apply to both remote and in-person interpreting, interpreters need to be aware of specific factors affecting remote interpreting.

Not having to travel and wait at appointments can be both a benefit and a challenge. As with all interpreting, you need to be aware of your own abilities and limitations. This way, you can assess whether remote interpreting is a good fit for you.

Lesson 18

Resources for Professional Growth

Goal

Support the continuing professional growth of medical interpreters by identifying resources and opportunities.

Knowledge Outcomes

- Identify areas of professional growth

- Identify a variety of resources available to support professional growth and development

Vocabulary
Interpreter networks and organizations
National Certification
State Certification

Introduction

This course will lay the groundwork for your work as an interpreter. Once the course is over, it is important to continue to develop your skills, knowledge, and experience, and to stay abreast of trends and developments in the field.

You can do this by joining professional organizations, taking continuing education courses, practicing your skills, and becoming certified. A good interpreter never stops learning and developing their skills and knowledge.

The following are some areas of professional development that many interpreters find it beneficial to work on:

- vocabulary development in both English and your non-English target language
- interpreting skills in consecutive and simultaneous interpreting
- memory development
- note-taking skills
- familiarity with the common medical procedures and specialists
- increased awareness of your own culture, including traditional health beliefs and the culture(s) of your patients
- communication skills
- community resources specific to your non-English language communities

There are many resources available to help you develop in the areas where you need the most growth.

Resources for Professional Growth

Appendix A provides a list of resources on various topics addressed throughout this curriculum. There, you will find names of books, instructional videos, and other resources for professional development. This appendix is a good starting point for research on specific topics of interest.

You may also want to pursue additional training and continuing education. If you become certified, you will be required to participate in a certain amount of continuing education to maintain your certification.

Interpreter Networks and Organizations

Interpreter networks and organizations are important tools for professional growth. Networking with other professional interpreters will provide an invaluable support system in this challenging and complex profession.

There are many professional interpreter and translator associations at the local, state, national, and international level. It is a good idea to join both a local or regional organization, as well as a larger, national organization. Attending conferences and workshops hosted by these organizations, as well as joining their mailing lists, is a good way to continue to develop professionally.

Local interpreter associations
Many states and regions have associations that serve and represent the interests of

interpreters in that area. Some examples include:

- NOTIS (Northwest Translators and Interpreters Society)
- CHIA (The California Health Interpreting Association)
- TAHIT (Texas Association of Healthcare Interpreters and Translators)
- many other state and regional organizations

National and international associations

- International Medical Interpreters Association (IMIA) is a national trade association committed to the "advancement of professional medical interpreters as the best practice to equitable language access to health care for linguistically diverse patients."

  Information on IMIA's activities, resources, and membership can be found at http://www.imiaweb.org/.

- National Council on Interpreting in Health Care (NCIHC) is a multidisciplinary professional organization whose mission is to "promote culturally competent professional health care interpreting as a means to support equal access to health care for individuals with limited English proficiency."

  Information on NCIHC's activities, resources and membership can be found at: www.ncihc.org.

Interpreter Certification Programs

The *Bridging The Gap* curriculum is recognized and utilized by many institutions across the United States. You receive a certificate of successful completion upon receiving a 70% score or better on the Post-Test. This is not to be confused with "certification." At the time of publication, there are two accredited, national certification programs for medical or healthcare interpreters in the United States.

National Certification

Interpreter organizations have continuously supported a national certification program. At the time of this publication, there are two organizations that have developed national certification programs: the Certification Commission

---

Vocabulary

Interpreter networks and organizations: professional organizations that represent and support interpreters

National Certification: nationally recognized professional certification for interpreters. Interpreters can be certified by taking a certification exam. A certificate of completion of an interpreter training course is not the same as being a certified interpreter.

State Certification: certification that is required by a specific state

for Healthcare Interpreters (CCHI) and the National Board of Certification for Medical Interpreters (NBCMI). The following section provides a brief overview of their efforts as well as resources to learn more.

Certification Commission for Healthcare Interpreters

CCHI was incorporated in 2009 as an independent certification agency. The purpose of CCHI is to create a single, unified national certification for health care interpreters to ensure the competency of interpreters through an accredited, professional certification program.

CCHI is governed by commissioners and advisors, some of whom began their careers with the National Council on Interpreting in Health Care (NCIHC) and were involved in developing national standards and the interpreter code of ethics.

CCHI released its first certification examination in the fall of 2010. More information about CCHI and their efforts towards national certification can be found at: www.healthcareinterpretercertification.org

National Board for Certification of Medical Interpreters (NBCMI or National Board):

Founded in 2009, the NBCMI is an independent non-profit organization. For NBCMI the purpose of certification is 'to ensure LEP patient safety by evaluating and assuring the competency of medical interpreters."

Governed by a board of leaders in the medical and interpreting industries, the NBCMI was created as the result of a proposal to the field of medical interpreting by the International Medical Interpreter Association (IMIA) and Language Line University (LLU).

NBCMI released its first certification examination in 2009. At the time of this publication, certification is offered in Spanish, Russian, Vietnamese, Korean, Cantonese, and Mandarin, with additional languages being developed. More information can be found at: www.certifiedmedicalinterpreters.org

State Certification

Some states have specific certification programs or requirements, in addition to national certification. You should become familiar with your state's requirements. The following are some examples of state-specific requirements:

Washington State
The Washington State Department of Social and Health Services (DSHS) provides a Language Testing and Certification program for state medical interpreters. The tests measure English language proficiency and interpreting skills in a second language. Certification is available in Spanish, Vietnamese, Russian, Cambodian, Laotian, Mandarin Chinese, Cantonese Chinese, and Korean. For other languages, DSHS provides screening tests. Certified interpreters are then eligible to

work either as DSHS employees or through other contracted agencies.

More information can be found through the Washington State DSHS site at: www.dshs.wa.gov/ltc/

Utah

Information about requirements for Medical Interpreter Licensing certification, plus the applicable Laws and Rules of Utah, can be found through the State of Utah Department of Commerce's Division of Occupational and Professional Licensing at:

https://dopl.utah.gov/mli/

Oregon

As part of a growing trend throughout the profession, the state of Oregon set new standards for medical interpreters that "raise the bar" for certification in Oregon. As of 2013, Oregon requires interpreters to have a minimum of 60 hours of basic training, including 8 hours of study of the codes of ethics for medical interpreters. The state also requires national certification by either of the two accredited national certification bodies, the National Board of Certification for Medical Interpreters (NBCMI) or the Certification Commission for Healthcare Interpreters (CCHI). When an interpreter can show proof of meeting both of these requirements and the equivalent of at least 80 hours of documented health care interpreting experience, the interpreter can apply with the state to become certified.

Finding a Job as a Medical Interpreter

Whether you are new to the interpreting profession, or already have some years of experience, the information in this section may provide some new ideas and suggestions on how to search for and secure a new medical interpreting job. The following are some suggestions on how to gain employment as a medical interpreter:

- determine the certification requirements in your state and develop a course of action to meet those requirements
- successfully complete well-recognized medical interpreter training programs to continue your professional development
- join a local interpreter association to network with other interpreters in your region
- join a national professional organization to stay connected to changes and developments in the profession
- volunteer with local organizations (see text box on the following page) that require interpreting services to gain experience
- consider which type of position will work for you - staff interpreter, bilingual staff, agency, remote or contract interpreter

- explore opportunities to work as a court, escort, conference or business interpreter, if you have the required qualifications
- find a mentor (an experienced interpreter) who can guide you through the process of finding and succeeding in your first job

Guidelines for Freelance or Contract Interpreters

A freelance or contract interpreter is also sometimes called an independent contractor. An independent contractor is someone who is an independent business person and is not a salaried employee of an institution or agency. The following is a set of guidelines that will help establish yourself as a professional independent contractor.

Setting up:
Acquire a business license (UBI) number, which can be obtained for a fee by registering with the Department of Revenue in the city and/or state where you work.

Determine the taxes you will be required to pay as an independent contractor. Since you are not an employee, you will be responsible for paying all of your own taxes; they will not be deducted automatically from your paycheck.

Determine if you will need professional liability insurance (Errors and Omissions Insurance). Some of the contracts you choose to sign may require it. Consult with an insurance broker or agent on the options available for your situation.

Gaining Experience

The following types of organizations may use interpreter services. Consider approaching them to volunteer or see if they offer paid interpreting work in order to gain experience. Organizations to consider include:

- state and local government
- public health departments
- college/university-based programs
- organizations that put on events with international participants (like sporting events)
- faith-based charities
- refugee resettlement/mutual assistance agencies that work with targeted populations
- nonprofit organizations
- independent community based organizations
- health care services like hospitals and clinics
- service organizations such as Red Cross and Mercy Corps

Considering different contracts
It is important to carefully determine the benefits of each contract you have the opportunity to sign. Some questions to consider are:

- What is the hourly pay rate for interpreters at this institution?
- What is the volume of work I can expect at this institution?

Consider that it might be better to be paid at a lower rate with more appointments than at a higher rate with only one appointment a week. Different organizations pay their interpreters differently, and it is important to recognize that small differences in pay can be offset by other important benefits.

- Will I be paid for travel time and wait time?
- Does the per-hour rate differ depending on the location of the assignment?
- What will I be paid if the patient does not show up?
- How long is the "minimum"? For example, a "one hour minimum" means that the interpreter will be paid for an hour whether the session lasts for one minute or sixty minutes.
- What is the cancellation policy? (How close to the time of the appointment can I, or the agency cancel without any responsibility?)
- By when do I need to complete the invoice after providing the interpreting service?
- How soon after invoicing can I expect to receive payment?
- Is professional liability insurance required for this contract?
- Will I be required to use a cell phone? If so, will the organization provide me with one or can I get reimbursed for the minutes I use from my own cell phone plan?
- Will I be required to participate in any specific training? If so, will the organization pay for all or part of the costs of the training?

When you are getting ready to sign a contract, remember that you are providing a valuable service. You may be contracting with multiple organizations, so make sure that you review each contract carefully.

Related Interpreting Work

Interpreting for Deaf, Deaf-Blind, and Hard of Hearing individuals

This area of interpreting is highly developed and well organized, with its own system for training, certifying, qualifying, and contracting interpreters. There are many available resources for more information about this branch of interpreting. If you are interested in becoming an interpreter for deaf, deaf-blind, and/or hard of hearing individuals, the following website is a good place to start your research:

Registry of Interpreters for the Deaf (RID): www.rid.org

RID is a national membership organization that represents professionals who facilitate communication between people who are deaf or hard of hearing and people who can hear.

Escort Interpreting

Escort interpreters accompany foreign dignitaries and business people who are in the U.S. on training programs or trade delegations. There interpreters provide interpretation for all aspects of the trip, virtually twenty four hours a day. Escort interpreters are contracted directly by the business or training organization that is organizing the visit. If you are interested in becoming an escort interpreter, the following website is a good place to start your research:

The State Department of the United States: www.languageservices.state.gov

The State Department contracts a large number of escort interpreters on a regular basis through the State Department Office of Language Services. In addition to escort interpreting, they also contract in conference interpreting. The state department has their own process of screening for qualified escort interpreters.

Business Interpreting

Business interpreters interpret for trade delegations or during international business negotiations. They are contracted either through interpreting agencies or directly by the business involved. No specific certification is available, but most agencies will require some type of screening test, which will focus largely on relevant vocabulary and technical knowledge.

Conference Interpreting

Conference interpreters provide language services from an isolated booth (area) using earphones and a microphone to reach conference attendees who are listening through earphones. Conference interpreting is typically done using the simultaneous mode of interpretation. Because continuous simultaneous interpretation requires tremendous concentration, conference interpreters usually work in teams and relieve each other every 20-30 minutes. Conference interpreters usually require specialized training and are contracted through agencies or directly by conference organizers.

Legal (Court) Interpreting

Court interpreters are utilized in a variety of venues, such as municipal courts, state courts, U.S. federal courts, immigration proceedings, attorney's offices, police interventions, etc. See Lesson 1, Section 6: *Interpreter Roles in Other Settings* (p.31) for an introductory discussion on the differences between medical interpreting and legal/court interpreting.

U.S. Federal Court System: www.uscourts.gov/interpretprog/interp_prog.html

The U.S. Federal Court System has an established procedure for contracting qualified court interpreters.

State Courts: www.ncsc.org

Contact state, municipal, and local courts directly to find opportunities for court interpreting. A database of state, municipal and local courts with their websites and contact information can be found in the Information and Resources section of the National Center for State Courts website.

National Association of Judiciary Interpreters and Translators (NAJIT): www.najit.org

The National Association of Judiciary Interpreters and Translators (NAJIT) was incorporated as a professional association to promote quality interpretation and translation services in the judicial system.

Translation

Interpretation and translation are related, but different fields. Becoming a translator requires different expertise and training. As previously discussed, interpreting is the oral rendition of a spoken communication from one language into another whereas translation is the rendition of written text in one language into a comparable written text in another language.

American Translators Association (ATA): www.atanet.org

More information about becoming a professionally certified translator can be found at the American Translators Association (ATA) website. The ATA is the largest professional association of translators and interpreters in the U.S.

Summary

There are many resources available for interpreters to continue their professional development. Interpreters should research applicable requirements to work as an interpreter in their area and take steps to meet these requirements. Medical interpreting is a specialized field, and there are other options for interpreters to branch out and develop professionally. As an interpreter, you should consider what type of work will best suit you and take steps to pursue those opportunities.

Appendix A: Additional Resources

The resources in this section have been categorized into the following groups:

1. General Interpreting Resources
2. Cultural Competence Resources
3. Professional Standards, Ethics and Skills Resources
4. Laws and Regulations Resources
5. U.S. Health Care System and History Resources
6. Health Disparities Resources
7. Anatomy and Physiology Resources
8. Research Tools and Resources

Information regarding access to resources was updated at the time of publication and some information may have changed since then.

1. GENERAL INTERPRETING RESOURCES

- Cross Cultural Health Care Program. (1998). Communicating Effectively Through an Interpreter: An Instructional DVD for Health Care Providers. Seattle, WA. This DVD is designed to help health care professionals choose appropriate interpreters, recognize the signs of professional and unprofessional interpretation, and work effectively with trained interpreters.

- Mikkelson, Holly (1994). The Interpreter's Rx: practical exercises in medical interpreting. Spreckels, CA: ACEBO.
- This book is for Spanish-English medical interpreting. More information about ordering can be found at: http://www.acebo.com/rx.htm

- Sampson, Alyssa. (2006). Language Services Resource Guide for Health Care Providers. Los Angeles, CA: The National Health Law Program. This text provides information on how to locate language services, interpreter training programs, Office of Civil Rights documents, multilingual health resources and many other topics. The full text can be found online at http://www.healthlaw.org (Search in the Language Access Library).

- Shackman, Jane. (1984). The Right to Be Understood: A Handbook on Working with, Employing and Training Community Interpreters. Cambridge, UK: National Extension College.

- The Bilingual Medical Interview I (1987), and The Bilingual Medical Interview II: The Geriatric Interview, Section of General Internal Medicine, Boston City Hospital, in collaboration with the Department of Interpreter Services and the Boston Area Health Education Center. Available from the BAHEC, 818 Harrison Ave., Boston, MA 02118; Phone (617)-534-5258.

2. CULTURAL COMPETENCY RESOURCES

- Andrews, A.M. & J.S. Boyle. (2003). Transcultural Concepts in Nursing Care. (4th ed.). Philadelphia, PA: Lippencott, Williams &Wilkins.

- CCHCP's Community Profile Series. Available for: Cambodian, Hmong, Japanese, Lao, Vietnamese. A Cross Cultural Health Care Publication.

- Cross, T., Bazron, B., Dennis, K., & Isaacs, M. (1989). Towards a Culturally Competent System of Care: A Monograph on Effective Services for Minority Children who are Severely Emotionally Disturbed. Washington DC: CASSP Technical Assistance Center, Georgetown University Child Development Center.

- Galanti, Geri-Ann. (1997). Caring for Patients from Different Cultures: Case Studies from American Hospitals. Philadelphia, PA: University of Pennsylvania Press.

- A description and information on ordering this book can be found at http://www.xculture.org/NWRCrec_books.php

- Gropper, R.C. (1996). Culture and the Clinical Encounter. An Intercultural Sensitizer for the Health Professions. Yarmouth, ME: Intercultural Press.

- Grossman, D.C., Putsch, R.W. & Inui, T.S. (1993). The Meaning of Death to Adolescents in an American Indian Community. Family Medicine, 1993; 25:593-7.

- Kaufert, J.M. & Putsch, R.W. (1997) Communication through Interpreters in Health Care: Ethical Dilemmas Arising from Differences in Class, Culture, Language, and Power. Journal of Clinical Ethics, Vol. 8, No. 1.

- Lonner, Thomas D. (2000). Constructing the Middle Ground: Cultural Competence in Medicaid Managed Care. Seattle, WA: A Cross Cultural Health Care Program Publication. This book examines the relationships among best organizational, clinical, consumer service practices, and perceived outcomes as found among several community and migrant health centers.

- Pediatric Pulmonary Centers Cultural Health Care – Case Studies: http://ppc.mchtraining.net/

- Putsch, R.W. (1998). Language and Meaning in Health Care: What's in the Message. Originally published in Across Cultures, the Newsletter of the Cross Cultural Health Care Program.

- Putsch, R.W. (1997). Truth Telling, Disclosure, and Informed Consent. Originally published in Across Cultures, the Newsletter of the Cross Cultural Health Care Program.

- Putsch, R.W. & Joyce, M. (1990). Dealing with Patients from Other Cultures: Methodology in Cross Cultural Care. Clinical Methods, 3rd Edition. Boston, MA: Butterworths.

- Putsch, R. W. (1988). Ghost illness: A cross-cultural experience with the expression of a non-Western tradition in clinical practice. American Indian & Alaska Native Mental Health Research, 2(2), 6–26.

- Solomon, N.R.Z., & Langford, J. (2000). Death and Dying in Ethnic America. Seattle, WA: A Cross Cultural Health Care Program Publication.

- Transcultural Nursing Basic Concepts and Case Studies: http://www.culturediversity.org/cases.htm

3. **PROFESSIONAL STANDARDS, ETHICS AND SKILLS RESOURCES**

- California Healthcare Interpreters Association. (2002). California Standards for Healthcare Interpreters: Ethical Principles, Protocols and Guidance on Roles and Interventions (2nd ed.). Woodland Hills, CA.

- International Medical Interpreters Association. (2007). Medical Interpreting Standards of Practice.

- International Medical Interpreters Association. (2006). IMIA Code of Ethics.

- National Council on Interpreting in Health Care. (2009). Sight Translation and Written Translation: Guidelines for Healthcare Interpreters.

- Full text can be found at http://www.ncihc.org/

- National Council on Interpreting in Health Care. (2005). National Standards of Practice for Interpreters in Health Care.

- National Council on Interpreting in Health Care. (2004). A National Code of Ethics for Interpreters in Health Care, 24.

- National Council on Interpreting in Health Care. (2003). Guide to Interpreter Positioning in Health Care Settings.

- Txabarriaga, Rocio. (2009). IMIA Guide on Medical Translation. International Medical Interpreters Association. The full text of this document can be found at: www.imiaweb.org/uploads/pages/438.pdf

4. **LAWS AND REGULATIONS RESOURCES**

- Child Welfare Information Gateway: A summary of all the state laws regarding mandatory reporting: http://www.childwelfare.gov/systemwide/laws_policies/statutes/mandaall.pdf

- Department of Health and Human Services, U.S.A. (2009). A Health Care Provider's Guide to the HIPAA Privacy Rule: Communicating with a Patient's Family, Friends, or Others involved in the Patient's Care. The full text to this document can be found online at: http://www.hhs.gov/ocr/privacy/hipaa/understanding/coveredentities/provider_ffg.pdf

- National Center for Elder Abuse: Information on how to navigate the laws, and find out about the laws in your own state: http://www.ncea.aoa.gov/

Resources for Professional Growth

- National Health Law Program. (2005). HIPAA and Language Services in Health Care.

- Rodriguez, M.A., Wallace, S.P., Woolf, N.H., & Mangione, C.M. (2006). Mandatory Reporting of Elder Abuse: Between a Rock and Hard Place. Annals of Family Medicine, 4, (5), 403.The full text to this document can be found online at: http://www.annfammed.org/cgi/reprint/4/5/403

- Stiegal, L., & Klem, E. (2007). Information about Laws Related to Elder Abuse. American Bar Association Commission on Law and Aging. Retrieved from http://www.ncea.aoa.gov/

- Teaster, P.B. (2000). A Response to the Abuse of Vulnerable Adults: The 2000 Survey of State Adult Protective Services. Washington DC: National Center on Elder Abuse.

- The National Health Resource Center on Domestic Violence. (2004). Health Care: Mandatory Reporting of Domestic Violence by Health Care Providers. Retrieved from http://www.endabuse.org/section/programs/health_care/_mandatory_reporting

- U.S. Department of Health and Human Services, (n.d.). Guidance to Federal Financial Assistance Recipients Regarding Title VI Prohibition Against National Origin Discrimination Affecting Limited English Proficient Persons. Retrieved from http://www.hhs.gov/ocr/civilrights/resources/specialtopics/lep/

- The full text of this document can be found at the official Federal Register website: http://www.gpoaccess.gov/fr/index.html

- U.S. Department of Health and Human Services Office of Civil Rights: www.hhs.gov/ocr

- U.S. Department of Labor. Health Plans and Benefits: Continuation of Health Coverage (COBRA).

- Information about COBRA and other governmental health care laws can be found at the United States Department of Labor website: http://www.dol.gov/

5. **U.S. HEALTH CARE SYSTEM and HISTORY RESOURCES**

- Boards of Trustees of the Federal Hospital Insurance and Federal Supplementary Medical Insurance Trust Funds. (2009) Annual Report of the Boards of Trustees of the Federal Hospital Insurance and Federal Supplementary Medical Insurance Trust Funds, 8. The full text to this document can be found online at the U.S. Department of Health and Human Services, Centers for Medicare and Medicaid Services: http://www.cms.hhs.gov/

- Centers for Disease Control and Prevention. (2008). Early Release of Selected Estimates Based on Data

- From the 2008 National Health Interview Survey. Retrieved from http://www.cdc.gov/nchs/fastats/hinsure.htm

- Centers for Medicare and Medicaid Services (2005). Medicaid At-A-Glance 2005: A Medicaid Information Source. The full text to this document can be found online at the U.S. Department of Health and Human Services, Centers for Medicare and Medicaid Services: http://www.cms.hhs.gov/

- Davis, K., Schoen, C., Schoenbaum, S.C., Doty, M.M., Holmgren, A.L., Kriss, J.L., & Shea, K.K. (2007). Mirror, Mirror on the Wall: An International Update on the Comparative Performance of American Health Care. The Commonwealth Fund, 59.

- The full text to this document can be found online in the Publications Section of the Commonwealth Fund website at: http://www.commonwealthfund.org/Publications.aspx

- Park, Yoosun. (2000). Chronology of United States Immigration History 1790-1998. Seattle, WA: A Cross Cultural Health Care Program Publication.

- The Henry J. Kaiser Family Foundation. (2008). Managed Care and Health Insurance: Total HMO Enrollment, Healthleaders, Inc., Special Data Request. Retrieved from http://www.statehealthfacts.org/

- The Henry J. Kaiser Family Foundation. (2003). The Kaiser Commission on Key Facts: Medicaid and the Uninsured. Retrieved from http://www.kff.org/uninsured/immigrantcare_linguisticaccess.cfm

- Tufts Managed Care Institute. (1998). A Brief History of Managed Care. Retrieved from http://www.thci.org/downloads/briefhist.pdf

6. HEALTH DISPARITIES RESOURCES

National Partnership for Action to End Health Disparities: From the U.S. Department of Health and Human Services:
http://minorityhealth.hhs.gov/npa/

Office of Minority Health and Health Disparities (OMHD):
http://www.cdc.gov/omhd/

The Henry J. Kaiser Family Foundation – Minority Health and Health Disparities:
http://www.kff.org/minorityhealth/

7. ANATOMY AND PHYSIOLOGY RESOURCES

- An Interpreter's Guide to Common Medications. (2008). Seattle WA: Cross Cultural Health Care Program.

- Baggaley, Ann (Eds.). (2001). Human Body: An Illustrated Guide to Every Part of the Human Body and How it Works. New York, NY: Dorling Kindersley Limited.

- Bilingual Medical Glossaries. The following bilingual medical glossaries are available from the Cross Cultural Health Care Program: Amharic, Arabic, Bengali, Bosnian, Cambodian, Chinese, English, French, Haitian Creole, Hindi, Japanese, Korean, Lao, Polish, Portuguese, Russian, Somali, Spanish, Tigrigna, Urdu and Vietnamese.

Helpful Websites for Learning Medical Terminology

- Merck Manual: www.merckmanuals.com. The Merck Manual webpages can be found in multiple languages at www.merckmanuals.com/languages.html

- Medline Plus: www.nlm.nih.gov/medlineplus Government website that contains basic health information.

8. RESEARCH TOOLS and RESOURCES

- Journal of the American Medical Association: Free access to full text of archived journal articles going back to 1996. Articles published prior to 1996 require subscription fees.
- Available at: jama.ama-assn.org/

- Journal of the National Medical Association: Free access to current articles online. Available at: www.nmanet.org/index.php/Publications_Sub/jnma

- Medline Plus: A service of the National Library of Medicine and the National Institutes of Health, this website provides a variety of resources on many health care topics. Available at: www.nlm.nih.gov/medlineplus/

- Pub Med Online: Free access to the full text of articles in the U.S. National Library of Medicine's digital archive. Available at: www.pubmedonline.com/

- The National Health Law Program: In addition to information about health law, this website provides access to articles on a variety of relevant topics, from language access to managed care. Available at: www.healthlaw.org

References

American Medical Association. "Health Literacy Video." 2001.

Andrews, A.M. & Boyle, J.S. *Transcultural Concepts in Nursing Care (4th Edition)*. Philadelphia, PA: Lippencott, Williams, & Wilkins, 2003.

Center for Disease Control (n.d). "[Image# 410, Operating Room Scene]." n.d. <http://phil.cdc.gov/phil.asp>.

CHIA. *http://www.chiaonline.org/?page=CHIAStandards&hhSearchTerms=standards*. n.d. 3 February 2014.

Craig Locatis, PhD,corresponding author1 Deborah Williamson, DHA, Carrie Gould-Kabler, BSW, Laurie Zone-Smith, PhD, Isabel Detzler, BA, Jason Roberson, MA, Richard Maisiak, PhD, and Michael Ackerman, PhD. *National Institutes of Health*. April 2010. <http://www.ncbi.nlm.nih.gov/pmc/articles/PMC2842540/>.

Cross, T., Bazron, B. Dennis, K., & Issacs, M. "Toward a Culturally Competent System of Care: A Monograph on Effective Services for Minority Children who are Severely Emotionally Disturbed." Washington, DC: CASSP Technical Assistance Center, Georgetown University Child Development Center, 1989.

Department of Health and Human Services. "A Health Care Provider's Guide to the HIPAA Privacy Rule: Communicating with a Patient's Family, Friends, or Others Involved in the Patient's Care." U.S.A, 2009.

—. "Guidance to Federal Financial Recipients Regarding Title VI Prohibition Against National Origin Discrimination Affecting Limited English Proficient Persons." n.d. <www.hhs.gov/ocr/civilrights/resources/specialtopics/lep>.

Galanti, Geri-Ann. *Caring for Patients from Different Cultures: Case Studies from American Hospitals*. Philadelphia, PA: University of Pennsylvania Press, 128, (1997).

Gropper, R.C. *Culture and the Clinical Encounter. An Intercultural Sensitizer for the Health Professions*. Yarmouth, ME: Intercultural Press, 1996.

—. *Culture and the Clinical Encounter: An Intercultural Sensitizer for the Health Professions*. Yarmouth, ME: Intercultural Press, 1996.

Hodos, Adrian, and SenGupta, Ira. *Connecting To Care: Patient Guide Training Program*. Seattle, WA: The Cross Cultural Health Care Program, 2014.

IMIA. *IMIA*. 2006. 3 February 2014. <http://www.imiaweb.org/code/>.

—. "Medical Interpreting Standards of Practice." 2007.

Kelly, Nataly. *Telephone Interpreting*. Victoria, BC, Canada: Trafford Publishing, 2008.

Locatis, Craig, et al. *National Institute of Health*. April 2010. 27 March 2013. <http://www.ncbi.nlm.nih.gov/pmc/articles/PMC2842540/>.

MJ Hockenberry, D Wilson. *Wong's Essentials of Pediatric Nursing, 8th Edition*. St. Louis: Mosby, 2009.

National Council on Interpreting in Health Care. "Guide to Interpreter Positioning in Health Care Settings." 2003.

NCHIC. *NCIHC*. July 2004. 3 February 2014. <http://www.ncihc.org/assets/documents/publications/NCIHC%20National%20Code%20of%20Ethics.pdf>.

NCIHC. "National Standards of Practice for Interpreters in Health Care." 2005.

—. *NCHIC*. 2005. 3 February 2014. <http://www.ncihc.org/assets/documents/publications/NCIHC%20National%20Standards%20of%20Practice.pdf>.

Office of Minority Health, HHS Office of Minority. "Standard 1: Provide Effective, Equitable, Understandable, and Respectful Quality Care and Services." *The National Standards for*

Culturally and Linguistically Appropriate Services in Health and Health Care: A Blueprint for Sustaining CLAS Policy and Practice (The Blueprint) 2013.

The National Office of Civil Rights. *Title VI of the Civil Rights Act of 1964: Policy Guidance on the Prohibition Against National Origin Discrimination As It Affects Persons With Limited English Proficiency.* Federal Register, 2000. <www.gpoaccess.gov/fr/>.

Youdelman, Maria. *National Health Law Program.* 1 July 2009. 3 February 2014.

—. *National Health Law Program.* 1 July 2009. 3 February 2014.

Part 2

Medical Terminology

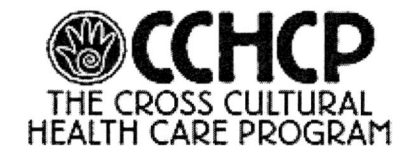

Section 1

LEARNING MEDICAL TERMINOLOGY

Introduction

A medical interpreter is not a licensed physician, nor are they required to know every aspect of the human body. However, the more technical vocabulary an interpreter knows, the more smoothly the interpreted session will go. This part of the curriculum provides medical interpreters with content knowledge and the skills to learn the necessary technical vocabulary.

This section is not intended to be used to diagnose or treat a medical condition. The definitions of the medical terms used are adapted from Medline Plus (http://www.nlm.nih.gov/medlineplus/), which is a good source for further study on medical terminology. The definitions and diagrams found in Part B, Section 2: *Body Systems Terminology* are adapted from *A Handbook for Interpreters in Health,* Part II: Body Systems and Their Problems, published by Territorial Government of the Northwest Territories, Canada.

Strategies for Learning Medical Terminology

Even though interpreters are always encouraged to ask the speaker for more clarification when unfamiliar terms are used, the more technical terminology an interpreter knows, the more smoothly the interpreted session will go.

The following are some best practices and techniques to use when learning new medical terminology.

Multiple exposures: In order to fully learn the meaning of a word and commit it to long term memory, multiple exposures to the word are necessary. This means that using one strategy today is not enough. You will need to repeat and see and use the word many times before it belongs in your long term memory.

The first time you see a certain medical term may be through the exercises in this curriculum. The next time you see the word might be when you encounter it in an interpreting session and have to ask the provider for clarification. The third time you encounter the word might be when you return to your study of medical terminology and approach the word using another technique.

Through this process of multiple exposures, the meaning of the word will become a part of your long term memory. When you encounter the word in an interpreting session, you will be comfortable and confident as you interpret the word.

Learn words with all your senses: When learning a new term, use your visual, auditory, and kinesthetic senses to learn the new word. This technique also provides you with multiple exposures to the word.

Visual senses: Create diagrams of new medical terminology. When learning new words, it helps to have images associated with them. For example, draw a picture of the human body and label it with the names of the organs to learn the names of human organs.

Learning Medical Terminology

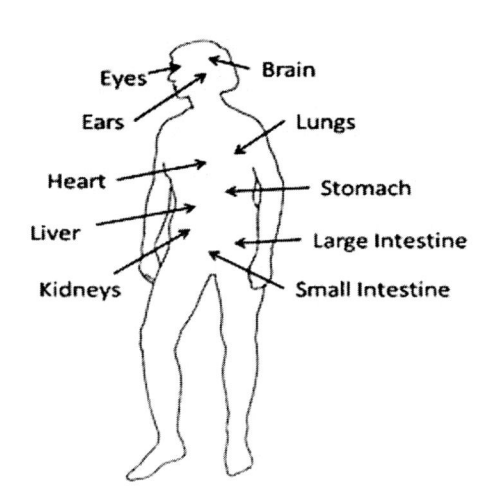

Auditory senses: This refers to the sense of hearing. Saying new terminology and their definitions out loud to yourself will help you retain the new information. It may seem strange, particularly if you are studying the new terms by yourself, but verbalizing your new knowledge out loud will help.

Kinesthetic senses: This refers to your sense of motion. Using this sense is a useful way to commit new information to your long term memory.

One way to use your kinesthetic sense is to write down the definitions you learn by hand. Writing the definitions of new terminology uses your kinesthetic sense because your hand has to physically make the motions of writing the definition.

For medical procedure vocabulary, acting out the procedure is another way to engage your kinesthetic senses. When learning about the body's organs, you can also point to the part of the body as a way to engage your kinesthetic senses.

Categorize: When you learn large amounts of new words, categorize them. Put your new list of words in an order that makes sense to you. You could categorize them in order of size, location on the body, or any other commonality between them.

Take the word "gargantuan" as an example. Gargantuan means huge, tremendous or immense in size. You could learn the word "gargantuan" by categorizing it with other similar words that have to do with "size".

Small

Medium

Large

Gargantuan

Finding categories for vocabulary words and listing them in a logical order that makes sense to you will help provide a context for your new vocabulary.

Link to prior knowledge: Define new medical terminology in your own words. When you define them in your own words, you begin to associate the new words with things that you already know. This is called linking new information to prior knowledge. Because you are associating the new term with things that you already know, you are more likely to remember the new term as well.

Study the word structure: Learn the structure of new terminology. Most medical words are a combination of roots, prefixes, and suffixes. Knowing what these roots, prefixes, and suffixes will allow you to be able to decipher the meaning of new words that you encounter. More information on roots, prefixes, and suffixes will be provided in the next section.

Use mnemonic devices: A strategy to remember groups of words is to use mnemonic devices. A mnemonic device is a short word or phrase used to remember key terms. To some people, it may seem childish, but the simpler and funnier it is, the more likely you are to remember the device, and thus remember the new terminology.

For example, you are trying to remember that air/oxygen goes through the nose and trachea, to the lungs, and then through the bronchi and then the alveoli, and then the oxygen is transferred to the blood vessels. The mnemonic device you decide to remember is:

NTLBAB

Never Think Little Balls of Air Bounce

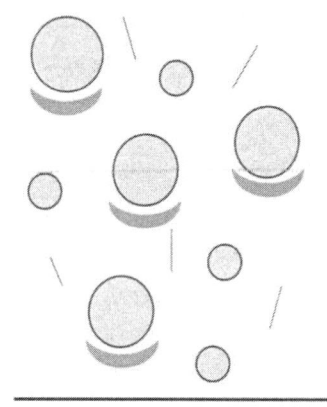

This mnemonic device will help you remember that instead of bouncing, they go from the **N**ose and **T**rachea to the **L**ungs, and then to the **B**ronchi, **A**lveoli and **B**lood vessels (NTLBAB).

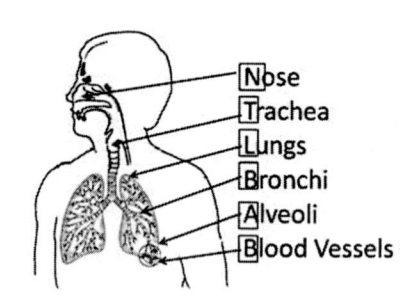

Roots, Prefixes and Suffixes

One of the keys to medical terminology is in the structure of the words. Knowledge of a number of common roots, prefixes, and suffixes will give an interpreter important clues as to the meaning of the word and will make it easier to learn and remember new words.

English is a language that often builds words from three kinds of parts. The three parts are called the:

- root = the basic part of the word
- prefix = the beginning of a word
- suffix = the end of a word

The prefixes and suffixes added to the root can change the meaning of the word. Often, the meaning of a word can be determined just by knowing the meaning of the roots, prefixes, and suffixes that are found in the word.

Consider the following combinations of roots, prefixes, and suffixes. By analyzing the prefixes, roots, and suffixes of the word, we can gain an understanding of its meaning.

Cardiology (study of the heart)

Prefix	Root	Suffix
-	cardi-	-logy
-	"heart"	"study of"

Dermatology (study of the skin)

Prefix	Root	Suffix
-	dermat-	-logy
-	"skin"	"study of"

Dermatosis (disease or condition of the skin)

Prefix	Root	Suffix
-	dermat-	-osis
-	"skin"	"disease, or condition of"

Hypodermis (lowest skin layer, below the epidermis and dermis)

Prefix	Root	Suffix
hypo-	dermis	-
"under, decreased"	"skin"	-

See the chart on the following pages for a list of roots, prefixes, and suffixes that are commonly used in medical terminology. As you study them, try matching them up to form new words. If you come up with a word you are not sure of, check the dictionary to make sure the word really exists, and what it means.

Common Prefixes Used in Medical Terminology

Prefixes	Meaning	Example
an-	without	*an*emia
anti-	against	*anti*toxin
auto-	self	*auto*immune
contra-	against	*contra*indication
dys-	abnormal, difficult	*dys*functional
endo-	within, inside	*endo*scopy
extra-	outside of	*extra*ventricular
hemi-	half	*hemi*glossectomy
hyper-	above, increased	*hyper*plasia
hypo-	under, decreased	*hypo*dermic
infra-	below, beneath	*infra*red
inter-	between	*inter*costals
intra-	within	*intra*venous
mal-	bad, poor	*mal*nutrition
macro-	large	*macro*cephalia
micro-	small	*micro*scope
multi-	many	*multi*parous
neo-	new	*neo*natal
peri-	around	*peri*natal
poly-	many	*poly*neuritis
post-	after	*post*partum
pre-	before	*pre*clampsia
pro-	before, for, on account of	*pro*lapse
pseudo-	false	*pseudo*cyesis
retro-	backward	*retro*peritoneal
sub-	under, beneath	*sub*cutaneous
uni-	one	*uni*lateral

Common Roots Used in Medical Terminology

Root	Meaning	Example
arthr	joint	*arthr*ocentesis
aden/o	having to do with glands	*adeno*pathy
carcin/o	cancerous	*carcin*oma
cardi/o	having to do with the heart	*cardio*graphy
cephal/o	head	*cephal*ic
dermat/o	skin	Hypo*dermic*
enter/o	intestines	*enter*itis
gastr/o	related to the digestive tract	*gastr*itis
gynec/o	woman, female	*gyneco*logy
hem/o	having to do with blood	*hemo*dialysis
iatr/o	practice of healing	ped*iatric*
my/o	muscle	*myo*fibril
nephr/o	kidney	*nephro*logy
neur/o	having to do with nerves	*neur*algia
oste/o	bone	*osteo*pathy
orth/o	straight, normal	*ortho*tics
ophthalm/o	having to do with the eye	*ophthal*moscope
ot/o	having to do with the ear	*oto*scope
path/o	disease	*path*ology
ped/o	child	*ped*iatrics
psych/o	mind	*psych*iatrist
ur/o	urine	*ur*ic acid
therm/o	heat	*thermo*meter

Common Suffixes Used in Medical Terminology

Suffixes	Meaning	Example
-algia	pain	neur*algia*
-cide	destructive, killing	bacter*icide*
-ectomy	surgical removal of	tonsill*ectomy*
-emia	blood	an*emia*
-graphy	process of recording	cardio*graphy*
-gram	record	angio*gram*
-itis	inflammation	bronch*itis*
-ist	person who practices something	nephrolog*ist*
-logy	study of	dermato*logy*
-oma	tumor	sarc*oma*
-opsy	to view	bi*opsy*
-osis	disease, condition	lymphcyt*osis*
-ostomy	opening to form a mouth	col*ostomy*
-pathy	disease	neuro*pathy*
-phobia	fear	hydro*phobia*
-plasia	formation, growth	dys*plasia*
-plegia	paralysis	para*plegia*
-scope	instrument for visual examination	oto*scope*
-tomy	incision of	lapar*otomy*

Vocabulary Development

Define the following terms using only your knowledge of roots, prefixes and suffixes. Check your answers with a dictionary.

Ophthalmologist:

Prefix	Root	Suffix
-	'opthalmo-'	'- logy' and '- ist'

Electrocardiogram:

Prefix	Root	Suffix
'electro-'	'cardio-'	'- gram'

Define the following terms using only your knowledge of roots, prefixes, and suffixes. Check your answers with a dictionary. This time, you will have to determine which parts of the words are prefixes, roots, and suffixes.

Myalgia
Hypoglycemia
Arthritis
Osteoporosis
Endocardial
Dermatosis
Dermatology
Cardiology
Hypodermis

Section 2

BODY SYSTEMS TERMINOLOGY

Introduction

Section 2: *Body Systems Terminology* has ten sections devoted to each system in the body. The systems discussed are:

- Cardiovascular system
- Digestive system
- Endocrine system
- Musculoskeletal system
- Nervous system
- Respiratory system
- Skin system
- Urinary system
- Female reproductive system
- Male reproductive system

Each system includes:
- important vocabulary words related to the system
- some of the major anatomical parts of the system
- common problems related to the system (descriptions taken from the non-copyrighted Health Topics pages of Medline Plus)
- specialists of the system
- common procedures related to the system

Remember that this section is meant to provide an overview of some of the vocabulary you may work with as a medical interpreter. It is not intended to diagnose or treat any illness.

Anatomy and Physiology

Anatomy and physiology are two of the basic areas of vocabulary development that are important to medical interpreters.

Human anatomy is the study of the structure and the design of the human body. Human physiology is the study of the function of the different parts of the human body. Here is one way to think about these two terms:

- **Anatomy** is the list of vocabulary words of the various parts of the body. These are the words that you can use to label various diagrams of the body.
- **Physiology** is where you define the function of each anatomical part.

Why Study Anatomy and Physiology?

Almost all providers refer to anatomy and physiology. It is difficult, if not impossible, to interpret correctly if you do not know the right word for the parts of the body in question. However, you do not need to know the name of every bone, every nerve, and every muscle.

Still, familiarity with basic anatomy and physiology is absolutely mandatory for a medical interpreter. In biomedicine, medical specialties are often defined by body system. Knowing what each specialist does will provide you with information about the topic and nature of the medical appointment.

Finally, familiarity with common medical procedures and health problems can help you do a better job of interpreting clearly and accurately what the doctor says. Since anatomy, physiology, specialists, procedures, and common problems are all related to each other, this lesson will integrate them so as to make them more interesting and easier to learn.

One of the more difficult things to interpret in a medical setting are the procedures that providers use. Often there is no clear linguistic equivalent, either for the name of the procedure, or for the explanation. While it is the job of the provider, not the interpreter, to explain medical procedures, the more familiar you are with the procedure, the easier it will be to interpret accurately.

Purposes of Procedures

Screening procedures are used to catch problems early on and to prevent future health problems.

Diagnostic procedures help providers discover what is wrong with a patient.

Therapeutic procedures help a patient become healthier.

Another way to distinguish procedures is by how "invasive" they are. Medical procedures that involve penetrating the body through the skin or one of the natural openings (like a biopsy or an endoscopy) are considered to be **invasive procedures**. Those that do not penetrate the body, like an ultrasound, are considered to be **non-invasive.**

Categorizing new vocabulary words is one of the strategies for learning medical terminology discussed in this curriculum. When studying medical procedure vocabulary, categorizing them by purpose or levels of invasiveness may aid your learning.

Body Systems Terminology

The Cardiovascular System

Cardiovascular System Vocabulary

Anemia
Aneurysm
Angina
Aorta
Arrythmia
Arteries
Blood tests
Bone marrow transplant
Capillaries
Cardiologist
Cholesterol
Congenital heart defect
Congestive heart failure
Diastolic pressure
Echocardiogram (Echo)
Electrocardiogram (EKG)
Exercise tolerance test
Heart
Heart attack
High blood pressure
Hypertension
Hypothermia
Inferior vena cava
Left Atrium
Left Ventricle
Lymph nodes
Lymphatic system
Myocardial infarction
Pulmonary artery
Pulmonary veins
Right atrium
Right ventricle
Sickle-cell anemia
Spleen
Superior vena cava
Systolic pressure
Valves
Varicose veins
Veins

Function and Major Anatomical Parts of the Cardiovascular System

The cardiovascular system moves blood within our bodies. Blood carries food and oxygen that our bodies need to keep going. It also carries waste materials produced by our bodies and helps to keep our body temperatures stable.

The heart

The **heart** is a muscle that is at the center of the circulatory system. It keeps the blood moving at all times. The heart works with two pumps side by side. Each side (or pump) has two parts - one part at the top to take in the blood (**right and left atriums**) and one part at the bottom to pump it out (**right and left ventricles**). The ventricles are bigger than the atriums. Unlike other muscles in our body, the heart does not tire easily. The heart uses a lot of blood, delivered through blood vessels to keep itself going.

Blood vessels

There are three main kinds of blood vessels - arteries, capillaries, and veins.

Arteries carry blood away from the heart. They have strong, flexible walls. The blood traveling in the arteries is high in oxygen and looks red.

Capillaries are very tiny, thin-walled blood vessels. All parts of the body contain capillaries. Nutrients (food) and oxygen move through the capillary walls into the body cells. Waste products and carbon dioxide move from the cells into the blood.

© 2014 The Cross Cultural Health Care Program

Major Anatomical Parts of the Heart

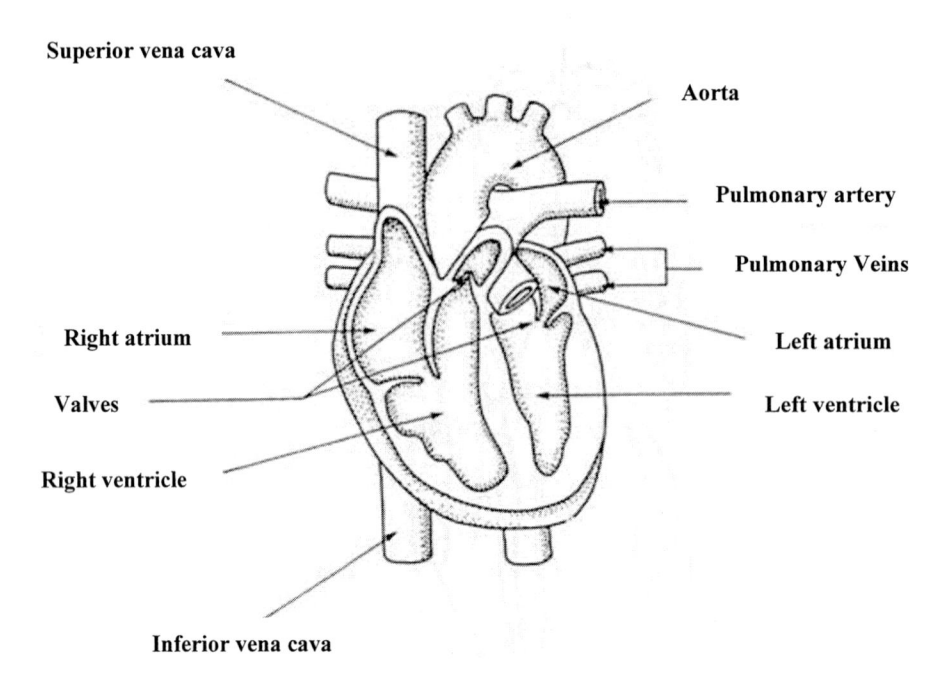

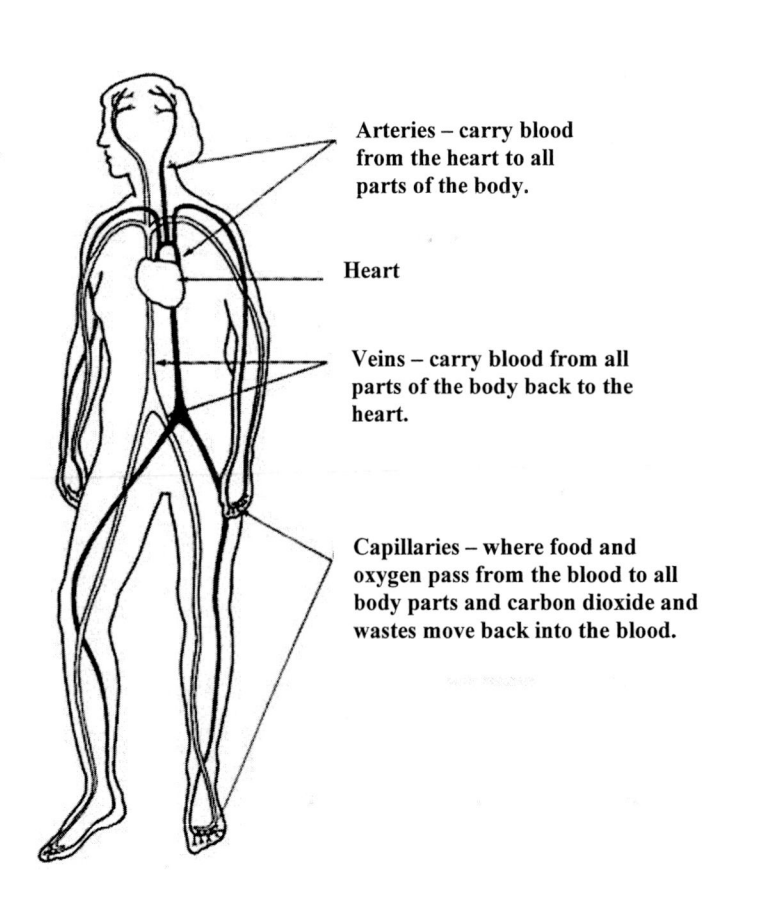

- Superior vena cava
- Aorta
- Pulmonary artery
- Pulmonary Veins
- Right atrium
- Left atrium
- Valves
- Left ventricle
- Right ventricle
- Inferior vena cava

- **Arteries** – carry blood from the heart to all parts of the body.
- **Heart**
- **Veins** – carry blood from all parts of the body back to the heart.
- **Capillaries** – where food and oxygen pass from the blood to all body parts and carbon dioxide and wastes move back into the blood.

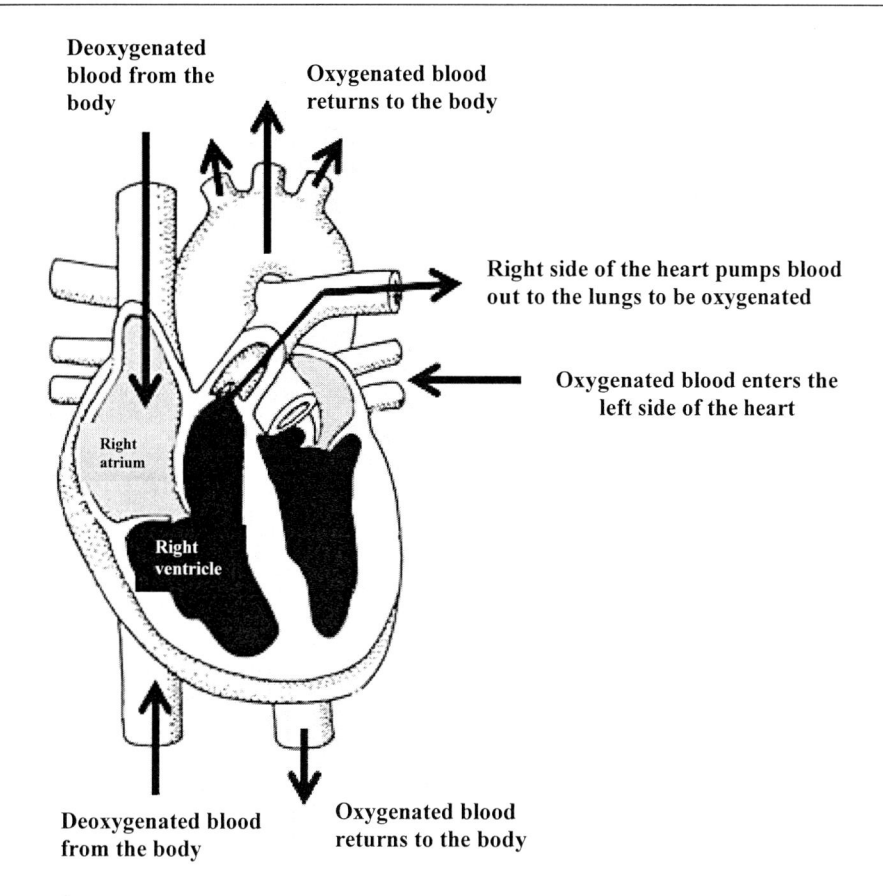

Diagram of the heart showing:
- Deoxygenated blood from the body
- Oxygenated blood returns to the body
- Right side of the heart pumps blood out to the lungs to be oxygenated
- Oxygenated blood enters the left side of the heart
- Right atrium
- Right ventricle
- Deoxygenated blood from the body
- Oxygenated blood returns to the body

Veins take blood from the capillaries and carry it back to the heart. The walls of the veins are thinner and less flexible than artery walls. Veins have **valves,** or doors, that allow the blood to move in only one direction.

When we move, our muscles push against the veins, and because the blood can only move in one direction (back to the heart), this moving helps our circulation. The blood traveling in the veins is low in oxygen and looks blue.

The **aorta** is the largest artery that carries blood away from the heart to other arteries throughout the body.

The **pulmonary artery** is an artery that carries blood away from the heart to the lungs.

The **pulmonary veins** return blood from the lungs to the heart.

The **superior vena cava** brings blood from the head and the shoulders to the heart, and the **inferior vena cava** brings blood from the abdomen and lower part of the body to the heart.

Blood Pressure
The blood circulating in our bodies creates pressure on the inside of our blood vessels. This is called blood pressure. Most of us have a normal blood pressure.

Our hearts normally produce just enough pressure to keep the blood flowing steadily. There are two measurements of blood pressure. **Systolic pressure** (the upper number) is created each time the heart beats. **Diastolic pressure** (the lower number) is created each time the heart relaxes between beats. A normal blood pressure range for a healthy young adult is about 120 over 80.

Blood flowing in your arteries can be felt in the pulse that results each time the heart beats. By feeling your pulse, you can tell how fast or how slow your heart is beating. To feel your pulse, place your fingers on the inside of the wrist or on the front part of the neck, just below the jaw. Each pulse measures one heartbeat.

Blood

Our blood is made up of two basic parts, blood cells and plasma (fluid). The cells float in the plasma. Cells are the very small parts that go together to make up the body. We are made up of many different kinds of cells (like skin cells, muscle cells, bone cells, etc.).

There are three different kinds of blood cells. Red blood cells carry oxygen from the lungs to the body and the waste product of carbon dioxide from the body to the lungs. The oxygen is carried by a substance in the red blood cell called hemoglobin. White blood cells fight infections by destroying bacteria and making antibodies. Platelets are the third kind of blood cell and they help to stop bleeding whenever a blood vessel is injured. Nutrients, antibodies, and other body substances are also carried in the fluid part of the blood.

Common Problems of the Cardiovascular System

Anemia: If you have anemia, your blood does not carry enough oxygen to the rest of your body. The most common cause of anemia is not having enough iron. Your body needs iron to make hemoglobin. Hemoglobin is an iron-rich protein that gives the red color to blood. It carries oxygen from the lungs to the rest of the body.

Anemia can make you feel tired, cold, dizzy, and irritable. You may be short of breath or have a headache. Your doctor will diagnose anemia with a physical exam and blood tests. Treatment depends on the kind of anemia you have.

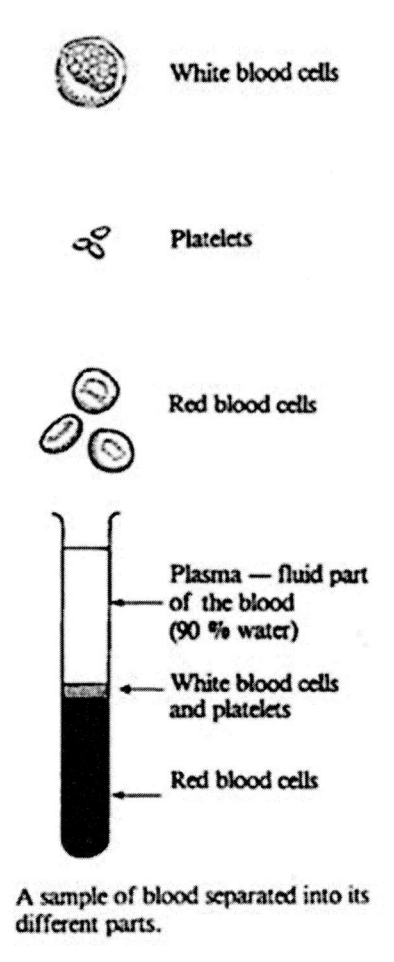

Aneurysm: An aneurysm is a bulge or "ballooning" in the wall of an artery. Arteries are blood vessels that carry oxygen-rich blood from the heart to other parts of the body. If an aneurysm grows large, it can burst and cause dangerous bleeding or even death.

Most aneurysms occur in the aorta, the main artery that runs from the heart through the chest and abdomen. Aneurysms also can happen in arteries in the brain, heart and other parts of the body. If an aneurysm in the brain bursts, it causes a stroke.

Aneurysms can develop and become large before causing any symptoms. Often doctors can stop aneurysms from bursting if they find and treat them early. They use imaging tests to find aneurysms. Often aneurysms are found by chance during tests done for other reasons. Medicines and surgery are the two main treatments for aneurysms.

Angina pectoris: Angina is chest pain or discomfort you feel when there is not enough blood flow to your heart muscle. Your heart muscle needs the oxygen that the blood carries. Angina may feel like pressure or a squeezing pain in your chest. It may feel like indigestion. You may also feel pain in your shoulders, arms, neck, jaw, or back.

Angina is a symptom of coronary artery disease (CAD), the most common heart disease. CAD happens when a sticky substance called plaque builds up in the arteries that supply blood to the heart, reducing blood flow.

Arrhythmia: An arrhythmia is a problem with the rate or rhythm of your heartbeat. It means that your heart beats too quickly, too slowly, or with an irregular pattern. When the heart beats faster than normal, it is called tachycardia. When the heart beats too slowly, it is called bradycardia. The most common type of arrhythmia is atrial fibrillation, which causes an irregular and fast heartbeat.

Many factors can affect your heart's rhythm, such as having had a heart attack, smoking, congenital heart defects, and stress. Some substances or medicines may also cause arrhythmias.

Symptoms of arrhythmias include
- Fast heartbeat (tachycardia)
- Slow heartbeat (bradycardia)
- Skipping beats
- Lightheadedness or dizziness
- Chest pain
- Shortness of breath
- Sweating

Cholesterol: Cholesterol is a waxy, fat-like substance that occurs naturally in all parts of the body. Your body needs some cholesterol to work properly. But if you have too much in your blood, it can combine with other substances in the blood and stick to the walls of your arteries. This is called plaque. Plaque can narrow your arteries or even block them. High levels of cholesterol in the blood can increase your risk of heart disease. Your cholesterol levels tend to rise as you get older. There are usually no signs or symptoms that you have high blood cholesterol, but it can be detected with a blood test. You are likely to have high cholesterol if members of your family have it, if you are overweight or if you eat a lot of fatty foods.

You can lower your cholesterol by exercising more and eating more fruits and vegetables. You also may need to take medicine to lower your cholesterol.

Congenital heart defects: A congenital heart defect is a problem with the structure of the heart. It is present at birth. Congenital heart defects are the most common type of birth defect. The defects can involve the walls of the heart, the valves of the heart, and the arteries and veins near the heart. They can disrupt the normal flow of blood through the heart. The blood flow can slow down, go in the wrong direction or to the wrong place, or be blocked completely.

Many children with congenital heart defects don't need treatment, but others do. Treatment can include medicines, catheter procedures, surgery, and heart transplants. The treatment depends on the type of the defect, how severe it is, and a child's age, size, and general health.

Congestive heart failure: Heart failure is a condition in which the heart can't pump enough blood to meet the body's needs. Heart failure does not mean that your heart has stopped or is about to stop working. It means that your heart is not able to pump blood the way it should. It can affect one or both sides of the heart.
The weakening of the heart's pumping ability causes blood and fluid to back up into the lungs, a buildup of fluid in the feet, ankles and legs - called edema, and tiredness and shortness of breath.

Common causes of heart failure are coronary artery disease, high blood pressure and diabetes. It is more common in people who are over 65 years old, overweight, and people who have had a heart attack. Men have a higher rate of heart failure than women.

Your doctor will diagnose heart failure by doing a physical exam and heart tests. Treatment includes treating the underlying cause of your heart failure, medicines, and heart transplantation if other treatments fail.

High blood pressure: Blood pressure is the force of your blood pushing against the walls of your arteries. Each time your heart beats, it pumps blood into the arteries. Your blood pressure is highest when your heart beats, pumping the blood. This is called systolic pressure. When your heart is at rest, between beats, your blood pressure falls. This is called diastolic pressure.

Your blood pressure reading uses these two numbers. Usually the systolic number comes before or above the diastolic number. A reading of 119/79 or lower is normal blood pressure; 140/90 or higher is high blood pressure.

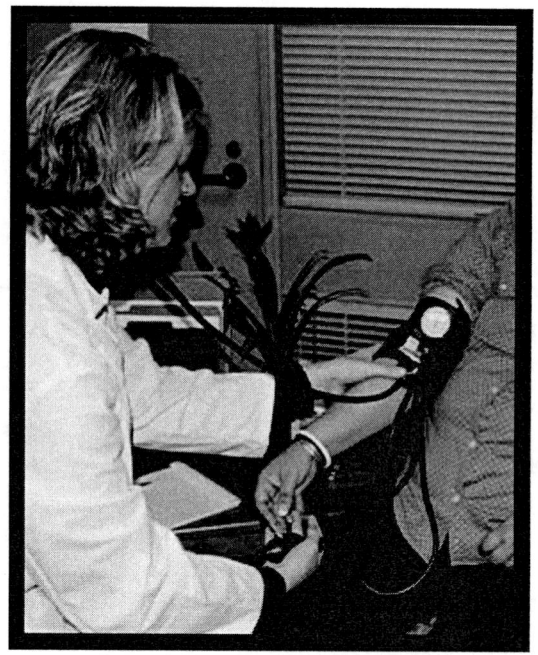

A provider taking a patient's blood pressure

Between 120 and 139 for the top number, or between 80 and 89 for the bottom number is called **prehypertension**. Prehypertension means you may end up with high blood pressure, unless you take steps to prevent it.

High blood pressure usually has no symptoms, but it can cause serious problems such as stroke, heart failure, heart attack and kidney failure.
You can control high blood pressure through healthy lifestyle habits and taking medicines, if needed.

Hypothermia: Cold weather can affect your body in different ways. You can get frostbite, which is frozen body tissue. Your body can also lose heat faster than you can produce it. The result is hypothermia, or abnormally low body temperature. It can make you sleepy, confused and clumsy. Because it happens gradually and affects your thinking, you may not realize you need help. That makes it especially dangerous. A body temperature below 95°

F is a medical emergency and can lead to death if not treated promptly.

Anyone who spends much time outdoors in cold weather can get hypothermia. You can also get it from being cold and wet, or under cold water for too long. Babies and old people are especially at risk. Babies can get it from sleeping in a cold room.

Myocardial infarction (MI) (heart attack): Each year over a million people in the U.S. have a heart attack. About half of them die. Many people have permanent heart damage or die because they don't get help immediately. It's important to know the symptoms of a heart attack and call 9-1-1 if someone is having them. Those symptoms include:
- Chest discomfort - pressure, squeezing, or pain
- Shortness of breath
- Discomfort in the upper body - arms, shoulder, neck, back
- Nausea, vomiting, dizziness, lightheadedness, sweating

These symptoms can sometimes be different in women.

What exactly is a heart attack? Most heart attacks happen when a clot in the coronary artery blocks the supply of blood and oxygen to the heart. Often this leads to an irregular heartbeat - called an arrhythmia - that causes a severe decrease in the pumping function of the heart. A blockage that is not treated within a few hours causes the affected heart muscle to die.

Sickle cell anemia: Sickle cell anemia is a disease in which your body produces abnormally shaped red blood cells. The cells are shaped like a crescent or sickle. They don't last as long as normal, round red blood cells. This leads to anemia. The sickle cells also get stuck in blood vessels, blocking blood flow. This can cause pain and organ damage.

A genetic problem causes sickle cell anemia. People with the disease are born with two sickle cell genes, one from each parent. If you only have one sickle cell gene, it's called sickle cell trait. About 1 in 12 African Americans has sickle cell trait. The most common symptoms are pain and problems from anemia. Anemia can make you feel tired or weak. In addition, you might have shortness of breath, dizziness, headaches, or coldness in the hands and feet.

A blood test can show if you have the trait or anemia. Most states test newborn babies as part of their newborn screening programs.

Sickle cell anemia has no widely available cure. Treatments can help relieve symptoms and lessen complications. Researchers are investigating new treatments such as blood and marrow stem cell transplants, gene therapy, and new medicines.

Varicose veins: Varicose veins are swollen, twisted veins that you can see just under the skin. They usually occur in the legs, but also can form in other parts of the body. Hemorrhoids are a type of varicose vein.

Your veins have one-way valves that help keep blood flowing toward your heart. If the valves are weak or damaged, blood can back up and pool in your veins. This causes the veins to swell, which can lead to varicose veins.

Varicose veins are very common. You are more at risk if you are older, a female, obese, don't exercise or have a family history. They can also be more common in pregnancy.

Doctors often diagnose varicose veins from a physical exam. Sometimes you may need additional tests.

Exercising, losing weight, elevating your legs when resting, and not crossing them when sitting can help keep varicose veins from getting worse. Wearing loose clothing and avoiding long periods of standing can also help. If varicose veins are painful or you don't like the way they look, your doctor may recommend procedures to remove them.

Cardiovascular System Specialists

The medical specialist who handles the health of the heart and the cardiovascular system is called a **cardiologist**.

Cardiovascular System Procedures

Blood Tests: Blood is drawn with a needle, usually from one of the veins in the inside of the elbow. The number of vials of blood drawn will depend on what kind of tests the provider has requested. Blood tests check for the number and function of normal parts of the blood, such as the red blood cells or platelets, or for the presence of invaders in the blood, such as viruses.

Blood Transfusion: In this procedure, blood (or some part of it) is taken from a donor, tested for a match of blood type, and then injected into the patient. Before being injected, the blood is tested for various diseases to make sure it is safe for the patient.

Bone Marrow Transplant: This transplant is done when a patient's own bone marrow can no longer produce the blood he needs. First, the patient receives chemotherapy (radiation) to kill his own diseased bone marrow. An intravenous line injects substances directly into the veins. The bone marrow will find and lodge in the space where the old bone marrow was. This is a very dangerous procedure and can result in serious infection, a rejection by the body of the new bone marrow, or a return of the original disease.

Echocardiogram (Echo): Pulses of ultrasound (a specific frequency of sound waves) are directed through the patient's chest, and the returning echoes are recorded. This test shows the structure and movement of the heart.

Electrocardiogram (EKG): An EKG is a recording of the electricity flowing through the heart. Small discs connected to a machine by wires are attached to the patient's chest. The patient feels nothing during the recording. The discs are easily removed.

Exercise Tolerance Test (ETT): While a patient is walking or jogging on a treadmill, a technician measures blood pressure, pulse, and takes an EKG. This procedure determines how the heart responds under stress and helps identify areas of weakness.

The Digestive System

Digestive System Vocabulary

Abdomen
Acid reflux
Appendicitis
Appendix
Bowel
Bowel movement
Cirrhosis
Constipation
Diarrhea
Duodenum
Endoscopy
Epiglottis
Esophagus
Gallbladder
Gallstones
Gastroenteritis
Gastroenterologist
Gum disease
Gums
Heartburn
Hemorrhoids
Hiatal hernia
Irritable bowel syndrome
Large intestine
Liver
Mouth
Pancreas
Peptic ulcer
Rectum
Saliva glands
Sigmoid colon
Small intestine
Stomach
Teeth
Trachea
Upper GI Series (Barium Swallow)

Function and Major Anatomical Parts of the Digestive System

The main function of the digestive system is the digestion and absorption of food. The food we eat is digested (broken down) in stages. It gets broken down slowly as it moves through the system and the different organs and parts described in this section.

Food and nutrients enter the body through the **mouth**. The **teeth and gums** begin the process of digesting food. When we chew food, our saliva glands add saliva to aid the process of digestion.

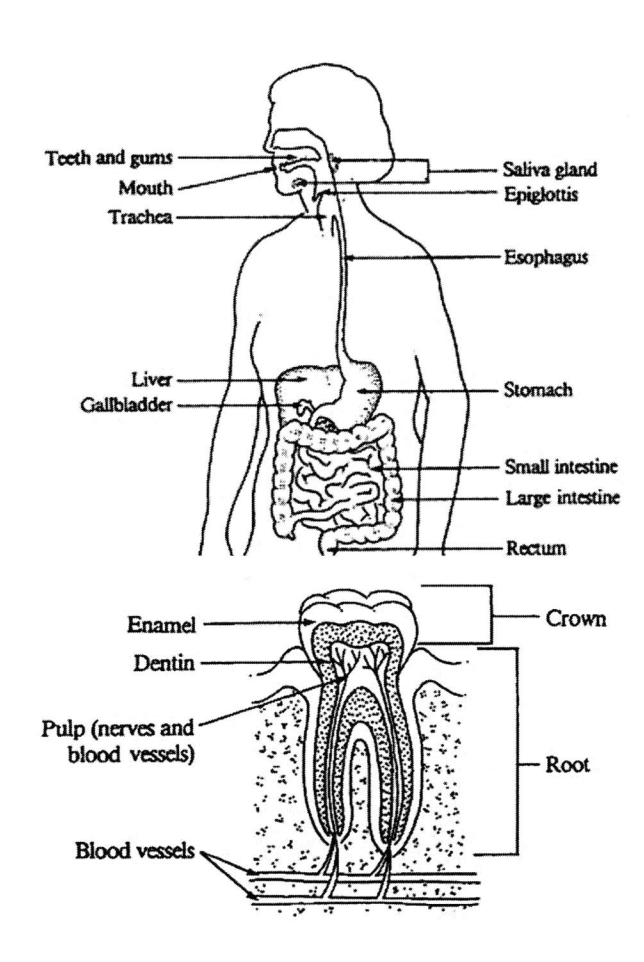

Teeth are a part of the digestive system. Blood vessels carry food to them, and nerves inside them sense heat, cold, pressure, and pain. We use our teeth to break food into small pieces. Teeth also help to shape our faces. The following diagram shows the structure of a tooth.

After passing through the mouth, food enters the **esophagus** on the way to the **stomach.** The **epiglottis** is a flap of skin that is controlled by the brain. The epiglottis can open and close and is able to prevent food from entering the trachea by mistake. The **trachea, also called** the windpipe, is a tube that carries air to the lungs.

In the stomach, food is mixed with stomach juices that contain enzymes that aid in the digestion of food. From the stomach, the food enters the **small intestine.** The small intestine adds more digestive enzymes, or juices, that aid the body in breaking down and absorbing nutrients. The small intestine is composed of three parts - the **duodenum,** jejunum, and ileum. In the duodenum, juices from the **liver** and **pancreas,**[1] two other digestive organs, are added.

As food travels through the small intestine, the body absorbs the nutrients found within the food, leaving mostly waste. This waste then reaches the **large intestine.** As food travels through the large intestine it is turned into feces and is prepared to be removed from the body. The digested food goes through the different parts of the large intestine. It enters the ascending colon, then the transverse colon, then the descending colon, and finally the **sigmoid colon** before entering the **rectum.** The rectum is where the solid waste is finally expelled from the body. Another term that is often used to describe the process of expelling solid waste is called a **bowel movement**, and sometimes the large intestine is commonly referred to as the **bowel**.

The liver, gallbladder, and pancreas are three organs that are a very important part of the digestive system.

The liver is the largest internal organ in the body. (The largest organ of the human

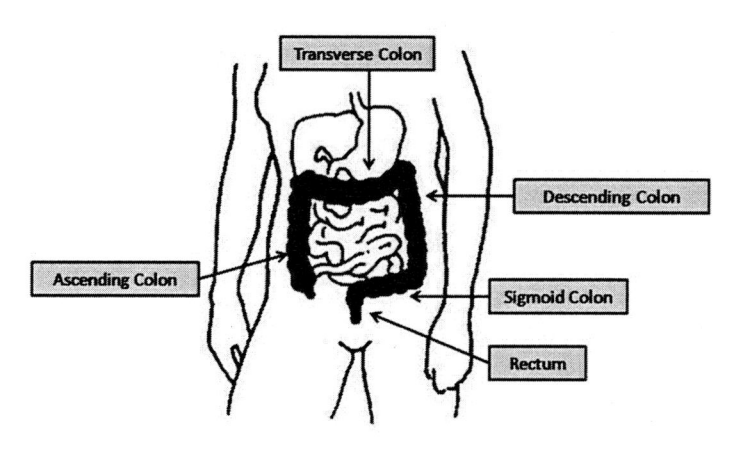

---

[1] The pancreas is also a part of the endocrine glands system and is listed as a vocabulary word in that section.

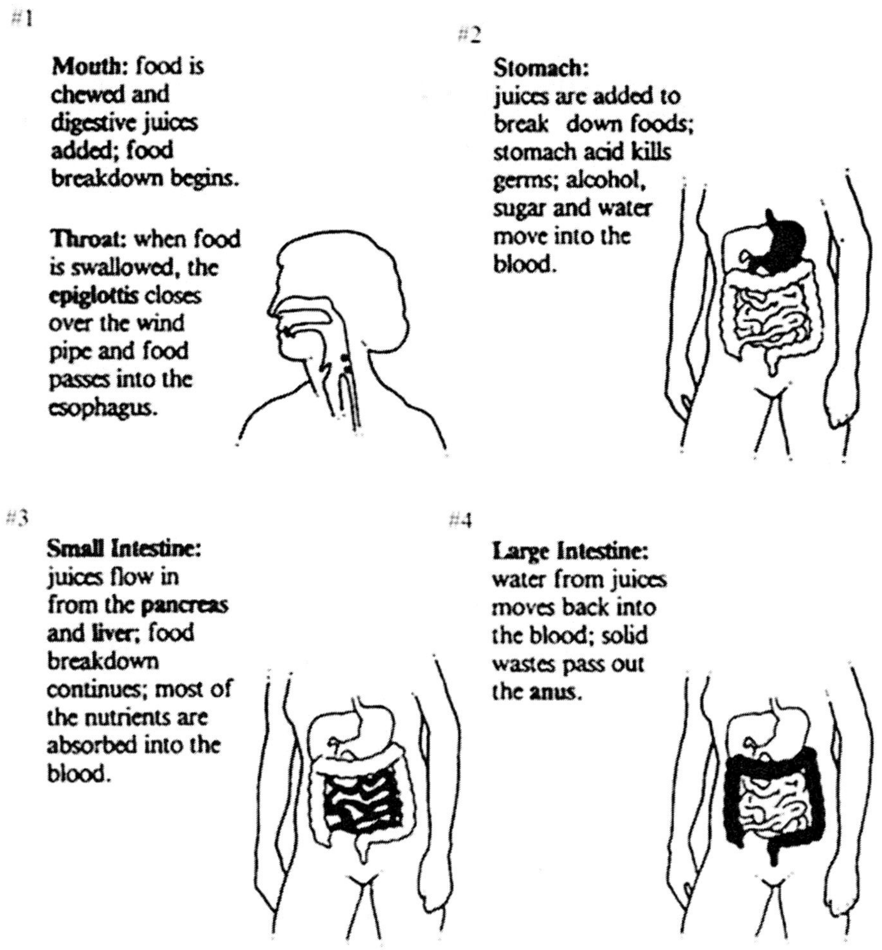

#1 **Mouth:** food is chewed and digestive juices added; food breakdown begins.

Throat: when food is swallowed, the **epiglottis** closes over the wind pipe and food passes into the esophagus.

#2 **Stomach:** juices are added to break down foods; stomach acid kills germs; alcohol, sugar and water move into the blood.

#3 **Small Intestine:** juices flow in from the **pancreas** and **liver**; food breakdown continues; most of the nutrients are absorbed into the blood.

#4 **Large Intestine:** water from juices moves back into the blood; solid wastes pass out the anus.

Steps in the digestive process.

body is the skin. It carries out many complex jobs related to controlling what is in the blood. For example, it gets rid of alcohol and poisonous chemicals. The liver also makes a digestive juice called bile. Bile collects in a sac called the gallbladder. When we eat, the **gallbladder** empties bile into the small intestine to help break down fatty foods. Bile also replaces acid from the stomach so that it doesn't burn the inside of the intestine.

The pancreas makes digestive juices that drain into the small intestine. It also makes hormones (chemical messengers) that control many body functions. The pancreas is a part of the digestive system and the endocrine system. We will discuss the pancreas more in the section on the endocrine system.

Common Problems of the Digestive System

Appendicitis: The **appendix** is a small, tube-like organ attached to the first part of the large intestine. It is located in the lower right part of the abdomen. It has no known function. A blockage inside of the appendix causes appendicitis. The blockage leads to increased pressure, problems with blood flow, and inflammation. If the blockage is not treated, the appendix can burst and spread infection into the abdomen. This causes a condition called peritonitis.

The main symptom of appendicitis is pain in the **abdomen**, often on the right side. It is usually sudden and gets worse over time. Other symptoms may include:
- swelling in the abdomen
- loss of appetite
- nausea and vomiting
- constipation or diarrhea
- inability to pass gas
- low fever

Not everyone with appendicitis has all these symptoms.

Appendicitis is a medical emergency. Treatment almost always involves removing the appendix. Anyone can get appendicitis, but it is more common among people between 10 and 30 years old.

Cirrhosis: Cirrhosis is scarring of the liver. Scar tissue forms because of injury or long-term disease. Scar tissue cannot do what healthy liver tissue does - make protein, help fight infections, clean the blood, help digest food and store energy. Cirrhosis can lead to**:**
- easy bruising or bleeding, or nosebleeds
- swelling of the abdomen or legs
- extra sensitivity to medicines
- high blood pressure in the vein entering the liver
- enlarged veins called varices in the esophagus and stomach; varices can bleed suddenly
- kidney failure
- jaundice
- severe itching
- gallstones

A small number of people with cirrhosis get liver cancer.

Your doctor will diagnose cirrhosis with blood tests, imaging tests, or a biopsy.

Cirrhosis has many causes. In the United States, the most common causes are chronic alcoholism and hepatitis. Nothing will make the scar tissue disappear but treating the cause can keep it from getting worse. If too much scar tissue forms, you may need to consider a liver transplant.

Diarrhea and constipation: Diarrhea means that you have loose, watery stool more than three times in one day. You may also have cramps, bloating, nausea and an urgent need to have a bowel movement. Causes of diarrhea include bacteria, viruses or parasites, certain medicines, food intolerances and diseases that affect the stomach, small intestine or colon. In many cases, no cause can be found.

Although usually not harmful, diarrhea can become dangerous or signal a more serious problem. You should talk to your doctor if you have a strong pain in your abdomen or rectum, a fever, blood in your stool, severe diarrhea for more than three days or symptoms of dehydration. If your child has diarrhea, do not hesitate to call the doctor for advice. Diarrhea can be dangerous in children.

Constipation means that a person has three or fewer bowel movements in a week. The stool can be hard and dry. Sometimes it is painful to pass. At one time or another, almost everyone gets constipated. In most cases, it lasts a short time and is not serious.

There are many things you can do to prevent constipation. They include
- eating more fruits, vegetables and grains, which are high in fiber
- drinking plenty of water and other liquids
- getting enough exercise
- taking time to have a bowel movement when you need to

- using laxatives only if your doctor says you should
- asking your doctor if medicines you take may cause constipation

Gallstones: Your gallbladder is a pear-shaped organ under your liver. It stores bile, a fluid made by your liver to digest fat. As your stomach and intestines digest food, your gallbladder releases bile through a tube called the common bile duct. The duct connects your gallbladder and liver to your small intestine.

Your gallbladder is most likely to give you trouble if something blocks the flow of bile through the bile ducts. That is usually a gallstone. Gallstones form when substances in bile harden. Gallstone attacks usually happen after you eat. Signs of a gallstone attack may include nausea, vomiting, or pain in the abdomen, back, or just under the right arm.

Gallstones are most common among older adults, women, overweight people, Native Americans and Mexican Americans.

Gallstones are often found during imaging tests for other health conditions. If you do not have symptoms, you usually do not need treatment. The most common treatment is removal of the gallbladder. Fortunately, you can live without a gallbladder. Bile has other ways to reach your small intestine.

Heartburn/acid reflux: Heartburn is a painful burning feeling in your chest or throat. It happens when stomach acid backs up into your esophagus, the tube that carries food from your mouth to your stomach.

If you have heartburn more than twice a week, you may have GERD (gastroesophageal reflux disease/acid reflux). But you can have GERD without having heartburn.

Pregnancy, certain foods, alcohol, and some medications can bring on heartburn. Treating heartburn is important because over time reflux can damage the esophagus. Over-the-counter medicines may help. If the heartburn continues, you may need prescription medicines or surgery.

If you have other symptoms such as crushing chest pain, it could be a heart attack. Get help immediately.

Gastroenteritis: Have you ever had the "stomach flu"? What you probably had was gastroenteritis - not a type of flu at all. Gastroenteritis is an inflammation of the lining of the intestines caused by a virus, bacteria or parasites. Viral gastroenteritis is the second most common illness in the U.S. The cause is often a norovirus infection. It spreads through contaminated food or water and contact with an infected person. The best prevention is frequent hand washing.

Symptoms of gastroenteritis include diarrhea, abdominal pain, vomiting, headache, fever and chills. Most people recover with no treatment.

The most common problem with gastroenteritis is dehydration. This happens if you do not drink enough fluids to replace what you lose through vomiting and diarrhea. Dehydration is most common in babies, young children, the elderly and people with weak immune systems.

Hemorrhoids: Hemorrhoids are swollen, inflamed veins around the anus or lower rectum. They are either inside the anus or under the skin around the anus. They often result from straining to have a bowel movement. Other factors include pregnancy, aging and chronic constipation or diarrhea.

Hemorrhoids are very common in both men and women. About half of all people have hemorrhoids by age 50. The most common symptom of hemorrhoids inside the anus is bright red blood covering the stool, on toilet paper or in the toilet bowl. Symptoms usually go away within a few days.

If you have rectal bleeding, you should see a doctor. You need to make sure bleeding is not from a more serious condition such as colorectal or anal cancer. Treatment may include warm baths and a cream or other medicine. If you have large hemorrhoids, you may need surgery and other treatments.

Hepatitis
Your liver is the largest organ inside your body. It helps your body digest food, store energy, and remove poisons. Hepatitis is an inflammation of the liver.

Viruses cause most cases of hepatitis. The type of hepatitis is named for the virus that causes it; for example, hepatitis A, hepatitis B or hepatitis C. Drug or alcohol use can also cause hepatitis. In other cases, your body mistakenly attacks healthy cells in the liver.

Some people who have hepatitis have no symptoms. Others may have:
- loss of appetite
- nausea and vomiting
- diarrhea
- dark-colored urine and pale bowel movements
- stomach pain
- jaundice, yellowing of skin and eyes

Some forms of hepatitis are mild, and others can be serious. Some can lead to scarring, called cirrhosis, or to liver cancer.

Sometimes hepatitis goes away by itself. If it does not, it can be treated with drugs. Sometimes hepatitis lasts a lifetime. Vaccines can help prevent some viral forms.

Irritable bowel syndrome (IBS)
Irritable bowel syndrome (IBS) is a problem that affects the large intestine. It can cause abdominal cramping, bloating, and a change in bowel habits. Some people with the disorder have constipation. Some have diarrhea. Others go back and forth between the two. Although IBS can cause a great deal of discomfort, it does not harm the intestines.

IBS is common. It affects about twice as many women as men and is most often found in people younger than 45 years. No one knows the exact cause of IBS. There is no specific test for it. Your doctor may run tests to be sure you don't have other diseases. These tests may include stool sampling tests, blood tests, and x-rays. Your doctor may also do a test called a sigmoidoscopy or colonoscopy. Most people diagnosed with IBS can control their symptoms with diet, stress management, probiotics, and medicine.

Peptic ulcer
A peptic ulcer is a sore in the lining of your stomach or your duodenum, the first part of your small intestine. A burning stomach pain is the most common symptom. The pain:
- starts between meals or during the night
- briefly stops if you eat or take antacids
- lasts for minutes to hours
- comes and goes for several days or weeks

Peptic ulcers happen when the acids that help you digest food damage the walls of the stomach or duodenum. The most common cause is infection with a bacterium called Helicobacter pylori. Another cause is the long-term use of nonsteroidal anti-inflammatory medicines (NSAIDs) such as aspirin and ibuprofen. Stress and spicy foods do not cause ulcers but can make them worse.

To see if you have an H. pylori infection, your doctor will test your blood, breath, or stool. Your doctor also may look inside your stomach and duodenum by doing an endoscopy or x-ray.

Peptic ulcers will get worse if not treated. Treatment may include medicines to reduce stomach acids or antibiotics to kill H. pylori. Antacids and milk can't heal peptic ulcers. Not smoking and avoiding alcohol can help. You may need surgery if your ulcers don't heal.

Digestive System Specialists

The medical specialist that handles the health of the digestive system is called a **gastroenterologist.**

Dentists are also medical specialists who handle the health of the digestive system; they focus on the teeth and the gums.

Digestive System Procedures

Endoscopy: A thin fiber-optic tube with a scope on the end is inserted into the digestive tract. This allows the provider to see the inside of the tract on a TV monitor. An endoscopy may be recommended to investigate symptoms, diagnose diseases and conditions, and treat problems.

Upper endoscopy (also called esophagogastroduodenoscopy or EGD): the scope is used to examine the esophagus, stomach, and duodenum (the first part of the small intestine).

Colonoscopy: a scope is used to examine the entire colon (large intestine).

Sigmoidoscopy: a scope is used to examine the lower part of the large intestine, including the sigmoid colon.

Upper GI Series (Barium Swallow): The patient swallows a substance called barium sulfate that acts like a dye. Next, an x-ray method called fluoroscopy tracks how the barium moves through the esophagus, stomach, and small intestine.

The Endocrine System

Endocrine System Vocabulary

Adrenal glands
Cushing's syndrome
Diabetes
Endocrinologist
Hormone imbalance
Hormones
Hyperthyroidism
Ovaries
Pancreas
Parathyroid gland
Pituitary gland
Testicles
Thyroid gland
Ultrasound

Function of the Endocrine System

The endocrine system (also known as ductless glands system) makes **hormones** that are put directly into the blood stream and carried to all parts of the body. Hormones are chemical messengers that help control how the body works. Hormones control many different body functions. Certain hormones act only on certain parts of the body. They work with the nervous system to keep the various parts of the body working together. The amount of a hormone that is made is balanced with the amount the body needs.

Pituitary Gland

This gland makes a number of hormones that control other endocrine glands and specific body functions. The pituitary gland makes a hormone that controls how we grow. It also produces another hormone that controls how our kidneys work.

Thyroid and Parathyroid Glands: The thyroid gland makes a hormone that controls how fast the metabolic processes work. The metabolic process is the body's chemical process of creating, using, and storing energy from nutrients. The parathyroid glands make a hormone that controls the level of calcium in the body. Calcium is an important substance in our bones and teeth.

Adrenal Glands: The adrenal glands produce hormones that act on heart rate and blood pressure. It also controls the amount of salt in the body. It influences the development of sex organs and controls other body functions.

Pancreas: The pancreas makes two hormones: insulin and glucagon. Insulin makes our body's cells absorb glucose (sugar) from the blood and store extra glucose in the liver. As a result, insulin lowers the amount of glucose in the blood. Glucagon raises the level of glucose in the blood by causing the liver to release glucose back into the blood.

Ovaries: The ovaries produce two female sex hormones: progesterone and estrogen. These hormones control female physical changes during the menstrual cycle (menstruation and menopause). It also controls other changes associated with the menstrual cycle.

Testicles (Testes): The testicles produce a male sex hormone, called testosterone. This controls the development of male sex characteristics such as a deep voice, pubic hair, and male body shape.

Common Problems of the Endocrine System

Too much or too little of a hormone will result in medical problems. Although each gland has a specific function, over activity or under activity on the part of one gland usually affects the other glands as well. In general, common problems of the endocrine system can be considered **hormone imbalances.** All of the following endocrine system problems are examples of hormone imbalances.

Cushing's syndrome: Cushing's syndrome is a hormonal disorder. The cause is long-term exposure to too much cortisol, a hormone that your adrenal gland makes. Sometimes, taking synthetic hormone medicine to treat an inflammatory disease leads to Cushing's. Some kinds of tumors produce a hormone that can cause your body to make too much cortisol.

Cushing's syndrome is rare. Some symptoms are
- upper body obesity
- thin arms and legs

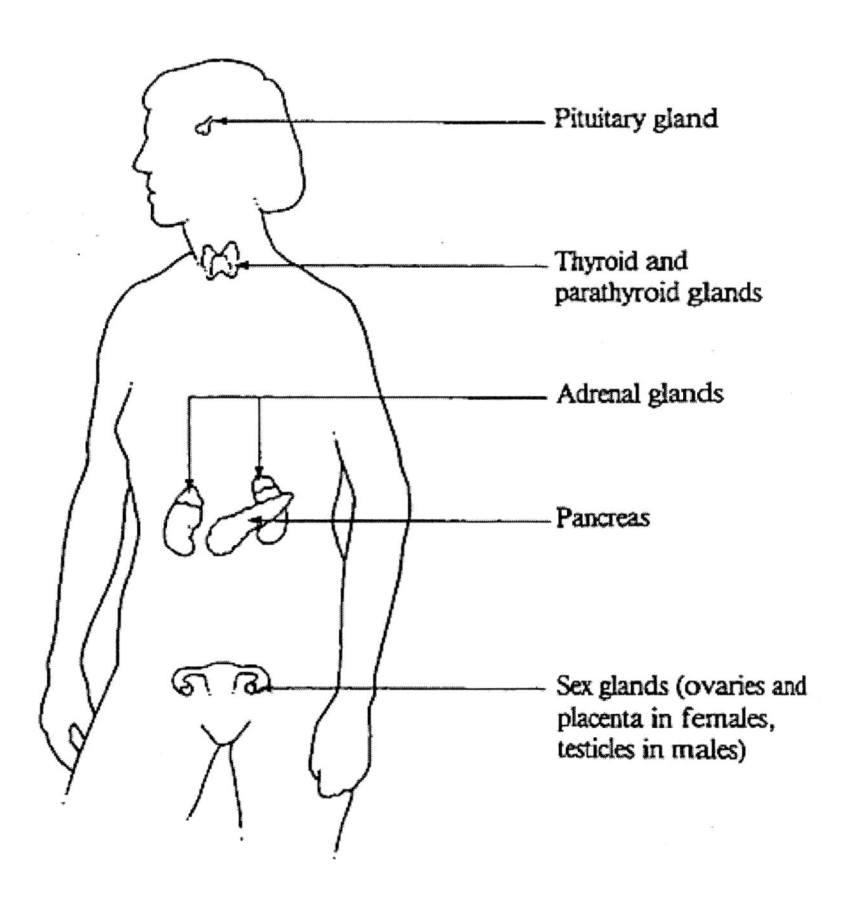

Hormone Producing Glands

- severe fatigue and muscle weakness
- high blood pressure
- high blood sugar
- easy bruising

Lab tests can show if you have it and find the cause. Your treatment will depend on why you have too much cortisol. If it is because you have been taking synthetic hormones, a lower dose may control your symptoms. If the cause is a tumor, surgery and other therapies may be needed.

Diabetes mellitus: Diabetes is a disease in which your blood glucose, or blood sugar, levels are too high. Glucose comes from the foods you eat. Insulin is a hormone that helps the glucose get into your cells to give them energy. With type 1 diabetes, your body does not make insulin. With type 2 diabetes, the more common type, your body does not make or use insulin well. Without enough insulin, the glucose stays in your blood.

Over time, having too much glucose in your blood can cause serious problems. It can damage your eyes, kidneys, and nerves. Diabetes can also cause heart disease, stroke and even the need to remove a limb. Pregnant women can also get diabetes, called gestational diabetes.
A blood test can show if you have diabetes. Exercise, weight control and sticking to your meal plan can help control your diabetes. You should also monitor your glucose level and take medicine if prescribed.

Hyperthyroidism: Your thyroid is a butterfly-shaped gland in your neck, just above your collarbone. It is one of your endocrine glands, which make hormones. Thyroid hormones control the rate of many activities in your body. These include how fast you burn calories and how fast your heart beats. All of these activities are your body's metabolism. If your thyroid is too active, it makes more thyroid hormones than your body needs. This is called hyperthyroidism.

Hyperthyroidism is more common in women, people with other thyroid problems, and those over 60 years old. Grave's disease, an autoimmune disorder, is the most common cause. Other causes include thyroid nodules, thyroiditis, consuming too much iodine, and taking too much synthetic thyroid hormone.
The symptoms can vary from person to person. They may include
- being nervous or irritable
- mood swings
- fatigue or muscle weakness
- heat intolerance
- trouble sleeping
- hand tremors
- rapid and irregular heartbeat
- frequent bowel movements or diarrhea
- weight loss
- goiter, which is an enlarged thyroid that may cause the neck to look swollen

To diagnose hyperthyroidism, your doctor will look at your symptoms, blood tests, and sometimes a thyroid scan. Treatment is with medicines, radioiodine therapy, or thyroid surgery. No single treatment works for everyone.

Hypothyroidism: Your thyroid is a butterfly-shaped gland in your neck, just above your collarbone. It is one of your endocrine glands, which make hormones. Thyroid hormones control the rate of many activities in your body. These include how fast you burn calories and how fast your heart beats. All of these activities are your body's metabolism. If your thyroid gland is not active enough, it does not make enough thyroid hormone to meet your body's needs. This condition is hypothyroidism.

Hypothyroidism is more common in women, people with other thyroid problems, and those over 60 years old. Hashimoto's disease, an autoimmune disorder, is the most common cause. Other causes include thyroid nodules, thyroiditis, congenital hypothyroidism, surgical removal of part or all of the thyroid, radiation treatment of the thyroid, and some medicines.

The symptoms can vary from person to person. They may include:
- fatigue
- weight gain
- a puffy face
- cold intolerance
- joint and muscle pain
- constipation
- dry skin
- dry, thinning hair
- decreased sweating
- heavy or irregular menstrual periods and fertility problems
- depression
- slowed heart rate

To diagnose hypothyroidism, your doctor will look at your symptoms and blood tests. Treatment is with synthetic thyroid hormone, taken every day.

Endocrine System Specialists

Endocrinologists are the medical specialists who treat hormone imbalances and other problems of the endocrine system.

Endocrine System Procedures

Blood Tests: Blood tests can be used to check for specific hormone levels. For example, it can be used to determine the level of cortisol in the blood, which may lead to a diagnosis of Cushing's Syndrome.

CT Scan: See Musculoskeletal System Procedures

Ultrasound: Pulses of sound (that are at a frequency higher than humans have the ability to hear directly) are directed at the patient and the returning echoes are recorded and used to create images of specific portions of the body.

X rays: See Musculoskeletal System Procedures

The Musculoskeletal System

Musculoskeletal System Vocabulary
Arthritis
Back pain
Bone
Carpal tunnel syndrome
Cartilage
Coccyx
CT Scan
Fibromyalgia
Fracture
Hernia
Hip bone (Pelvis)
Joint
Kneecap (Patella)
Ligament
MRI
Muscle
Muscle fiber
Orthopedist
Osteoporosis
Podiatrist
Rheumatologist
Skull
Strain
Tendon
Vertebra
X-Ray

Function and Major Anatomical Parts of the Musculoskeletal System

The musculoskeletal system is made up of **bones, joints**, and **muscles**.

There are about 206 major bones in the adult human body (the exact number may vary slightly from person to person). The purpose of our bones is to support our bodies and protect our vital organs. For example, humans have twelve pairs of rib bones to protect the heart and lungs. The **skull** is another example; its purpose is to protect the brain.

A **joint** is where two or more bones come together, like the knee, hip, elbow, or shoulder.

Your **muscles** help you move and help your body work. Different types of muscles have different jobs. On average, muscles account for about half the weight of the human body.

Our skeletal muscles work when we move around. Muscles in our organs work to move things around inside the body. Some of these muscles work automatically, like the heart and stomach muscle.

The diagram on the following page shows some of the major bones that support the human body. Of these major bones, pay close attention to the location and function of the following bones: **skull, vertebra, coccyx, pelvis (hip bone),** and **patella (kneecap).** There are thirty three **vertebrae** (singular: vertebra) which compose the spine (or backbone). The **coccyx** is the lowest part of the vertebrae and is often known as the tailbone.

Bones: Bones are made of flexible fibers and a solid material formed from calcium. Children's bones contain lots of fibers and are less likely to break than those of older people. As we get older our bones lose

Body Systems Terminology

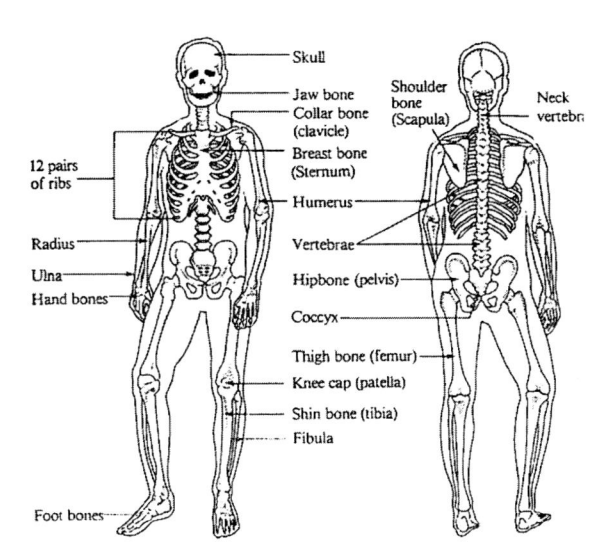

some of their flexibility and become more brittle. Down the center of a bone is a hollow part filled with tissues (bone marrow) where red blood cells are made. A woman's skeleton and a man's skeleton are only slightly different. A man's bones may be larger and heavier. A woman's hip bones may have a wider opening in the center for a baby's head to pass during childbirth.

A detailed view of a human bone

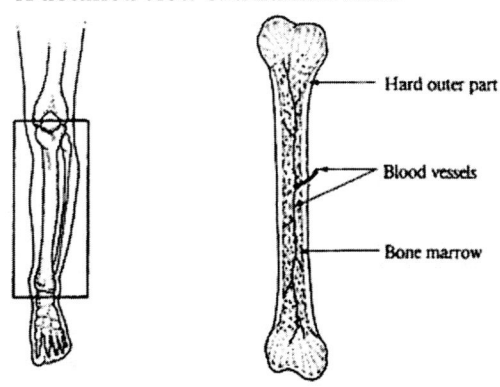

Joints: Individual bones are connected by joints. A joint is padded by a flexible substance called **cartilage** and held together by **ligaments**. Major joints, like the knee, hip, elbow, and shoulder joints are filled with a fluid that helps them move easily. There are several kinds of joints. Solid joints hold bones firmly together, like the skull. Partly moveable joints allow for some movement, like the spine. Very moveable joints allow a wide range of motion, like the shoulder.

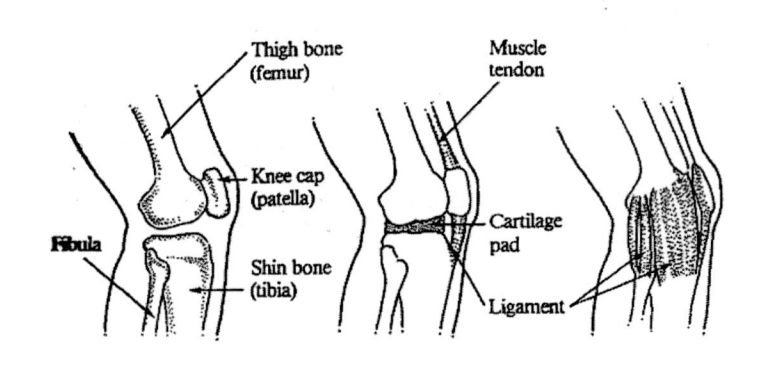

Knee joint showing typical structure of a joint.

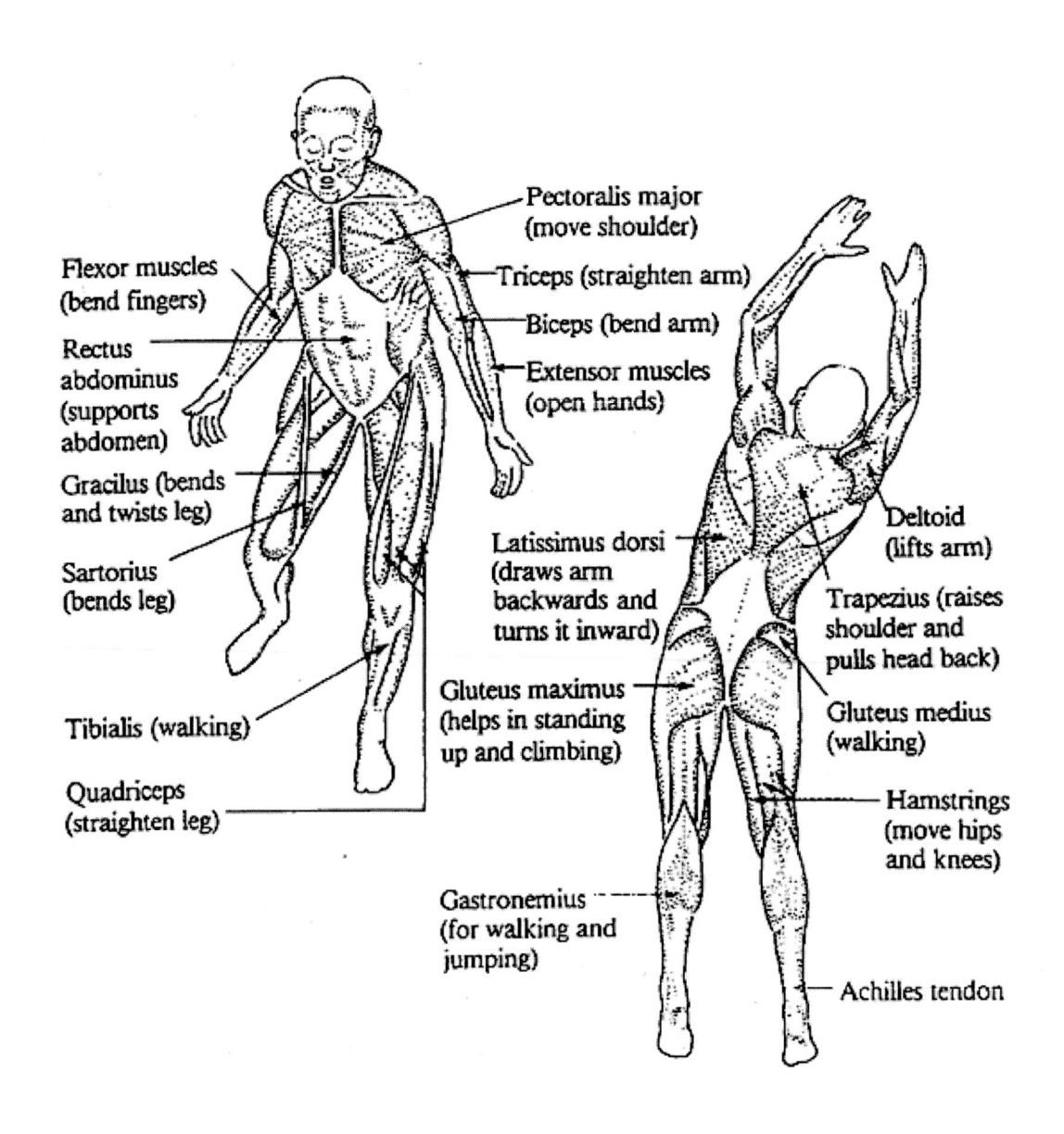

- Flexor muscles (bend fingers)
- Rectus abdominus (supports abdomen)
- Gracilus (bends and twists leg)
- Sartorius (bends leg)
- Tibialis (walking)
- Quadriceps (straighten leg)
- Pectoralis major (move shoulder)
- Triceps (straighten arm)
- Biceps (bend arm)
- Extensor muscles (open hands)
- Latissimus dorsi (draws arm backwards and turns it inward)
- Gluteus maximus (helps in standing up and climbing)
- Gastronemius (for walking and jumping)
- Deltoid (lifts arm)
- Trapezius (raises shoulder and pulls head back)
- Gluteus medius (walking)
- Hamstrings (move hips and knees)
- Achilles tendon

Body Systems Terminology

Muscles: The body has many groups of major muscles. Each of these muscles is attached to two or more bones by **tendons**. When the muscle contracts, the bone to which it is attached moves. The major muscle groups are also sometimes called skeletal muscles.

Skeletal muscles work in pairs, or in coordinated groups. When one muscle contracts, another muscle, working in the opposite direction, relaxes. Joints that are not being used can also be held steady by other muscles.

All the parts of our bodies are made up of a variety of types of cells. Muscle cells are called fibers. They are long and thin. **Muscle fibers** are arranged in small bundles, each one controlled by a nerve. Bundles of muscle fibers contract (shorten) when they are stimulated by nerve impulses. When the impulses stop, the muscles relax. We control our body movements by controlling this contraction of our muscles.

Some muscles can be controlled voluntarily, such as the muscles that move our arms and legs. Other muscles, like the ones that control our heart, are involuntary, meaning that we cannot control them. Our brain and our motor nerves control which ones contract, how much they contract, and which ones relax. See the section on the Nervous System for more information on this topic.

Common Problems of the Musculoskeletal System

Arthritis: If you feel pain and stiffness in your body or have trouble moving around, you might have arthritis. Most kinds of arthritis cause pain and swelling in your joints. Joints are places where two bones meet, such as your elbow or knee. Over time, a swollen joint can become severely damaged. Some kinds of arthritis can also cause problems in your organs, such as your eyes or skin.

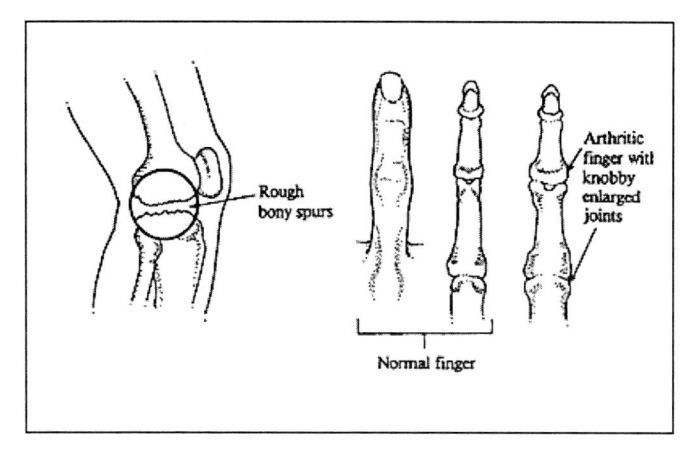

Types of arthritis include the following.

- Osteoarthritis is the most common type of arthritis. It's often related to aging or to an injury.
- Autoimmune arthritis happens when your body's immune system attacks healthy cells in your body by mistake. Rheumatoid arthritis is the most common form of this kind of arthritis. Juvenile rheumatoid arthritis is a form of the disease that happens in children.
- Infectious arthritis is an infection that has spread from another part of the body to the joint.
- Psoriatic arthritis affects people with psoriasis.
- Gout is a painful type of arthritis that happens when too much uric acid builds up in the body. It often starts in the big toe.

Back pain: If you've ever groaned, "Oh, my aching back!" you are not alone. Back pain is one of the most common medical problems, affecting 8 out of 10 people at some point during their lives. Back pain can range from a dull, constant ache to a sudden, sharp pain. Acute back pain comes on suddenly and usually lasts from a few days to a few weeks. Back pain is called

© 2014 The Cross Cultural Health Care Program

chronic if it lasts for more than three months.

Most back pain goes away on its own, though it may take a while. Taking over-the-counter pain relievers and resting can help. However, staying in bed for more than 1 or 2 days can make it worse.

If your back pain is severe or doesn't improve after three days, you should call your health care provider. You should also get medical attention if you have back pain following an injury.

Treatment for back pain depends on what kind of pain you have, and what is causing it. It may include hot or cold packs, exercise, medicines, injections, complementary and alternative treatments, and sometimes surgery.

Carpal tunnel syndrome: You're working at your desk, trying to ignore the tingling or numbness you've had for some time in your hand and wrist. Suddenly, a sharp, piercing pain shoots through the wrist and up your arm. Just a passing cramp? It could be carpal tunnel syndrome.

The carpal tunnel is a narrow passageway of ligament and bones at the base of your hand. It contains nerve and tendons. Sometimes, thickening from irritated tendons or other swelling narrows the tunnel and causes the nerve to be compressed. Symptoms usually start gradually. As they worsen, grasping objects can become difficult.

Often, the cause is having a smaller carpal tunnel than other people do. Other causes include performing assembly line work, wrist injury, or swelling due to certain diseases, such as rheumatoid arthritis. Women are three times more likely to have carpal tunnel syndrome than men.
Early diagnosis and treatment are important to prevent permanent nerve damage. Your doctor diagnoses carpal tunnel syndrome with a physical exam and special nerve tests. Treatment includes resting your hand, splints, pain and anti-inflammatory medicines, and sometimes surgery.

Fibromyalgia (FMS): Fibromyalgia is a disorder that causes muscle pain and fatigue. People with fibromyalgia have "tender points" on the body. Tender points are specific places on the neck, shoulders, back, hips, arms, and legs. These points hurt when pressure is put on them.

People with fibromyalgia may also have other symptoms, such as:
- trouble sleeping
- morning stiffness
- headaches
- painful menstrual periods
- tingling or numbness in hands and feet
- problems with thinking and memory (sometimes called "fibro fog")

No one knows what causes fibromyalgia. Anyone can get it, but it is most common in middle-aged women. People with rheumatoid arthritis and other autoimmune diseases are particularly likely to develop fibromyalgia. There is no cure for fibromyalgia, but medicine can help you manage your symptoms. Getting enough sleep, exercising, and eating well may also help.

Fracture: A fracture is a break, usually in a bone. If the broken bone punctures the skin, it is called an open or compound fracture. Fractures commonly happen because of car accidents, falls or sports injuries. Other causes are low bone density and osteoporosis, which cause weakening of the bones. Overuse can cause stress fractures, which are very small cracks in the bone.

Symptoms of a fracture are:
- out-of-place or misshapen limb or joint

- swelling, bruising or bleeding
- intense pain
- numbness and tingling
- limited mobility or inability to move a limb

You need to get medical care right away for any fracture. You may need to wear a cast or splint. Sometimes you need surgery to put in plates, pins or screws to keep the bone in place.

Some types of fractures include:
- simple or complex fracture
- closed or open fracture
- compound fracture

Hernia: A hernia happens when part of an internal organ or tissue bulges through a weak area of muscle. Most hernias are in the abdomen.
There are several types of hernias, including:
- inguinal, in the groin and is the most common type
- umbilical, around the belly button
- incisional, through a scar
- hiatal, a small opening in the diaphragm that allows the upper part of the stomach to move up into the chest
- congenital diaphragmatic, a birth defect that needs surgery

Hernias are common. They can affect men, women, and children. A combination of muscle weakness and straining, such as with heavy lifting, might contribute. Some people are born with weak abdominal muscles and may be more likely to get a hernia.

Treatment is usually surgery to repair the opening in the muscle wall. Untreated hernias can cause pain and health problems.

Osteoporosis: Osteoporosis makes your bones weak and more likely to break. Anyone can develop osteoporosis, but it is common in older women. As many as half of all women and a quarter of men older than 50 will break a bone due to osteoporosis.
Risk factors include:
- getting older
- being small and thin
- having a family history of osteoporosis
- taking certain medicines
- being a white or Asian woman
- having osteopenia, which is low bone density

Osteoporosis is a silent disease. You might not know you have it until you break a bone. A bone mineral density test is the best way to check your bone health. To keep bones strong, eat a diet rich in calcium and vitamin D, exercise and do not smoke. If needed, medicines can also help.

Strains and sprains: A sprain is a stretched or torn ligament. Ligaments are tissues that connect bones at a joint. Falling, twisting, or getting hit can all cause a sprain. Ankle and wrist sprains are common. Symptoms include pain, swelling, bruising, and being unable to move your joint. You might feel a pop or tear when the injury happens.

A strain is a stretched or torn muscle or tendon. Tendons are tissues that connect muscle to bone. Twisting or pulling these tissues can cause a strain. Strains can happen suddenly or develop over time. Back and hamstring muscle strains are common. Many people get strains playing sports. Symptoms include pain, muscle spasms, swelling, and trouble moving the muscle.

At first, treatment of both sprains and strains usually involves resting the injured area, icing it, wearing a bandage or device that compresses the area, and medicines. Later treatment might include exercise and physical therapy.

Musculoskeletal System Specialists

There are three medical specialists who focus on different parts of the health of the musculoskeletal system. An **orthopedist** specializes in bones. A **podiatrist** specializes in the health of the feet. A **rheumatologist** specializes specifically in the health problem known as arthritis.

Musculoskeletal System Procedures

X-Ray: X-rays are non-visible rays of energy produced by an energy source that can penetrate different materials to different degrees and then be used to create a photographic image. X-rays pass through tissue more than bone and so are very useful in diagnosing bone disorders.

Computed Tomography (CT Scan):
This is a type of X-ray that is directed through a patient at many different angles around a specific section of the body. A computer combines this information into a single picture of a "slice" of the section of the body (cross section). CT scans can detect problems in soft tissues that simple X-rays cannot.

Magnetic Resonance Imaging (MRI): This test does much the same as the CT scan without using X-rays at all, but by using magnetic and radio waves.
X-rays, CT Scans, and MRIs are used in many different medical specialties, in addition to the musculoskeletal system.

The Nervous System

Nervous System Vocabulary
Alzheimer's disease
Aqueous Humor
Cataract
Central nervous system
Cerebral palsy
Cochlea
Conjunctivitis
Cornea
Dementia
Ear
Ear drum
Electroencephalogram (EEG)
Epilepsy
Eustachian tube
Glaucoma
Headache
Inner ear
Iris
Lens muscle
Middle ear
Motor nerves
Nerve cells
Nerve impulses
Neurologist
Neurosurgeon
Ophthalmologist
Optic nerve
Optometrist
Otorhinolaryngologist
Outer ear
Parkinson's disease
Peripheral nervous system
Polio
Pupil
Refractive error
Retina
Sensory nerves
Spinal cord injury

Nervous System Vocabulary
Spinal tap
Stroke
Vitreous humor

Function of the Nervous System

All body systems are regulated and controlled through the nervous system. This system has two parts:

The **central nervous system** is made up of the brain and spinal cord. The **peripheral (or outer) nervous system** is made up of the nerves that connect the brain to all areas of the body. The nervous system works both automatically and under our direct control. Breathing, heart rate and digestion are mainly controlled automatically. Walking and running are directly controlled - this means we can stop and start these activities when we wish.

The nervous system is made up of many nerve cells connected together. **Nerve cells** are able to organize and conduct messages in the form of small electrical impulses called **nerve impulses**.

Motor nerves send messages from the brain and spinal cord to parts of the body. For example, messages go from our brains to our legs when we want to lift up one of our legs.

Sensory nerves pick up messages from the outside of the body and pass them to the brain. For example, sensory nerves in our tongue pass the taste and texture of food to our brain. Different parts of the

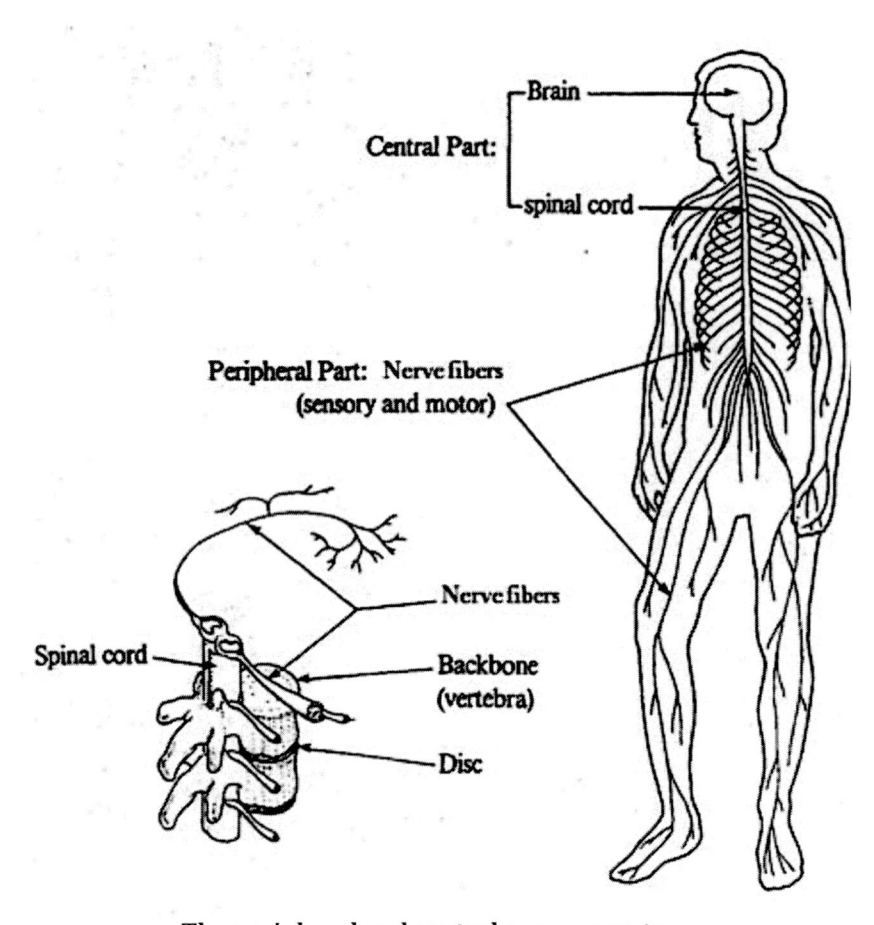

The peripheral and central nervous system

brain and spinal cord deal with different messages. For example, there are specific smell and taste centers in our brain. The part of the brain that we think with affects the entire nervous system. For example, if we are thinking about something sad, it can cause changes in the entire body.

The Eyes: The eye is like a television camera. The lens of the eye is where light passes through. The **lens muscles** in the eye can bend and change shape and contract, which allows it to further focus incoming light on the nerve endings at the back of the eye. This allows us to see objects at different distances.

The **cornea** is a transparent part of the eye that covers the lens muscle, iris, and pupil. The cornea is curved in a way that changes the direction of incoming light rays so that it can be focused into an image we can understand.

The **iris** is the colored part of the eye that controls the amount of light that is able to enter the eye. It is able to open the center part of the iris, known as the **pupil**, wider in dim light. The muscles of the iris can also make the pupil smaller in bright lights. This protects the eye from bright light and helps us to see better in dim light.

Fluids in the eye wash over the lens to keep it clean. The fluids also help to maintain the shape of the eye. **Aqueous humor** is one type of fluid found between the cornea and the lens. **Vitreous humor** is the other type of fluid and is found between the lens and the retina.

The **retina** is located at the back of the eye. The retina is where the light is focused. The retina contains retinal nerve fibers, which are connected to the **optic nerve.** Through these nerve fibers, the retina is able to send message to the brain, so that the brain can interpret what is being seen.

The Ears: The **ear** is another important part of the nervous system. The ear is for both hearing and balance. It has three parts: the outer, middle, and inner ear.

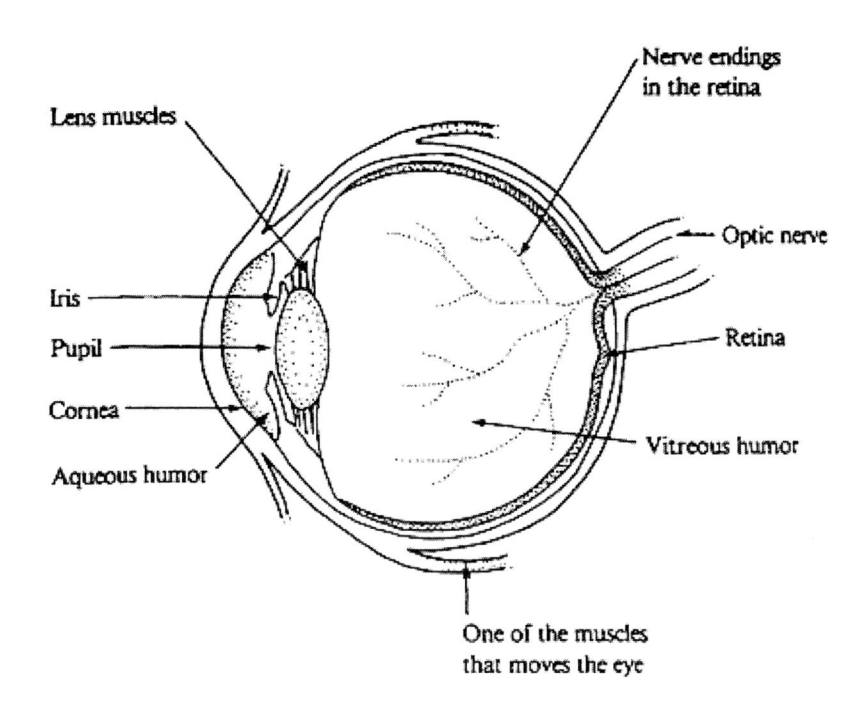

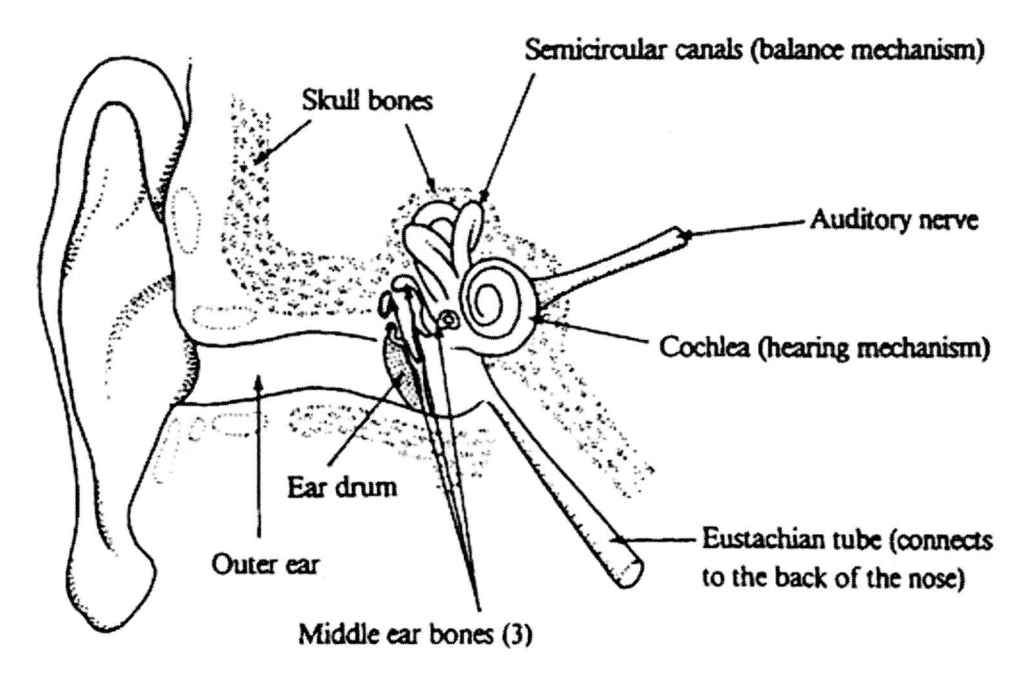

The **outer ear** is outside of the body and has an outer ear canal about ¾ of an inch long.

The **middle ear** is a small cavity between the **ear drum** (a thin membrane that stretches across the ear canal) and the inner ear. Three small bones bridge this cavity. A tube (**Eustachian tube**) connects the inner ear to the back of the nose. The **inner ear** is filled with fluid and contains auditory nerve endings for hearing and balance.

Sounds make vibrations in the air which move or vibrate the eardrum. The middle ear bones pass these vibrations to the fluid in the ear. The **cochlea** is the actual hearing organ of the ear. It turns the sound vibrations into signals that get sent through the auditory nerves. Nerve endings in the cochlea pick up these vibrations in the fluid and send nerve impulses to the brain. The brain processes these nerve impulses into the sounds that we hear.

The ear is important for balancing. When we move, the fluids in our inner ear also move. Nerve endings pick up this movement and send out balance messages to the brain. Our eyes also help us balance.

Common Problems of the Nervous System

Alzheimer's disease: Alzheimer's disease (AD) is the most common form of dementia among older people. Dementia is a brain disorder that seriously affects a person's ability to carry out daily activities.

AD begins slowly. It first involves the parts of the brain that control thought, memory and language. People with AD may have trouble remembering things that happened recently or names of people they know. A related problem, mild cognitive impairment (MCI), causes more memory problems than normal for people of the same age. Many, but not all, people with MCI will develop AD.

In AD, over time, symptoms get worse. People may not recognize family members or have trouble speaking, reading or writing. They may forget how to brush their teeth or comb their hair. Later on, they may become anxious or aggressive, or wander away from home. Eventually, they need total care. This can cause great stress for family members who must care for them.

AD usually begins after age 60. The risk goes up as you get older. Your risk is also higher if a family member has had the disease.

No treatment can stop the disease. However, some drugs may help keep symptoms from getting worse for a limited time.

Cataract: A cataract is a clouding of the lens in your eye. It affects your vision. Cataracts are very common in older people. By age 80, more than half of all Americans either have a cataract or have had cataract surgery.

A cataract can occur in either or both eyes. It cannot spread from one eye to the other. Common symptoms are:

- blurry vision
- colors that seem faded
- glare - headlights, lamps or sunlight may seem too bright. You may also see a halo around lights.
- not being able to see well at night
- double vision

- frequent prescription changes in your eye wear

Cataracts usually develop slowly. New glasses, brighter lighting, anti-glare sunglasses or magnifying lenses can help at first. Surgery is also an option. It involves removing the cloudy lens and replacing it with an artificial lens. Wearing sunglasses and a hat with a brim to block ultraviolet sunlight may help to delay cataracts.

Cerebral palsy: Cerebral palsy is a group of disorders that affect a person's ability to move and to maintain balance and posture. The disorders appear in the first few years of life. Usually they do not get worse over time. People with cerebral palsy may have difficulty walking. They may also have trouble with tasks such as writing or using scissors. Some have other medical conditions, including seizure disorders or mental impairment.

Cerebral palsy happens when the areas of the brain that control movement and posture do not develop correctly or get damaged. Early signs of cerebral palsy usually appear before 3 years of age. Babies with cerebral palsy are often slow to roll over, sit, crawl, smile, or walk. Some babies are born with cerebral palsy; others get it after they are born.

There is no cure for cerebral palsy, but treatment can improve the lives of those who have it. Treatment includes medicines, braces, and physical, occupational and speech therapy.

Conjunctivitis: Conjunctivitis is the medical name for pink eye. It involves inflammation of the outer layer of the eye and inside of the eyelid. It can cause swelling, itching, burning, discharge, and redness. Causes include:

- bacterial or viral infection
- allergies
- substances that cause irritation
- contact lens products, eye drops, or eye ointments

Pinkeye usually does not affect vision. Infectious pink eye can easily spread from one person to another. The infection will clear in most cases without medical care, but bacterial pinkeye needs treatment with antibiotic eye drops or ointment.

Cerebrovascular Accident (CVA) (stroke): A stroke is a medical emergency. Strokes happen when blood flow to your brain stops. Within minutes, brain cells begin to die. There are two kinds of stroke. The more common kind, called ischemic stroke, is caused by a blood clot that blocks or plugs a blood vessel in the brain. The other kind, called hemorrhagic stroke, is caused by a blood vessel that breaks and bleeds into the brain. "Mini-strokes" or transient ischemic attacks (TIAs), occur when the blood supply to the brain is briefly interrupted.

Symptoms of stroke are:

- sudden numbness or weakness of the face, arm or leg (especially on one side of the body)
- sudden confusion, trouble speaking or understanding speech
- sudden trouble seeing in one or both eyes

- sudden trouble walking, dizziness, loss of balance or coordination
- sudden severe headache with no known cause.

If you have any of these symptoms, you must get to a hospital quickly to begin treatment. Acute stroke therapies try to stop a stroke while it is happening by quickly dissolving the blood clot or by stopping the bleeding. Post-stroke rehabilitation helps individuals overcome disabilities that result from stroke damage. Drug therapy with blood thinners is the most common treatment for stroke.

Dementia: Dementia is the name for a group of symptoms caused by disorders that affect the brain. It is not a specific disease. People with dementia may not be able to think well enough to do normal activities, such as getting dressed or eating. They may lose their ability to solve problems or control their emotions. Their personalities may change. They may become agitated or see things that are not there.

Memory loss is a common symptom of dementia. However, memory loss by itself does not mean you have dementia. People with dementia have serious problems with two or more brain functions, such as memory and language. Although dementia is common in very elderly people, it is not part of normal aging.

Many different diseases can cause dementia, including Alzheimer's disease and stroke. Drugs are available to treat some of these diseases. While these drugs cannot cure dementia or repair brain damage, they may improve symptoms or slow down the disease.

Epilepsy: Epilepsy is a brain disorder that causes people to have recurring seizures. The seizures happen when clusters of nerve cells, or neurons, in the brain send out the wrong signals. People may have strange sensations and emotions or behave strangely. They may have violent muscle spasms or lose consciousness.

Epilepsy has many possible causes, including illness, brain injury, and abnormal brain development. In many cases, the cause is unknown.

Doctors use brain scans and other tests to diagnose epilepsy. It is important to start treatment right away. There is no cure for epilepsy, but medicines can control seizures for most people. When medicines are not working well, surgery or implanted devices such as vagus nerve stimulators may help. Special diets can help some children with epilepsy.

Seizures: Seizures are symptoms of a brain problem. They happen because of sudden, abnormal electrical activity in the brain. When people think of seizures, they often think of convulsions in which a person's body shakes rapidly and uncontrollably. Not all seizures cause convulsions. There are many types of seizures and some have mild symptoms. Seizures fall into two main groups. Focal seizures, also called partial seizures, happen in just one part of the brain. Generalized seizures are a result of abnormal activity on both sides of the brain.

Most seizures last from 30 seconds to 2 minutes and do not cause lasting harm.

However, it is a medical emergency if seizures last longer than 5 minutes or if a person has many seizures and does not wake up between them. Seizures can have many causes, including medicines, high fevers, head injuries and certain diseases. People who have recurring seizures due to a brain disorder have epilepsy.

Glaucoma: Glaucoma is a group of diseases that can damage the eye's optic nerve. It is a leading cause of blindness in the United States. It usually happens when the fluid pressure inside the eyes slowly rises, damaging the optic nerve. Often there are no symptoms at first. Without treatment, people with glaucoma will slowly lose their peripheral, or side vision. They seem to be looking through a tunnel. Over time, straight-ahead vision may decrease until no vision remains.

A comprehensive eye exam can tell if you have glaucoma. People at risk should get eye exams at least every two years. They include:

- African Americans over age 40
- people over age 60, especially Mexican Americans
- people with a family history of glaucoma

There is no cure, but glaucoma can usually be controlled. Early treatment can help protect your eyes against vision loss. Treatments usually include prescription eye drops and/or surgery.

Headaches: Almost everyone has had a headache. Headache is the most common form of pain. It's a major reason people miss days at work or school or visit the doctor.

The most common type of headache is a tension headache. Tension headaches are due to tight muscles in your shoulders, neck, scalp and jaw. They are often related to stress, depression or anxiety. You are more likely to get tension headaches if you work too much, don't get enough sleep, miss meals, or use alcohol.

Other common types of headaches include migraines, cluster headaches, and sinus headaches. Most people can feel much better by making lifestyle changes, learning ways to relax and taking pain relievers.

Not all headaches require a doctor's attention. But sometimes headaches warn of a more serious disorder. Let your health care provider know if you have sudden, severe headaches. Get medical help right away if you have a headache after a blow to your head, or if you have a headache along with a stiff neck, fever, confusion, loss of consciousness, or pain in the eye or ear.

Parkinson Disease: Parkinson's disease (PD) is a type of movement disorder. It happens when nerve cells in the brain don't produce enough of a brain chemical called dopamine. Sometimes it is genetic, but most cases do not seem to run in families. Exposure to chemicals in the environment might play a role.

Symptoms begin gradually, often on one side of the body. Later they affect both sides. They include:

- trembling of hands, arms, legs, jaw and face

- stiffness of the arms, legs and trunk
- slowness of movement
- poor balance and coordination

As symptoms get worse, people with the disease may have trouble walking, talking, or doing simple tasks. They may also have problems such as depression, sleep problems, or trouble chewing, swallowing, or speaking.

There is no lab test for PD, so it can be difficult to diagnose. Doctors use a medical history and a neurological examination to diagnose it.

PD usually begins around age 60, but it can start earlier. It is more common in men than in women. There is no cure for PD. A variety of medicines sometimes help symptoms dramatically. Surgery and deep brain stimulation (DBS) can help severe cases. With DBS, electrodes are surgically implanted in the brain. They send electrical pulses to stimulate the parts of the brain that control movement.

Poliomyelitis: Polio is an infectious disease caused by a virus. The virus lives in an infected person's throat and intestines. It is most often spread by contact with the stool of an infected person. You can also get it from droplets if an infected person sneezes or coughs. It can contaminate food and water if people do not wash their hands.

Most people have no symptoms. If you have symptoms, they may include fever, fatigue, nausea, headache, flu-like symptoms, stiff neck and back, and pain in the limbs. A few people will become paralyzed. There is no treatment to reverse the paralysis of polio.

Some people who've had polio develop post-polio syndrome (PPS) years later. Symptoms include tiredness, new muscle weakness, and muscle and joint pain. There is no way to prevent or cure PPS.

The polio vaccine has wiped out polio in the United States and most other countries.

Refractive errors: The cornea and lens of your eye helps you focus. Refractive errors are vision problems that happen when the shape of the eye keeps you from focusing well. The cause could be the length of the eyeball (longer or shorter), changes in the shape of the cornea, or aging of the lens. Four common refractive errors are

- Myopia, or nearsightedness - clear vision close up but blurry in the distance
- Hyperopia, or farsightedness - clear vision in the distance but blurry close up
- Presbyopia - inability to focus close up as a result of aging
- Astigmatism - focus problems caused by the cornea

The most common symptom is blurred vision. Other symptoms may include double vision, haziness, glare or halos around bright lights, squinting, headaches, or eye strain.

Glasses or contact lenses can usually correct refractive errors. Laser eye surgery may also be a possibility.

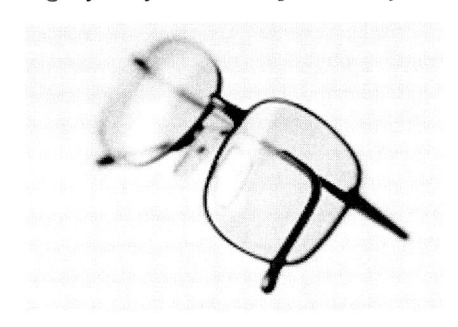

Spinal cord injuries: Your spinal cord is a bundle of nerves that runs down the middle of your back. It carries signals back and forth between your body and your brain. A spinal cord injury disrupts the signals. Spinal cord injuries usually begin with a blow that fractures or dislocates your vertebrae, the bone disks that make up your spine. Most injuries don't cut through your spinal cord. Instead, they cause damage when pieces of vertebrae tear into cord tissue or press down on the nerve parts that carry signals.

Spinal cord injuries can be complete or incomplete. With a complete spinal cord injury, the cord can't send signals below the level of the injury. As a result, you are paralyzed below the injury. With an incomplete injury, you have some movement and sensation below the injury.

A spinal cord injury is a medical emergency. Immediate treatment can reduce long-term effects. Treatments may include medicines, braces or traction to stabilize the spine, and surgery. Later treatment usually includes medicines and rehabilitation therapy. Mobility aids and assistive devices may help you to get around and do some daily tasks.

Nervous System Specialists

A **neurologist** is the medical specialist that takes care of the health of the nervous system and the brain. A **neurosurgeon** performs surgery on parts of the nervous system.

An **ophthalmologist** takes care of the health of the eyes. When there are specific problems with a person's vision, the medical specialist involved is called an **optometrist.**

A medical specialist known as an **otorhinolaryngologist** works with the ears, nose, and throat. This specialist works in both the nervous system and the respiratory system because the ear, nose, and throat are all connected and often have connected problems.

Nervous System Procedures

Electroencephalogram (EEG): This procedure provides a recording of the electrical activity of the brain. It can detect seizure activity in the brain, tumors, or injuries to the brain.

Lumbar Puncture (LP), also called spinal tap: Cerebrospinal fluid (CSF) is the fluid that encases the brain and fills the spinal cord. It can be removed through an incision between two vertebrae. The pressure of the fluid can be measured, contrast materials can be injected, or medicines can be administered this way. The CSF can be tested for various infections and problems in the nervous system.

The Respiratory System

Respiratory System Vocabulary
Alveoli
Asthma
Bronchi
Bronchitis
Bronchoscopy
Chronic Obstructive Pulmonary Disorder (COPD)
Common cold
Diaphragm
Emphysema
Epiglottis
Esophagus
Influenza
Larynx
Lung cancer
Lungs
Mouth
Mucous membrane
Nose passage
Pleura
Pneumonia
Pulmonary function test
Pulmonologist
Sinuses
Trachea
Tuberculosis (TB)

Function and Major Anatomical Parts of the Respiratory System

Like all living things, humans need energy to keep our body systems alive and working. We get this energy from the combination of the foods we eat and the air we breathe. When we eat, food is broken down in the digestive system so the elements we need to live can move into the blood stream and be carried to all parts of the body.

When we breathe, air enters the **respiratory system,** and oxygen moves into the blood stream to be carried to all parts of the body. Oxygen is part of the air and is an element essential for life; we cannot live without it. When oxygen is combined with elements from the food, we eat to make energy, waste products are also made. One of those waste products that our bodies cannot use is carbon dioxide. Our bodies get rid of carbon dioxide when we breathe out. Other elements we cannot use are removed by the urinary system (in our urine) and the digestive system (in our feces).

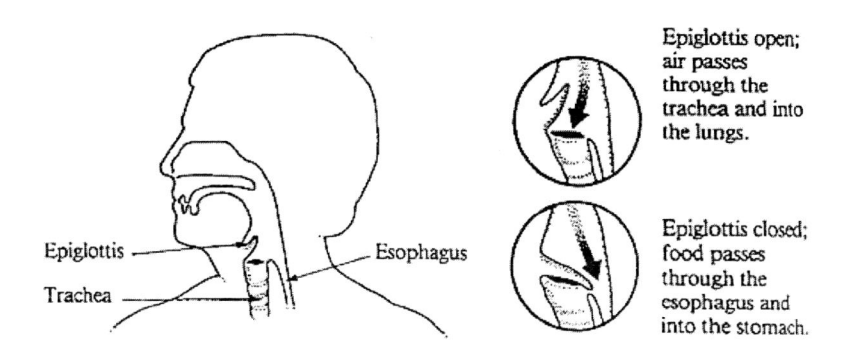

Body Systems Terminology

Epiglottis open; air passes through the trachea and into the lungs.

Epiglottis closed; food passes through the esophagus and into the stomach.

Air enters the **lungs** through the **nose passage** or the **mouth** and the **trachea**. The trachea is sometimes called the **windpipe**, and it leads to the lungs.

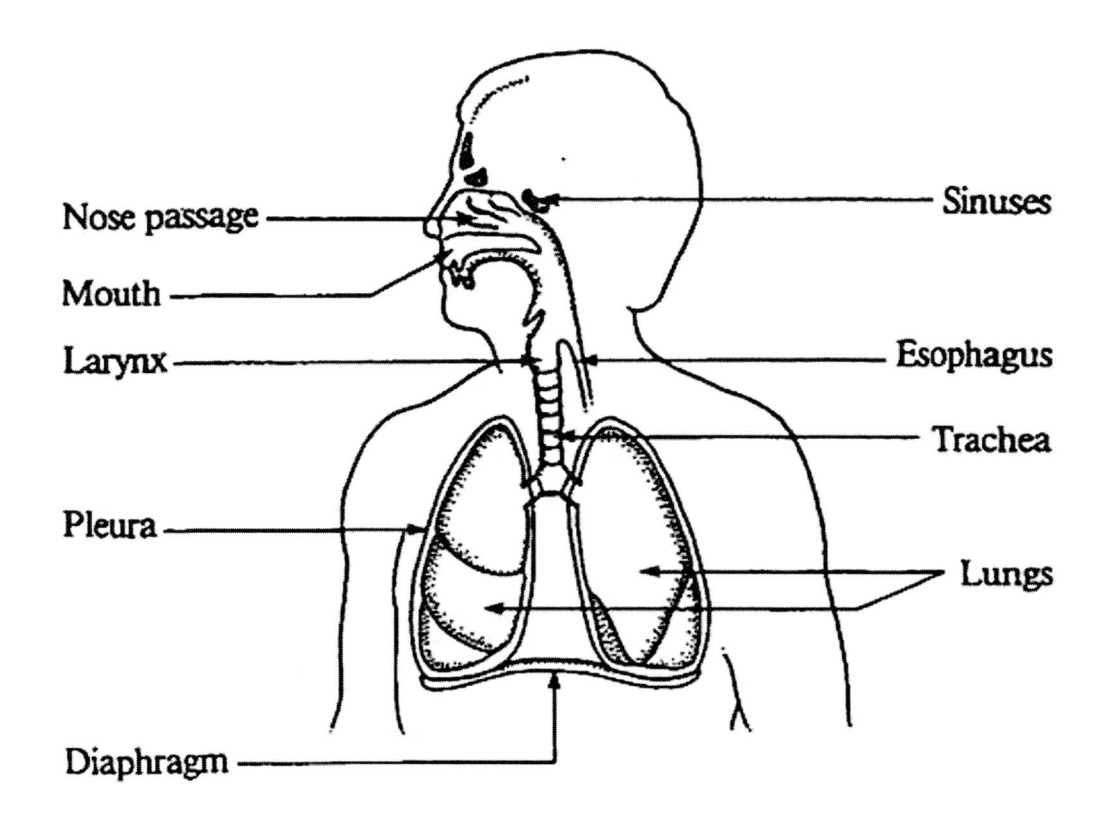

passage to the throat, and through the trachea to the lungs. In several places, the nose passage connects with spaces in the bones of the head called **sinus cavities**

The **nose passage** is the main opening into the lungs. It is lined with a wet layer of tissue (**mucous membrane**) that contains many tiny blood vessels. This lining moistens air as it passes through the nose

(sinuses). In the throat, air passes through the **larynx** (the larynx is also known as a voice box) to the lungs. When a person breathes out through the mouth, air passes over the vocal cords in the **larynx** and

© 2014 The Cross Cultural Health Care Program

279

produces sounds that are formed into words by the lips and tongue.

When a person swallows, the **epiglottis** (a flap of tissue) closes over the trachea (windpipe) to keep food and water from entering the lungs. Food and water pass down the **esophagus** (food pipe) to the stomach. When breathing, the epiglottis stays open and allows air to pass into the lungs.

Each lung is held in a smooth, thin lining **(pleura)** which allows it to expand and contract inside the chest when breathing. Inside the lungs, the trachea divides like the branches of a tree. Air passes through these branches, called **bronchi,** to all parts of the lungs. These branches get smaller and smaller through the lungs.

At the end of each branch of the bronchi are **alveoli**, small air sacks. The air in the alveoli is very close to the bloodstream. Here, oxygen from the air moves through a thin layer of cells into the blood, and carbon dioxide moves back from the blood into the air. Blood vessels branch out to all parts of the lungs. They bring blood that is low in oxygen to the lungs and carry blood that is high in oxygen back to the body. Chemicals (like those in cigarette smoke and air pollution) can also enter the body in this way.

Several muscles are used to draw air into the lungs. The main one is the **diaphragm** (breathing muscle). This is a dome-shaped muscle that lies under the lungs and is attached to the lower ribs. Chest muscles between the ribs also help us breathe.

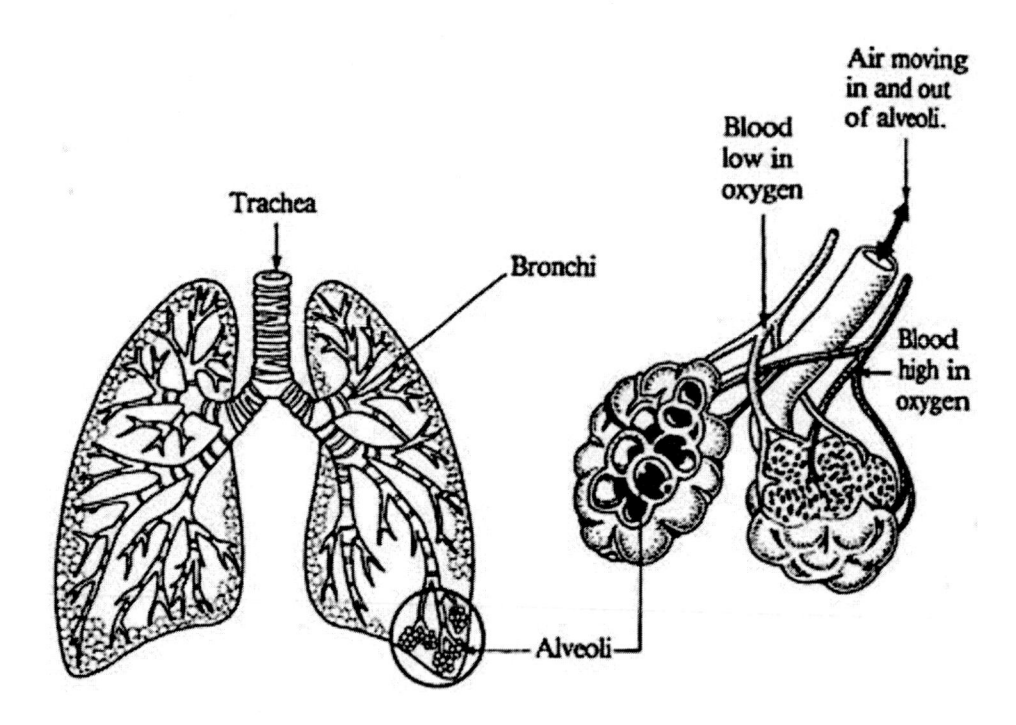

When you breathe in, the diaphragm is pulled flat and the chest muscles pull your ribs upwards. This opens up the inside of the chest and air is drawn in to fill up this bigger space. When you breathe out, these muscles relax, the space inside the chest gets smaller, and the air is pushed out.

Common Problems of the Respiratory System

Asthma: Asthma is a chronic disease that affects your airways. Your airways are tubes that carry air in and out of your lungs. If you have asthma, the inside walls of your airways become sore and swollen. That makes them very sensitive, and they may react strongly to things that you are allergic to or find irritating. When your airways react, they get narrower and your lungs get less air.

Symptoms of asthma include:
- wheezing
- coughing, especially early in the morning or at night
- chest tightness
- shortness of breath

Not all people who have asthma have these symptoms. Having these symptoms doesn't always mean that you have asthma. Your doctor will diagnose asthma based on lung function tests, your medical history, and a physical exam.

When your asthma symptoms become worse than usual, it's called an asthma attack. Severe asthma attacks may require emergency care and they can be fatal.

Asthma is treated with two kinds of medicines: quick-relief medicines to stop asthma symptoms and long-term control medicines to prevent symptoms

Bronchitis: Bronchitis is an inflammation of the bronchial tubes, the airways that carry air to your lungs. It causes a cough that often brings up mucus, as well as shortness of breath, wheezing, and chest tightness. There are two main types of bronchitis: acute and chronic.

The same viruses that cause colds and the flu often cause acute bronchitis. These viruses spread through the air when people cough, or through physical contact (for example, on unwashed hands). Being exposed to tobacco smoke, air pollution, dusts, vapors, and fumes can also cause acute bronchitis. Bacteria can also cause acute bronchitis, but not as often as viruses.

Most cases of acute bronchitis get better within several days. But your cough can last for several weeks after the infection is gone. If you think you have acute bronchitis, see your health care provider.

Treatments include rest, fluids, and aspirin (for adults) or acetaminophen to treat fever. A humidifier or steam can also help. You may need inhaled medicine to open your airways if you are wheezing. You probably do not need antibiotics. They don't work against viruses - the most common cause of acute bronchitis. If your health care provider thinks you have a bacterial infection, he or she may prescribe antibiotics.

Chronic Obstructive Pulmonary Disorder (COPD): COPD (chronic obstructive pulmonary disease) makes it hard for you to breathe. The two main types are chronic bronchitis and emphysema. The main cause of COPD is long-term exposure to substances that irritate and damage the lungs, usually cigarette smoke. Air pollution, chemical fumes, or dust can also cause it.

At first, COPD may cause no symptoms or only mild symptoms. As the disease gets worse, symptoms usually become more severe. They include:
- a cough that produces a lot of mucus;
- shortness of breath especially with physical activity
- wheezing
- chest tightness

Doctors use lung function tests, imaging tests, and blood tests to diagnose COPD. There is no cure. Treatments may relieve symptoms. They include medicines, oxygen therapy, surgery, or a lung transplant. Quitting smoking is the most important step you can take to treat COPD.

Common cold: Sneezing, sore throat, a stuffy nose, coughing - everyone knows the symptoms of the common cold. It is probably the most common illness. In the course of a year, people in the United States suffer 1 billion colds.

You can get a cold by touching your eyes or nose after you touch surfaces with cold germs on them. You can also inhale the germs. Symptoms usually begin 2 or 3 days after infection and last 2 to 14 days. Washing your hands and staying away from people with colds will help you avoid colds.

There is no cure for the common cold. For relief, try:
- getting plenty of rest
- drinking fluids
- gargling with warm saltwater
- using cough drops or throat sprays
- taking over-the-counter pain or cold medicines

However, do not give aspirin to children. And do not give cough medicine to children under four.

Emphysema: Emphysema is a type of COPD involving damage to the air sacs (alveoli) in the lungs. As a result, your body does not get the oxygen it needs. Emphysema makes it hard to catch your breath. You may also have a chronic cough and have trouble breathing during exercise.

The most common cause is cigarette smoking. If you smoke, quitting can help prevent you from getting the disease. If you already have emphysema, not smoking might keep it from getting worse. Treatment is based on whether your symptoms are mild, moderate or severe. Treatments include inhalers, oxygen, medications and sometimes surgery to relieve symptoms and prevent complications.

Influenza: Flu is a respiratory infection caused by a number of viruses. The viruses pass through the air and enter your body through your nose or mouth. Between 5% and 20% of people in the U.S. get the flu each year. The flu can be serious or even deadly for elderly people, newborn babies, and people with certain chronic illnesses.

Symptoms of the flu come on suddenly and are worse than those of the common cold. They may include:
- body or muscle aches
- chills
- cough

- fever
- headache
- sore throat

Most people with the flu recover on their own without medical care. People with mild cases of the flu should stay home and avoid contact with others, except to get medical care. If you get the flu, your health care provider may prescribe medicine to help your body fight the infection and lessen symptoms.

The main way to keep from getting the flu is to get a yearly flu vaccine. Good hygiene, including hand washing, can also help.

Pneumonia: Pneumonia is an infection in one or both of the lungs. Many germs, such as bacteria, viruses, and fungi, can cause pneumonia. You can also get pneumonia by inhaling a liquid or chemical. People most at risk are older than 65, younger than 2 years of age, or already have health problems.

Symptoms of pneumonia vary from mild to severe. See your doctor promptly if you:
- have a high fever
- have shaking chills
- have a cough with phlegm that doesn't improve or gets worse
- develop shortness of breath with normal daily activities
- have chest pain when you breathe or cough
- feel suddenly worse after a cold or the flu

Your doctor will use your medical history, a physical exam, and lab tests to diagnose pneumonia. Treatment depends on what kind you have. If bacteria are the cause, antibiotics should help. If you have viral pneumonia, your doctor may prescribe an antiviral medicine to treat it.

Preventing pneumonia is always better than treating it. Vaccines are available to prevent pneumococcal pneumonia and the flu. Other preventive measures include washing your hands frequently and not smoking.

Tuberculosis: Tuberculosis (TB) is a disease caused by bacteria called Mycobacterium tuberculosis. The bacteria usually attack the lungs, but they can also damage other parts of the body.

TB spreads through the air when a person with TB of the lungs or throat coughs, sneezes, or talks. If you have been exposed, you should go to your doctor for tests. You are more likely to get TB if you have a weak immune system.

Symptoms of TB in the lungs may include:
- a bad cough that lasts 3 weeks or longer
- weight loss
- loss of appetite
- coughing up blood or mucus
- weakness or fatigue
- fever
- night sweats

Skin tests, blood tests, x-rays, and other tests can tell if you have TB. If not treated properly, TB can be deadly. You can usually cure active TB by taking several medicines for a long period of time.

Respiratory System Specialists

A **pulmonologist** is a specialist in the respiratory system.

Respiratory System Procedures

Bronchoscopy: A light, flexible, fiberoptic tube is passed through the nose, throat, larynx and trachea into the lungs to examine the bronchial tubes. Biopsies can be performed or specimens of the mucus in the lungs can be obtained. See Skin System Procedures for more information on biopsies.

Pulmonary Function Test: The patient is asked to breathe in and then blow out as hard and long as he can into a tube connected to a machine. The machine determines how well the lungs are functioning.

The Skin System

Skin System Vocabulary

Acne
Athlete's foot
Biopsy
Blood vessels
Burns
Calluses
Corns
Dermatologist
Dermatologist
Dermis
Eczema
Epidermis
Hair follicles (Sacs)
Integumentary
Nerves
Shingles
Skin cancer
Sunburn
Sweat glands
Warts

Function of the Skin System

The skin system is also known as the **integumentary** system. The skin is the largest organ in the human body. (The liver is the largest internal organ).

The skin has three main purposes:

- It protects the body from germs.
- It keeps in heat and moisture.
- It contains nerves that sense temperature, pressure, and touch.

The skin is made up of two layers. The **epidermis** is the outer layer. The **dermis** is the inner layer.

The skin contains many glands, including oil glands and **sweat glands.** The skin also contains **hair follicles (sacs).** These follicles are found in the dermis. As hair cells develop and die, the dead cells build up, eventually pushing out of the dermis and through the epidermis to be seen as hair.

Skin Section

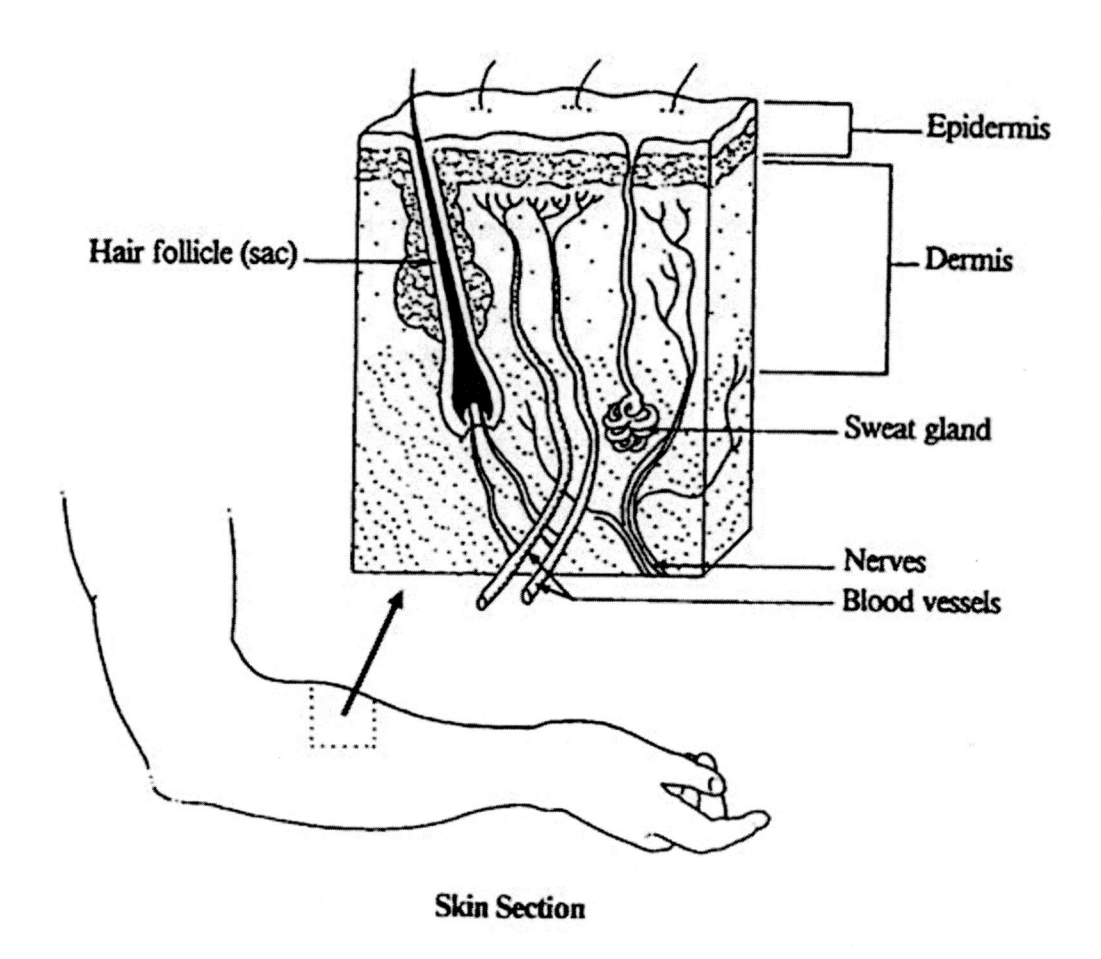

Cells grow from the dermis. It takes about a month for these cells to reach the surface. The dermis contains **blood vessels** which bring nutrients to nourish and develop the skin cells. As a result, the epidermis is always changing. It grows from the inside and gets worn away by the outside environment. The dermis also contains nerves. The **nerves** in the skin system communicate sensations of temperature, pressure, and touch to the brain.

Common Problems of the Skin System

Acne: Acne is a common skin disease that causes pimples. Pimples form when hair follicles under your skin clog up. Most pimples form on the face, neck, back, chest, and shoulders. Anyone can get acne, but it is common in teenagers and young adults. It is not serious, but it can cause scars.

No one knows exactly what causes acne. Hormone changes, such as those during the teenage years and pregnancy, probably play a role. There are many myths about what causes acne. Chocolate and greasy foods are often blamed, but there is little evidence that foods have much effect on acne in most people. Another common myth is that dirty skin causes acne; however, blackheads and pimples are not caused by dirt. Stress doesn't cause acne, but stress can make it worse.

If you have acne:
- clean your skin gently
- try not to touch your skin
- avoid the sun

Treatments for acne include medicines and creams.

Athlete's foot: Athlete's foot is a common infection caused by a fungus. It most often affects the space between the toes. Symptoms include itching, burning, and cracked, scaly skin between your toes.

You can get athlete's foot from damp surfaces, such as showers, swimming pools, and locker room floors. To prevent it:
- keep your feet clean, dry, and cool
- wear clean socks
- don't walk barefoot in public areas
- wear flip-flops in locker room showers
- keep your toenails clean and clipped short

Treatments include over-the-counter antifungal creams for most cases and prescription medicines for more serious infections. These usually clear up the infection, but it can come back.

Burns: A burn is damage to your body's tissues caused by heat, chemicals, electricity, sunlight, or radiation. Scalds from hot liquids and steam, building fires, and flammable liquids and gases are the most common causes of burns. Another kind is an inhalation injury, caused by breathing smoke.

There are three types of burns:
- first-degree burns damage only the outer layer of skin
- second-degree burns damage the outer layer and the layer underneath
- third-degree burns damage or destroy the deepest layer of skin and tissues underneath

Burns can cause swelling, blistering, scarring and, in serious cases, shock and even death. They also can lead to infections because they damage your skin's protective barrier. Antibiotic creams can prevent or treat infections. After a third-degree burn, you need skin or synthetic grafts to cover exposed tissue and encourage new skin to grow. First- and second-degree burns usually heal without grafts.

Calluses and corns: Corns and calluses are caused by pressure or friction on your skin. They often appear on feet where the bony parts of your feet rub against your shoes. Corns usually appear on the tops or sides of toes while calluses form on the soles of feet. Calluses also can appear on hands or other areas that are rubbed or pressed.

Wearing shoes that fit better or using non-medicated pads may help. While bathing, gently rub the corn or callus with a washcloth or pumice stone to help reduce the size. To avoid infection, do not try to shave off the corn or callus. See your doctor, especially if you have diabetes or circulation problems.

Eczema: Eczema is a term for several different types of skin swelling. Eczema is also called dermatitis. It is not dangerous, but most types cause red, swollen and itchy skin. Factors that can cause eczema include other diseases, irritating substances, allergies, and your genetic makeup. Eczema is not contagious.

The most common type of eczema is atopic dermatitis. It is an allergic condition that makes your skin dry and itchy. It is most common in babies and children.

Eczema is a chronic disease. You can prevent some types of eczema by avoiding irritants, stress, and the things you are allergic to.

Cold sores (herpes): Cold sores are caused by a contagious virus called herpes simplex. There are two types of herpes simplex virus. Type 1 usually causes oral herpes, or cold sores. Type 1 herpes virus infects more than half of the U.S. population by the time they reach their 20s. Type 2 usually affects the genital area

Some people have no symptoms from the infection. But others develop painful and unsightly cold sores that last for a week or more. Cold sores usually occur outside the mouth on the lips, chin, and cheeks, or in the nostrils. When they do occur inside the mouth, it is usually on the gums or the roof of the mouth.

There is no cure for cold sores. Medicines can relieve some of the pain and discomfort associated with the sores. These include ointments that numb the blisters, antibiotics that control secondary bacterial infections, and ointments that soften the crusts of the sores.

Shingles: Shingles is a disease caused by the varicella-zoster virus, the same virus that causes chickenpox. After you have chickenpox, the virus stays in your body. It may not cause problems for many years. As you get older, the virus may reappear as shingles. Although it is most common in people over age 50, anyone who has had chickenpox is at risk. Unlike chickenpox, you can't catch shingles from someone who has it.

Early signs of shingles include burning or shooting pain and tingling or itching, usually on one side of the body or face. The pain can be mild to severe. Rashes or blisters appear anywhere from one to 14 days later. If shingles appears on your face, it may affect your vision or hearing. The pain of shingles may last for weeks, months, or even years after the blisters have healed.

There is no cure for shingles. Early treatment with medicines that fight the virus may help. These medicines may also help prevent lingering pain.

A vaccine may prevent shingles or lessen its effects. The vaccine is recommended for people 60 or over. In some cases, doctors may give it to people ages 50 to 59.

Skin cancer: Skin cancer is the most common form of cancer in the United States. The two most common types are basal cell cancer and squamous cell cancer. They usually form on the head, face, neck, hands, and arms. Another type of skin cancer, melanoma, is more dangerous but less common.

Anyone can get skin cancer, but it is more common in people who:
- spend a lot of time in the sun or have been sunburned
- have light-colored skin, hair and eyes
- have a family member with skin cancer
- are over age 50

You should have your doctor check any suspicious skin markings and any changes in the way your skin looks. Treatment is more likely to work well when cancer is found early. If not treated, some types of skin cancer cells can spread to other tissues and organs. Treatments include surgery, radiation therapy, chemotherapy, photodynamic therapy (PDT), and biologic therapy. PDT uses a drug and a type of laser light to kill cancer cells. Biologic therapy boosts your body's own ability to fight cancer.

Sunburn: Ultraviolet (UV) rays are an invisible form of radiation. They can pass through your skin and damage your skin cells. Sunburns are a sign of skin damage. Suntans aren't healthy, either. They appear after the sun's rays have already killed some cells and damaged others. UV rays can cause skin damage during any season or at any temperature. They can also cause eye problems, wrinkles, skin spots, and skin cancer.

To protect yourself:
- stay out of the sun when it is strongest (between 10 a.m. and 2 p.m.)
- use sunscreen with an SPF of 15 or higher
- wear protective clothing
- wear wraparound sunglasses that provide 100 percent UV ray protection
- avoid sunlamps and tanning beds

Check your skin regularly for changes in the size, shape, color, or feel of birthmarks, moles, and spots. Such changes are a sign of skin cancer.

Warts: Warts are growths on your skin caused by an infection with human papillomavirus, or HPV. Types of warts include:
- common warts, which often appear on your fingers
- plantar warts, which show up on the soles of your feet
- genital warts, which are a sexually transmitted disease
- flat warts, which appear in places you shave frequently

In children, warts often go away on their own. In adults, they tend to stay. If they hurt or bother you, or if they multiply, you can remove them. Chemical skin treatments usually work. If not, various freezing, surgical and laser treatments can remove warts.

Skin system specialists

A **dermatologist** specializes in the health of the skin.

Skin System Procedures

Biopsy: A small sample of affected tissue is cut out and examined in the laboratory under a microscope. This procedure applies to many body systems, not just the skin system.

The Urinary System

Vocabulary
Bladder
Cystoscopy
Hemodialysis
Interstitial cystitis
Intravenous pyelogram (IVP)
Kidney failure
Kidney stones
Kidneys
Lithotripsy
Nephrologist
Peritoneal dialysis
Prostate diseases
Renal artery
Renal dialysis
Renal vein
Sphincter muscle
Ureter
Urethra
Urinary tract infection
Urine test
Urologist

Function of the Urinary System

The urinary system, also known as the urinary tract, removes wastes from the blood. These wastes are produced when the body makes energy from food. These wastes would poison the body if they were not taken away.

The urinary system is composed of the **kidneys, bladder, ureters,** and **urethra.** While the general function of the urinary system is the same for men and women, there are some differences between the male and female urinary systems.

The **kidneys** remove chemical wastes and excess water from the blood to make urine. They also help control blood pressure. Each kidney has over a million very small filters that remove wastes and other substances from the blood. Tiny blood vessels (capillaries) run through each of these filters. Each kidney is also attached to its own large blood vessels - the **renal artery** and the **renal vein**. Our blood is continually filtered by the kidneys. Urine is also being constantly produced by the kidneys and passes to the bladder through the **ureters.**

Body Systems Terminology

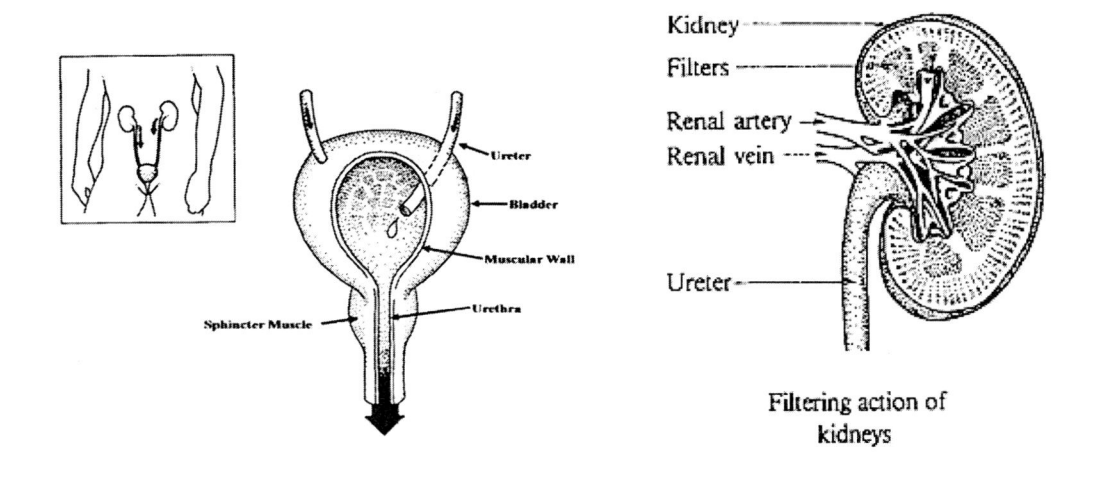

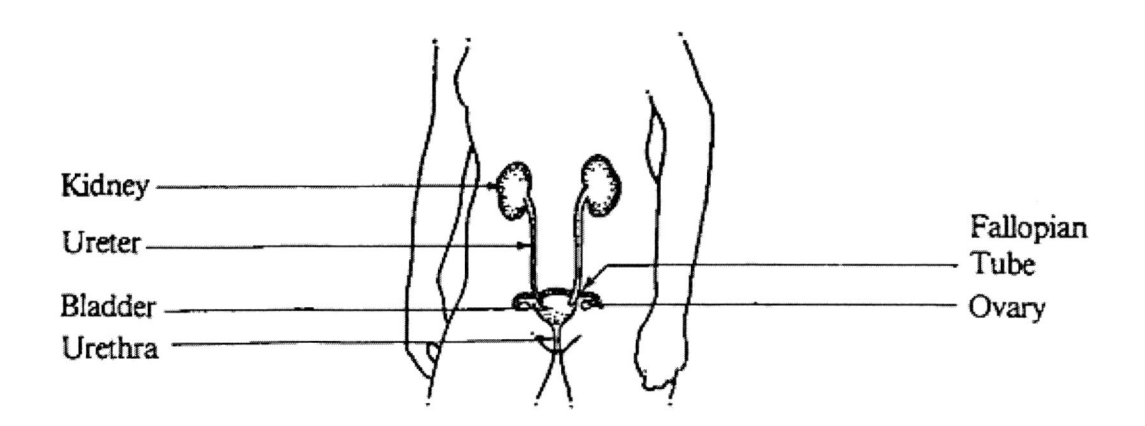

Filtering action of kidneys

Major Anatomical Parts of the Female Reproductive System

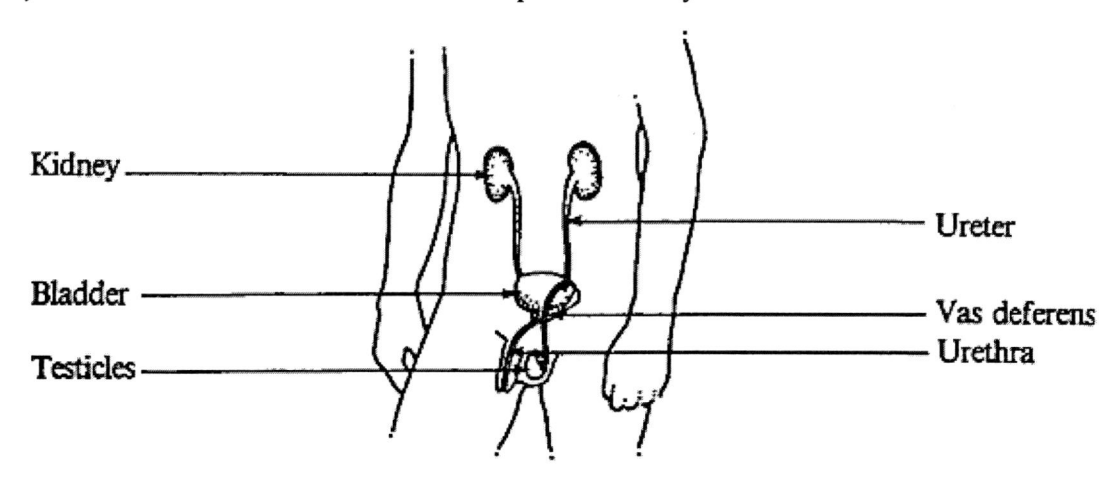

Major anatomical parts of the Male Reproductive System

The **bladder** holds the urine until the body is ready to get rid of it. It is an elastic muscular sac that expands as it fills up with urine. The **sphincter muscle** at the bottom of the bladder controls the release of urine. When we urinate, we relax the sphincter muscle and contract muscles in the walls of the bladder to push the urine out.

Tubes, known as **ureters,** pass urine from the kidneys to the bladder. Another tube, known as the **urethra,** passes urine from the bladder to the outside of the body.

In the male urinary system, the tube coming from the bladder (urethra) joins the tube coming from the testicles (the vas deferens). The testicle and the vas deferens are also a part of the male reproductive system.

Common Problems of the Urinary System

Interstitial Cystitis: Interstitial cystitis (IC) is a condition that causes discomfort or pain in the bladder and a need to urinate frequently and urgently. It is far more common in women than in men. The symptoms vary from person to person. Some people may have pain without urgency or frequency. Others have urgency and frequency without pain. Women's symptoms often get worse during their periods. They may also have pain during sexual intercourse.

The cause of IC isn't known. There is no one test to tell if you have it. Doctors often run tests to rule out other possible causes of symptoms. There is no cure for IC, but treatments can help most people feel better. They include:

- distending, or inflating, the bladder
- bathing the inside of the bladder with a drug solution
- oral medicines
- electrical nerve stimulation
- physical therapy
- lifestyle changes
- bladder training
- in rare cases, surgery

Kidney Failure: Healthy kidneys clean your blood by removing excess fluid, minerals, and wastes. They also make hormones that keep your bones strong and your blood healthy. But if the kidneys are damaged, they don't work properly. Harmful wastes can build up in your body. Your blood pressure may rise. Your body may retain excess fluid and not make enough red blood cells. This is called kidney failure.

If your kidneys fail, you need treatment to replace the work they normally do. The treatment options are dialysis or a kidney transplant. Each treatment has benefits and drawbacks. No matter which treatment you choose, you'll need to make some changes in your life, including how you eat and plan your activities. But with the help of health care providers, family, and friends, most people with kidney failure can lead full and active lives.

Kidney Stones: A kidney stone is a solid piece of material that forms in the kidney from substances in the urine. It may be as small as a grain of sand or as large as a pearl. Most kidney stones pass out of the body without help from a doctor, but sometimes a stone will not go away. It may get stuck in the urinary tract, block the flow of urine and cause great pain.

The following may be signs of kidney stones that need a doctor's help:

- extreme pain in your back or side that will not go away
- blood in your urine
- fever and chills
- vomiting
- urine that smells bad or looks cloudy
- a burning feeling when you urinate

Your doctor will diagnose a kidney stone with urine, blood, and imaging tests. If you have a stone that won't pass on its own, you may need treatment. It can be done with shock waves; with a scope inserted through the tube that carries urine out of the body, called the urethra; or with surgery.

Prostate Diseases: The prostate is a gland in the male urinary system. It helps make semen, the fluid that contains sperm. The prostate surrounds the tube that carries urine away from the bladder and out of the body. A young man's prostate is about the size of a walnut. It slowly grows larger with age. If it gets too large, it can cause problems. This is very common after age 50. The older men get, the more likely they are to have prostate trouble.

Some common problems are:
- prostatitis - an infection, usually caused by bacteria;
- benign prostatic hyperplasia (BPH) - an enlarged prostate, which may cause dribbling after urination or a need to go often, especially at night;
- prostate cancer - a common cancer that responds best to treatment when detected early.

Urinary tract infection: The urinary system is the body's drainage system for removing wastes and extra water. It includes two kidneys, two ureters, a bladder, and a urethra. Urinary tract infections (UTIs) are the second most common type of infection in the body.

You may have a UTI if you notice
- pain or burning when you urinate
- fever, tiredness, or shakiness
- an urge to urinate often
- pressure in your lower belly
- urine that smells bad or looks cloudy or reddish
- pain in your back or side below the ribs

People of any age or sex can get UTIs, but about four times as many women get UTIs as men. You're also at higher risk if you have diabetes, need a tube to drain your bladder, or have a spinal cord injury.

If you think you have a UTI it is important to see your doctor. Your doctor can tell if you have a UTI with a urine test. UTIs are treated is with antibiotics.

Urinary System Specialists

A **urologist** is the medical specialist of the urinary system and the male reproductive system. Women may see a urologist for issues relating to the urinary system or a gynecologist for the female reproductive system.

A **nephrologist** is the medical specialist who works with the kidneys.

Urinary System Procedures

Urine test: The patient urinates into a cup. The urine is then tested and examined under a microscope to identify bacteria or viruses.

Intravenous Pyelogram (IVP): Contrast material (dye) is injected into a vein. It travels to the kidneys, where it becomes part of the urine and then travels through the rest of the urinary tract. Meanwhile, X-rays are taken of this dye, which shows how the kidneys are functioning and if there are tumors, cysts, stones, etc.

Cystoscopy: A hollow metal tube (called a cystoscope) is passed into the urinary opening and up through the urethra into the bladder. By means of mirrors and a light source, the physician can examine the inside of the bladder. Urine samples can be withdrawn, and contrast materials injected into the bladder through the cystoscope.

Lithotripsy: As the patient is immersed in a tub of water, shock waves are used to break up stones in the kidneys so they can be passed out of the body through the urine.

Renal Dialysis: When the kidneys stop functioning, for example in cases of kidney failure, the waste materials in the blood build up. Dialysis is a procedure to artificially do the kidneys' work. There are two kinds of dialysis:

In **hemodialysis,** blood flows from the patient into an artificial kidney machine where it is filtered and then returned back into the patient.

In **peritoneal dialysis,** fluid is introduced into the cavity around the major organs (the peritoneal cavity). Waste passes from the blood to the fluid, which is then removed through a catheter.

The Female Reproductive System

Vocabulary
Amniotic sac
Breast cancer
Cervix
Cesarean section
Conception
Colposcopy
Dilation and curettage (D&C)
Ectopic (tubal) pregnancy
Ectopic pregnancy
Egg
Fallopian tubes
Female infertility
Fibroids
Gynecologist
Hysterectomy
Mammogram
Miscarriage
Obstetrician
Ovarian cysts
Ovary
Pap smear
Placenta
Sexually transmitted disease
Ultrasound
Umbilical cord
Uterus
Vagina
Vaginal infection
Vulva

Function and Major Anatomical Parts of the Female Reproductive System

The **fallopian tubes, eggs, ovaries, uterus, cervix, vagina,** and **vulva** are important parts of the female reproductive system.

The **ovaries** are an important organ that produces the hormones (chemical messengers) that control the female reproductive system.

The menstrual cycle is the name given to the monthly reproductive cycle that is controlled by hormones. At the beginning of each cycle an **egg** (usually just one) begins to ripen in one **ovary**. Then this egg is released from the ovary into a **fallopian tube.** This process is called ovulation.

The egg has the opportunity to be fertilized by male sperm in the fallopian tube. If fertilized, the egg moves down the fallopian tube and into the **uterus.** The uterus is where the fertilized egg (embryo) develops into a baby. To prepare for the potentially fertilized egg, the inside lining of the uterus begins to grow thick during each menstrual cycle. This lining is made up of a special mucous membrane called the endometrium. Also, the blood vessels in this area expand in preparation to receive a potentially fertilized egg.

If the egg is not fertilized by a sperm, it passes out of the body, along with the lining of the uterus. This is called a 'period' and usually looks like simple bleeding. This menstrual cycle is regulated by hormones that are produced in different

Major anatomical parts of the female reproductive system

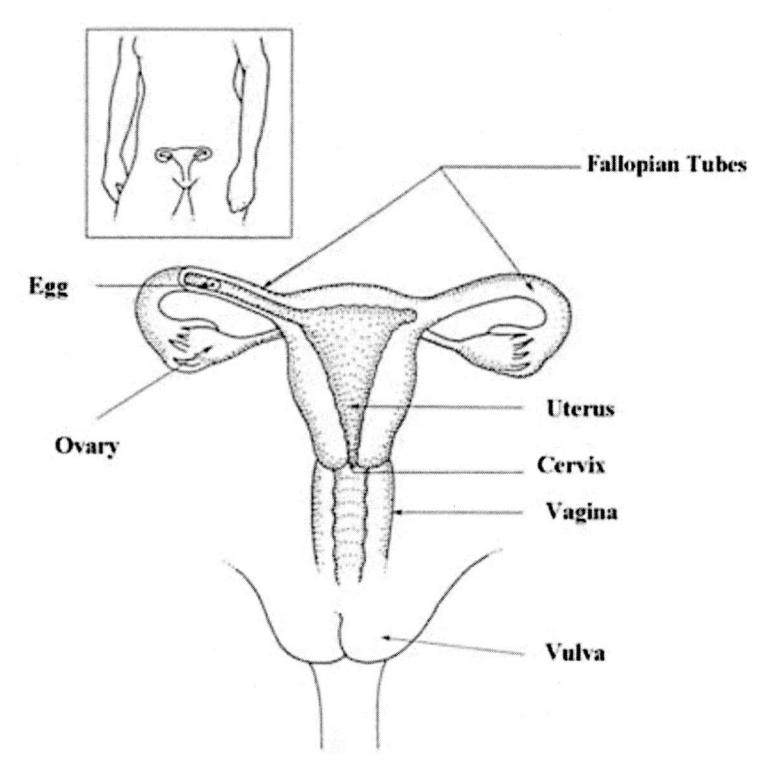

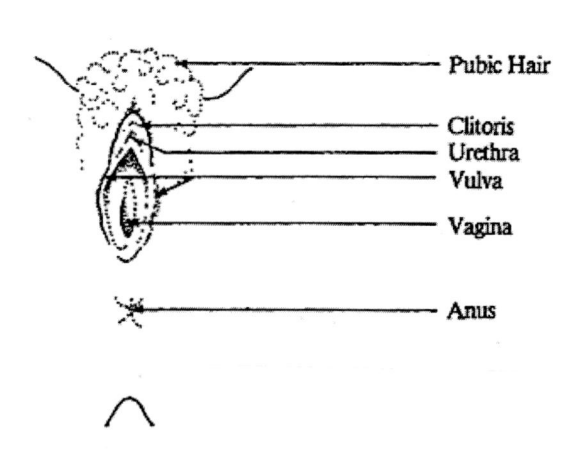

glands in the body. Many factors can affect the regularity of a woman's menstrual cycle such as emotional stress, medications, fatigue, and illness.

The **cervix** is the opening of the uterus. It is sometimes called the 'neck' of the uterus. The cervix expands and contracts during childbirth (called dilation). It is the opening that allows sperm, menstrual blood (from a period), and a baby to pass through.

The **vagina** is another important internal part of the female reproductive system. It is the structure between the cervix and the vulva. It contains mucus membranes that provide lubrication and allows it to stretch during sexual intercourse and childbirth.

The **vulva** is the term used to describe the external structure of the female reproductive system. It contains the inner and outer labia (folds of skin that are covered in pubic hair that cover the rest of the vulva), the clitoris (a female sexual organ with many nerve endings, making it sensitive to stimulation), the urethral opening, and the vaginal opening.

Pregnancy

Pregnancy happens when a female egg combines with a male sperm to produce an embryo. This process is called **conception**. The descriptions in this section are based on how pregnancy, fetal growth, and childbirth usually happen. However, each woman and each child is unique and will experience these processes differently.

Conception usually takes place while the egg is passing down the fallopian tube and when sperm are present as a result of intercourse. The lining of the uterus has already thickened to nourish the growing embryo as a part of the normal menstrual cycle. Once the embryo travels from the fallopian tube to the uterus, it attaches itself to the endometrium (the lining of the uterus). Once conception occurs, hormones stimulate changes in a woman's breasts. The nipples and the areola (area around the nipples) darken and the breasts produce milk.

The age of the growing fetus is calculated from the first day of the last period. From conception until twelve weeks the baby is called an embryo. From twelve weeks until birth, the baby is called a fetus.

The date when a baby is due to be born is determined by adding 280 days to the date of the first day of the last period. Although it is very small, the embryo develops very rapidly. It is very vulnerable to damage from alcohol, tobacco, drugs, and infections.

The fetus is nourished by the mother's blood, through the **placenta**. The placenta provides the oxygen and nutrients to the developing fetus. It is connected to the growing fetus through the **umbilical cord**. Within the uterus, the fetus floats in the **amniotic sac**. The amniotic sac is filled with a clear fluid and it provides protection for the fetus.

The following are normal signs that a baby will be born soon:
- Contractions begin in the uterus. These are felt as labor pains.
- The pains become progressively stronger, more regular, and closer together.
- The plug between the uterus and vagina is pushed out. This appears as a bloody discharge called "spotting."
- The sac surrounding the baby breaks, letting out fluid. This can happen slowly or all at once.

Labor normally has three stages: Stage 1 is from the beginning of labor until the cervix is opened up (fully dilated). With first babies, this stage may last 12 hours or longer. It usually happens faster the next time a woman has a child. Stage 2 is from the full dilation of the cervix to when the baby is born. Contractions are very strong as the baby moves down the birth canal. There is also an urge to push. This stage can last up to an hour, less with second babies. Stage 3 is from when the baby is born until the placenta is delivered. The uterus contracts to push out the placenta. Usually this stage lasts about 15 minutes.

Common Problems of the Female Reproductive System

This section is divided into two parts: Common Reproductive System Problems and Common Pregnancy and Childbirth Problems.

Common Reproductive System Problems

Cancer of the Reproductive Organs: Cancer refers to the abnormal growth of cells in the body. This abnormal cell growth can occur in tissues and organs throughout the body. If left untreated, often the cancer will spread.

Cancer of the reproductive organs include cancers such as cervical cancer, breast cancer, and ovarian cancer

Breast cancer: Breast cancer affects one in eight women during their lives. Breast cancer kills more women in the United States than any cancer except lung cancer. No one knows why some women get breast cancer, but there are a number of risk factors. Risks that you cannot change include:
- age - the chance of getting breast cancer rises as a woman gets older
- genes - there are two genes, BRCA1 and BRCA2, that greatly increase the risk
- personal factors - beginning periods before age 12 or going through menopause after age 55

Other risks include being overweight, using hormone replacement therapy (also called menopausal hormone therapy), taking birth control pills, drinking alcohol, not having children, having your first child after age 35, or having dense breasts.

Symptoms of breast cancer may include a lump in the breast, a change in size or shape of the breast or discharge from a nipple. Breast self-exam and mammography can help find breast cancer early when it is most treatable. Treatment may consist of radiation, lumpectomy, mastectomy, chemotherapy, and hormone therapy.

Men can have breast cancer, too, but the number of cases is small.

Fibroids: Uterine fibroids are the most common benign tumors in women of childbearing age. Fibroids are made of muscle cells and other tissues that grow in and around the wall of the uterus, or womb. The cause of fibroids is unknown. Risk factors include being African American or being overweight.

Many women with fibroids have no symptoms. If you do have symptoms, they may include:
- heavy or painful periods or bleeding between periods
- feeling "full" in the lower abdomen
- urinating often
- pain during sex
- lower back pain
- reproductive problems, such as infertility, multiple miscarriages or early labor

Your health care provider may find fibroids during a gynecological exam or by using imaging tests. Treatment includes drugs that can slow or stop their growth, or surgery. If you have no symptoms, you may not even need treatment. Many women with fibroids can get pregnant naturally. For those who cannot, infertility treatments may help.

Ovarian cysts: A cyst is a fluid filled sac. In most cases a cyst on the ovary does no harm and goes away by itself. Most women have them sometime during their lives. Cysts are rarely cancerous in women under 50. Cysts sometimes hurt, but not always. Often, a woman finds out about a cyst when she has a pelvic exam.

If you're in your childbearing years or past menopause, have no symptoms, and have a fluid filled cyst, you may choose to monitor the cyst. You may need surgery if you have pain, are past menopause, or if the cyst does not go away. Birth control pills can help prevent new cysts.

A health problem that may involve ovarian cysts is polycystic ovary syndrome (PCOS). Women with PCOS can have high levels of male hormones, irregular, or no periods and small ovarian cysts.

Vaginal infections:

Vaginal problems are some of the most common reasons women go to the doctor. They may have symptoms such as:
- itching
- burning
- pain
- abnormal bleeding
- discharge

Often, the problem is vaginitis, an inflammation of the vagina. The main symptom is smelly vaginal discharge, but some women have no symptoms. Common causes are bacterial infections, trichomoniasis, and yeast infections.

Some other causes of vaginal symptoms include sexually transmitted diseases, vaginal cancer, and vulvar cancer. Treatment of vaginal problems depends on the cause.

Common Pregnancy and Childbirth Problems

Ectopic pregnancy: The uterus, or womb, is an important female reproductive organ. It is the place where a baby grows when a woman is pregnant. If you have an ectopic pregnancy, the fertilized egg grows in an abnormal place, outside the uterus, usually in the fallopian tubes. The result is usually a miscarriage.

Ectopic pregnancy can be a medical emergency if it ruptures. Signs of ectopic pregnancy include:
- abdominal pain
- shoulder pain
- vaginal bleeding
- feeling dizzy or faint

Get medical care right away if you have these signs. Doctors use drugs or surgery to remove the ectopic tissue so it doesn't damage your organs. Many women who have had ectopic pregnancies go on to have healthy pregnancies later.

Female Infertility: Infertility is a term doctors use if a woman hasn't been able to get pregnant after at least one year of trying. If a woman keeps having miscarriages, it is also called infertility. Female infertility can result from physical problems, hormone problems, and lifestyle or environmental factors.

Most cases of infertility in women result from problems with producing eggs. One problem is premature ovarian failure, in which the ovaries stop functioning before natural menopause. In another, polycystic ovary syndrome (PCOS), the ovaries may not release an egg regularly or may not release a healthy egg.

About a third of the time, infertility is because of a problem with the woman. One third of the time, it is a problem with the man. Sometimes no cause can be found.

If you suspect you are infertile, see your doctor. There are tests that may tell if you have fertility problems. When it is possible to find the cause, treatments may include medicines, surgery, or assisted reproductive technologies. Happily, two-thirds of couples treated for infertility are able to have babies.

Miscarriage: A miscarriage is the loss of pregnancy from natural causes before the 20th week of pregnancy. Most miscarriages occur very early in the pregnancy, often before a woman even knows she is pregnant. There are many different causes for a miscarriage. In most cases, there is nothing you can do to prevent a miscarriage.

Factors that may contribute to miscarriage include:
- a genetic problem with the fetus
- problems with the uterus or cervix
- polycystic ovary syndrome

Signs of a miscarriage can include vaginal spotting or bleeding, abdominal pain or cramping, and fluid or tissue passing from the vagina. Although vaginal bleeding is a common symptom of miscarriage, many women have spotting early in their pregnancy but do not miscarry. But if you are pregnant and have bleeding or spotting, contact your health care provider immediately.

Women who miscarry early in their pregnancy usually do not need any treatment. In some cases, you may need a procedure called a dilatation and curettage (D&C) to remove tissue remaining in the uterus.

Counseling may help you cope with your grief. Later, if you do decide to try again, work closely with your health care provider to lower the risks. Many women who have a miscarriage go on to have healthy babies.

Female Reproductive System Specialists

A **gynecologist** takes care of the health of the female reproductive system.

An **obstetrician** is a medical specialist that handles pregnancy and birth.

Female Reproductive System Procedures

Amniocentesis: This test is done only if there is a suspected problem with the fetus. A sample of the amniotic fluid is taken and tested. Tests can determine if the baby has severe abnormalities (like down syndrome or spina bifida). The baby's sex can also be determined with this test; however, this can usually be determined from an ultrasound as well.

Caesarean Section (C-Section): A C-section is an operation to deliver a baby quickly if a vaginal delivery is not possible. An incision is made in the lower abdomen and through the outside of the uterus. The baby is delivered through this opening. It usually takes longer to recover from this operation than it does from normal childbirth.

Colposcopy: The physician uses a lighted, magnifying instrument to visually examine the cervix. This test is more accurate than a Pap Smear Test.

Dilation and Curettage (D&C): This is an operation that scrapes the lining of the uterus. It is done to treat heavy periods or after a miscarriage or abortion. The operation is usually done in a hospital under a general anesthetic.

Fetal Monitor: This is a machine used during labor to keep track of the baby's heart and the mother's contractions. It helps to keep track of how the baby is doing in general. It is a non-invasive procedure that involves placing electrodes on the abdomen of the mother that are sensitive to the baby's heart rate and the mother's contractions.

Hysterectomy: A hysterectomy is an operation to treat several conditions, such as cancer, fibroids, and cysts. In this operation, the uterus, and sometimes the ovaries and fallopian tubes, are removed. This is a fairly lengthy procedure and requires a long recovery time. Hormone pills may have to be taken after the surgery to replace the chemicals usually supplied by the ovaries.

Mammogram: A mammogram is a procedure that uses x-rays to take images of a woman's breast. It can be used to detect breast cancer, tumors and other abnormalities in the breast.

Pap smear: This test can show cancer before it spreads throughout the body. This is an important test for a woman to have on a regular basis as recommended by a primary care provider or gynecologist. The physician inserts a speculum into the vagina to hold the vaginal walls apart and then scrapes some material from the cervix (the entrance to the uterus). This material is examined in the laboratory under a microscope for abnormal cells that might suggest cancer. This test is named after Papaniccolao, the doctor who developed it.

Ultrasound: An ultrasound test is a way of seeing the baby inside the uterus. Sound waves are used to take an image of the baby. It is used to measure the size and shape of the baby. It is one way of seeing if the baby is growing normally.

Sexually Transmitted Diseases

Sexually transmitted diseases affect both men and women.

Sexually transmitted diseases (STDs) are infections that you can get from having sex with someone who has the infection. The causes of STDs are bacteria, parasites and viruses. There are more than 20 types of STDs, including:
- chlamydia
- gonorrhea
- genital herpes
- HIV/AIDS
- HPV
- syphilis
- trichomoniasis

Most STDs affect both men and women, but in many cases the health problems they cause can be more severe for women. If a pregnant woman has an STD, it can cause serious health problems for the baby.

If you have an STD caused by bacteria or parasites, your health care provider can treat it with antibiotics or other medicines.

If you have an STD caused by a virus, there is no cure. Sometimes medicines can keep the disease under control. Correct usage of latex condoms greatly reduces, but does not completely eliminate, the risk of catching or spreading STDs.

The Male Reproductive System

Vocabulary

Bladder
Erectile dysfunction
Male infertility
Penis
Prostate cancer
Prostate gland
Scrotum
Semen analysis
Seminal vesicles
Sexually transmitted disease
Testicles
Testicular cancer
Ureters
Urethra
Urologist
Vas deferens
Vasectomy

Function and Major Anatomical Parts of the Male Reproductive System

The **vas deferens, prostate gland, penis, testicles, scrotum,** and **seminal vesicles** are important parts of the male reproductive system. As discussed in the Urinary System Section, the male reproductive system is joined to the male urinary system. The **ureters, urethra,** and **bladder** are also included in the diagram of the male reproductive system on the following page.

The male reproductive system has two **testicles** (also called testes). When referring to just one, the term 'testis' is used. The testicles are the male sex glands that produce sperm. The testicles are located in an outer sac called a **scrotum.** The scrotum is located outside of the body.

The purpose of the scrotum is to keep the sperm at a temperature just lower than body temperature as this is necessary for the sperm to survive.

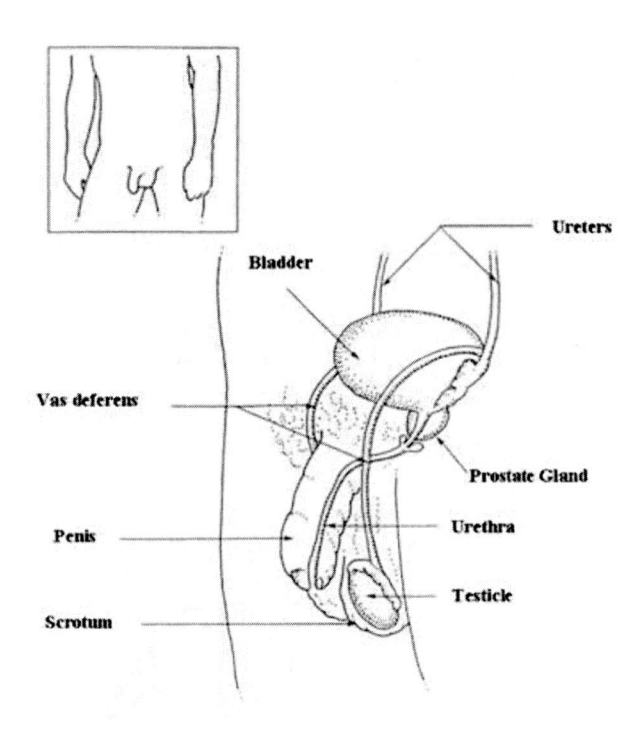

Major anatomical parts of the male reproductive system

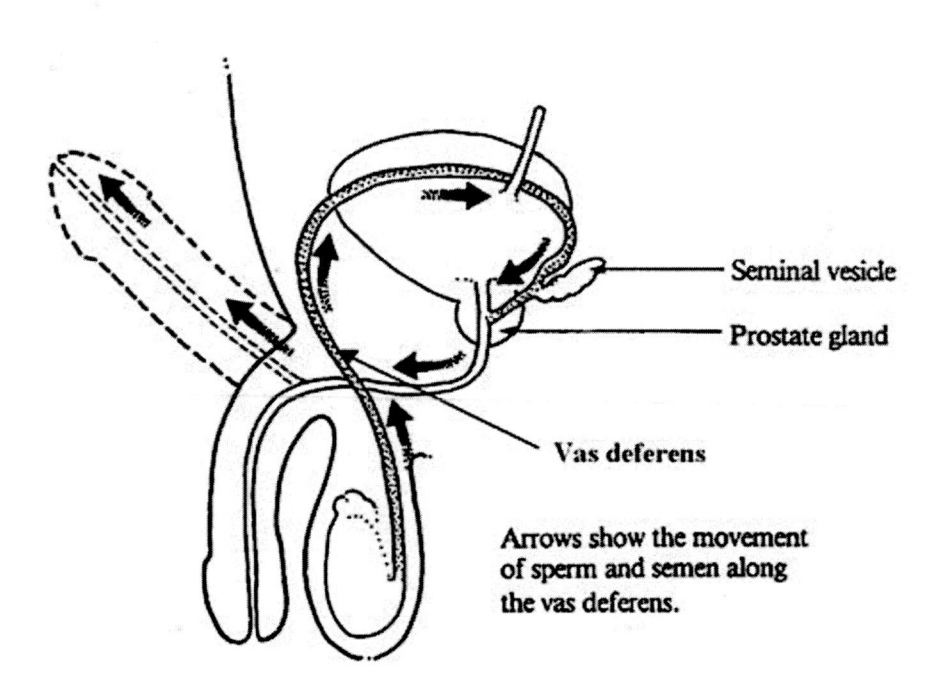

Arrows show the movement of sperm and semen along the vas deferens.

During ejaculation, the **vas deferens** (a long tube inside the body) carries the sperm to the **urethra,** which leads to the outside of the body. Before the sperm is ejaculated, seminal fluids are added through the **seminal vesicles** (glands located near the bladder and urethra) and the **prostate gland.** When sperm and seminal fluids are mixed together, it is called semen.

An ejaculation contains many sperm. When the semen is ejaculated and released into a female vagina, many of the sperm will not survive. However, one sperm may successfully fertilize an egg, resulting in conception.

Common Problems of the Male Reproductive System

Erectile dysfunction: Erectile dysfunction (also called impotence or ED) is a common type of male sexual dysfunction. It is when a man has trouble getting or keeping an erection. ED becomes more common as you get older. But it's not a natural part of aging.

Some people have trouble speaking with their doctors about sex. But if you have ED, you should tell your doctor. ED can be a sign of health problems. It may mean your blood vessels are clogged. It may mean you have nerve damage from diabetes. If you don't see your doctor, these problems will go untreated.

Your doctor can offer several new treatments for ED. For many men, the answer is as simple as taking a pill. Getting more exercise, losing weight, or stopping smoking may also help.

Male infertility: Infertility is a term doctors use if a man hasn't been able to get a woman pregnant after at least one year of trying. Causes of male infertility include:
- physical problems with the testicles
- blockages in the ducts that carry sperm
- hormone problems
- a history of high fevers or mumps
- genetic disorders
- lifestyle or environmental factors

About a third of the time, infertility is because of a problem with the man. One third of the time, it is a problem with the woman. Sometimes no cause can be found.

If you suspect you are infertile, see your doctor. There are tests that may tell if you have fertility problems. When it is possible to find the cause, treatments may include medicines, surgery, or assisted reproductive technologies. Happily, two-thirds of couples treated for infertility are able to have babies.

Testicular Cancer: Testicles, or testes, make male hormones and sperm. They are two egg-shaped organs inside the scrotum, the loose sac of skin behind the penis. You can get cancer in one or both testicles.

Testicular cancer mainly affects young men between the ages of 20 and 39. It is also more common in men who:
- have had abnormal testicle development;
- have had an undescended testicle;
- have a family history of the cancer.

Symptoms include pain, swelling, or lumps in your testicles or groin area. Doctors use a physical exam, lab tests, imaging tests, and a biopsy to diagnose testicular cancer. Most cases can be treated, especially if found early. Treatment options include surgery, radiation, and/or chemotherapy. Regular exams after treatment are important.

Treatments may also cause infertility. If you may want children later on, you should consider sperm banking before treatment.

Sexually transmitted diseases:
Sexually transmitted diseases affect both men and women. See the section on page 298 for more information.

Male Reproductive System Specialists

The male reproductive system is connected to the male urinary system. The same medical specialist works with the health of both systems. This medical specialist is called a **urologist.**

Male Reproductive System Procedures

Semen Analysis: The patient is asked to masturbate and ejaculate into a container. The sperm in the semen that is collected is then counted under a microscope. If the count is less than 20 million sperm/ml of semen, the man is usually sterile.

Vasectomy: The vas deferens tube, which carries sperm to the urethra, is cut. This sterilizes the patient, but, since it does not interfere with nerves or blood supply to the penis, it does not interfere with sexual function.

Section 3

MEDICAL TERMINOLOGY STUDY TOOLS

Medical Terminology Role-Plays

Medical Terminology Role-Plays are a great way to integrate all of the new kinds of vocabulary introduced in this curriculum (anatomy, physiology, common problems, procedures, and specialists).

How to create a Medical Terminology Role-Play:

1. The topic of your role-play will be one of the body systems assigned by your instructor. (Circulatory System, Digestive System, etc.)

2. With your group, read through the information on your assigned body system in Section 2. Be sure to read about the anatomical parts, their function, the common problems, the specialists, and the procedures. Make sure that <u>all</u> group members are able to define <u>all</u> the words in the System Vocabulary section.

3. Assign group members to play the following roles (or create roles of your own):

    a. Doctor
    b. Interpreter
    c. Patient
    d. Narrator

The doctor and the patient might be enacting a conversation about a topic relevant to the assigned body system. Be sure that the doctor and patient are using the vocabulary words from the System Vocabulary section.

The interpreter will demonstrate interpreting in their target language using the skills learned in this curriculum in Part A: *Interpreter Skills.* This is an excellent opportunity to start thinking about how to interpret new medical vocabulary into your target language.

The narrator's role will be to narrate the scene and introduce key information that may not be obvious in the role-play. For example, the narrator may help 'set up the scene' by introducing the audience to the type of medical specialist that is in the particular scene. The narrator may also 'pause' the scene to explain key concepts and emphasize main points.

4. During the role-play, audience members will take notes using the Note Taking Forms included in this curriculum. Review these forms as you prepare your Medical Terminology Role-Play.

At the end of the role-play, audience members should be able to identify the following:

    a. The name of the body system

    b. Five key points that describe the function of the body system

    c. Important anatomical parts in this body system

    d. At least one common problem associated with the body system (including information about common symptoms, procedures, cures, treatment plans, and prevention plans, when applicable)

    e. At least one medical specialist that works with the body system

5. Use the System Vocabulary as a guideline for which anatomical parts and common problems to emphasize in the role-play. You do not need to include information about *every* anatomical part and common problem associated with the body system.

6. Be creative in performing your Medical Terminology Role-Play. The more memorable your role-play, the more likely your audience will also be able to remember the key points about your body system.

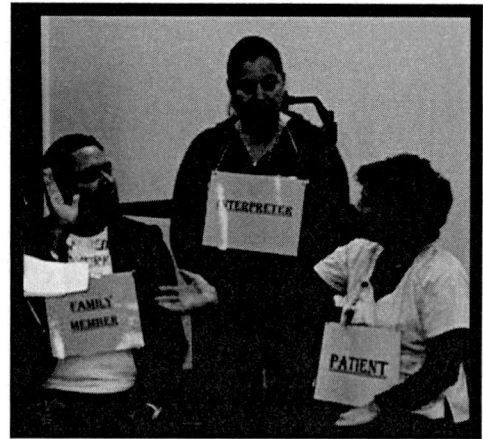

Hamilton Medical Center Interpreters, Dalton, GA

Note Taking Forms

Circulatory System

Five Key Points (FUNCTION):

1. _____

2. _____

3. _____

4. _____

5. _____

Common Problems:

Common Procedures:

Medical Specialists:

Circulatory System Word Bank

1. Right Ventricle	8. Pulmonary Veins
2. Capillaries	9. Left Atrium
3. Right Atrium	10. Pulmonary Artery
4. Valves	11. Inferior Vena Cava
5. Aorta	12. Heart
6. Left Ventricle	13. Veins
7. Arteries	14. Superior Vena Cava

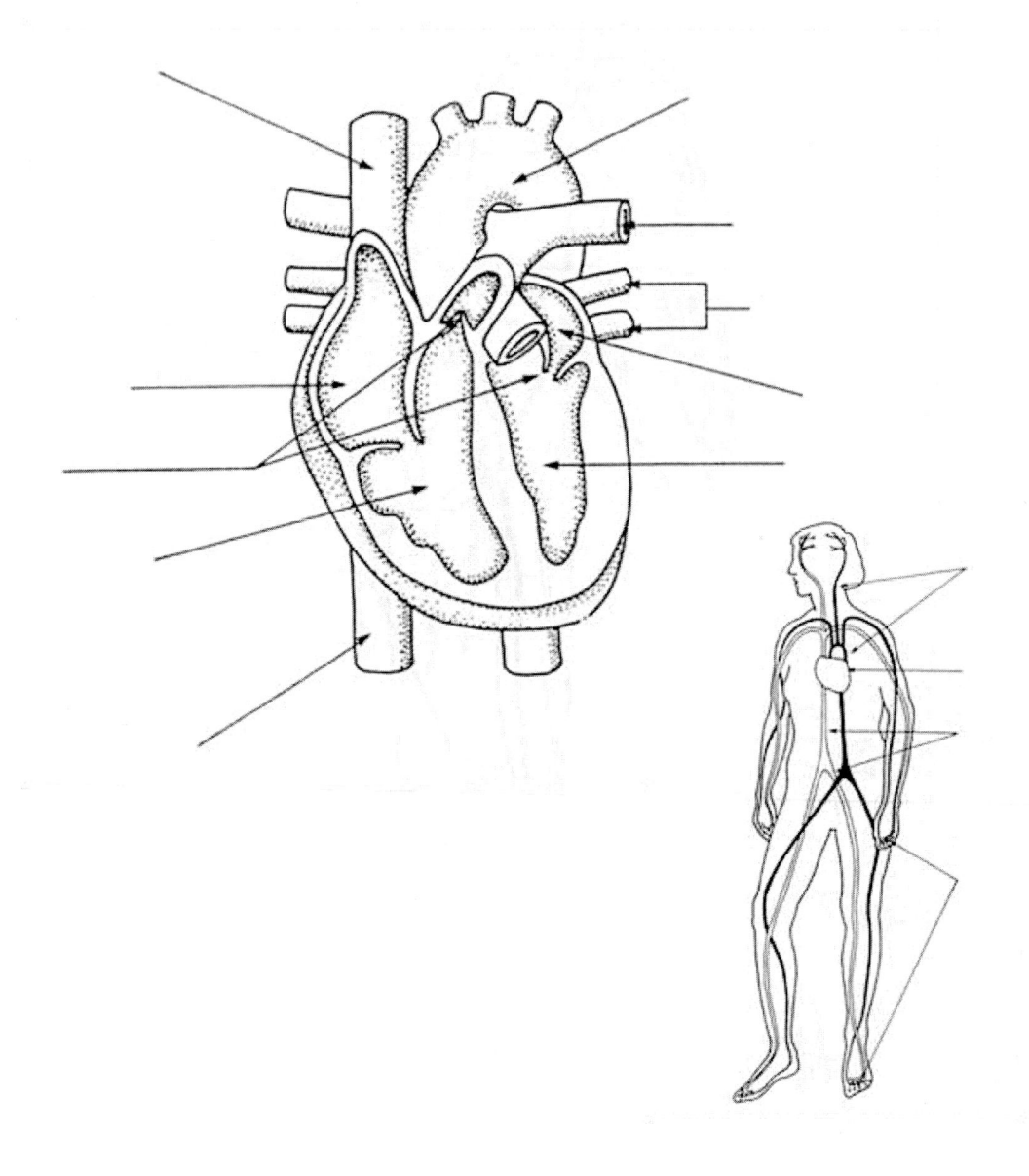

Medical Terminology Study Tools

Digestive System

Five Key Points (FUNCTION):

1. _____

2. _____

3. _____

4. _____

5. _____

Common Problems:

Common Procedures:

Medical Specialists:

© 2014 The Cross Cultural Health Care Program

Digestive System Word Bank

1. Rectum	8. Saliva Glands
2. Teeth	9. Liver
3. Small Intestine	10. Gums
4. Stomach	11. Esophagus
5. Mouth	12. Trachea
6. Gallbladder	13. Large Intestine
7. Epiglottis	

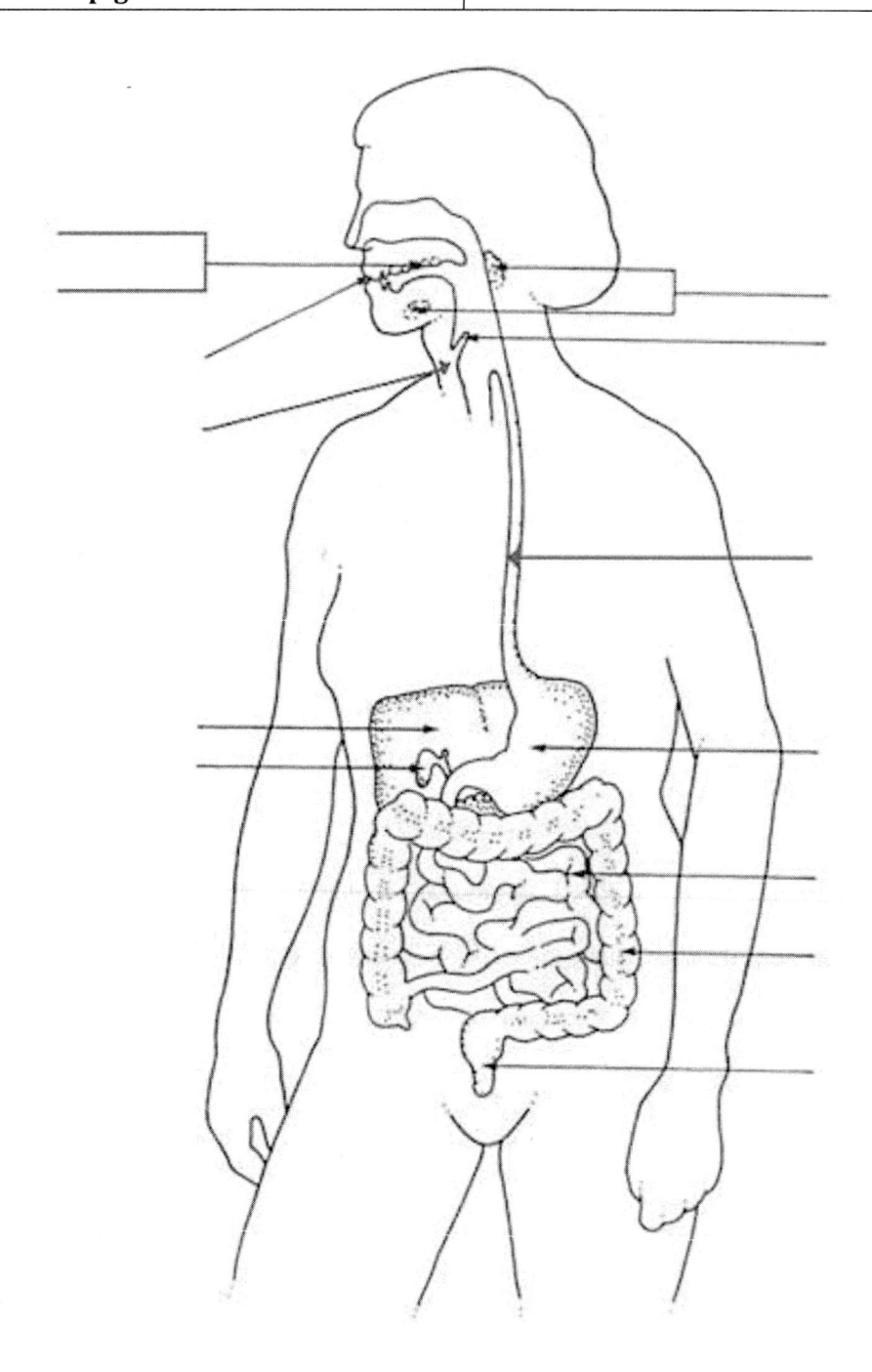

Medical Terminology Study Tools

Endocrine Glands System

Five Key Points (FUNCTION):

1. _____

2. _____

3. _____

4. _____

5. _____

Common Problems:

Common Procedures:

Medical Specialists:

© 2014 The Cross Cultural Health Care Program

Endocrine Glands System Word Bank

1. Thyroid Glands	4. Pancreas
2. Pituitary Gland	5. Adrenal Glands
3. Ovaries	6. Testicles

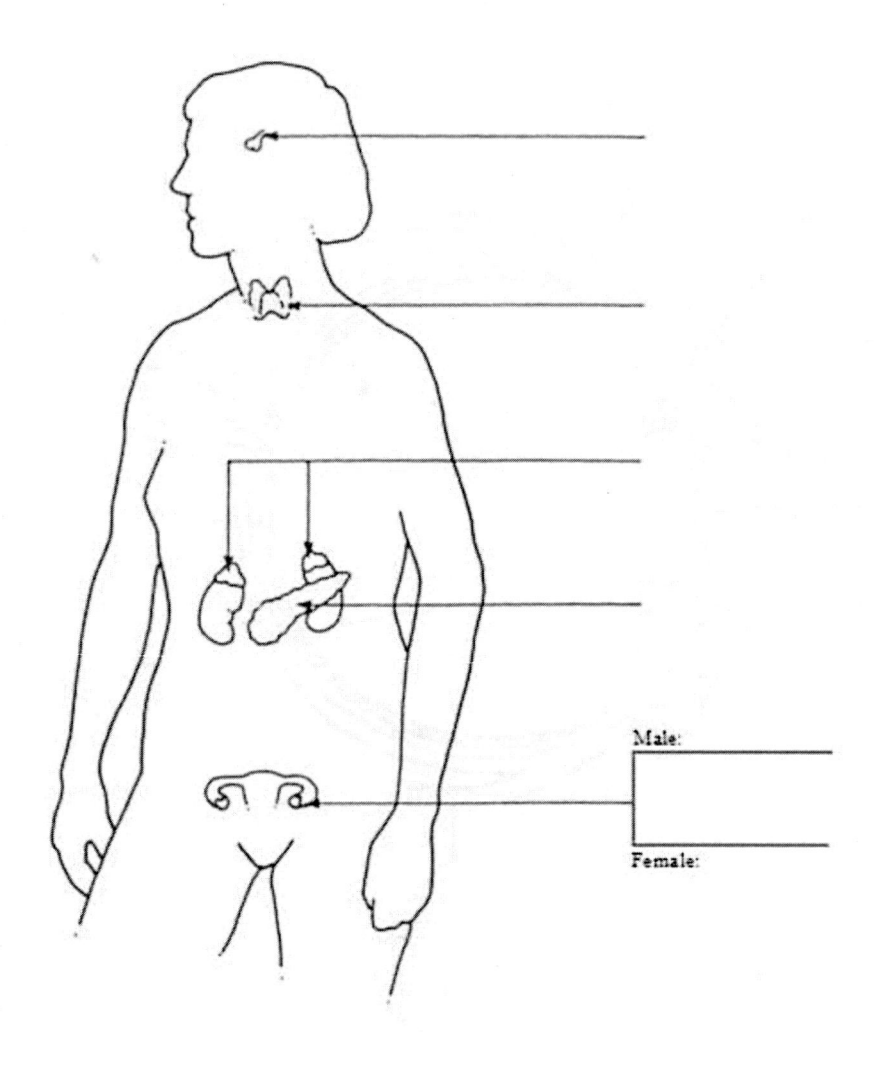

Male: _____

Female: _____

Musculoskeletal System

Five Key Points (FUNCTION):

1. _____

2. _____

3. _____

4. _____

5. _____

Common Problems:

Common Procedures:

Medical Specialists:

8 Musculoskeletal System Word Bank

1. Kneecap (Patella)	4. Hip bone (Pelvis)
2. Coccyx	5. Vertebra
3. Skull	

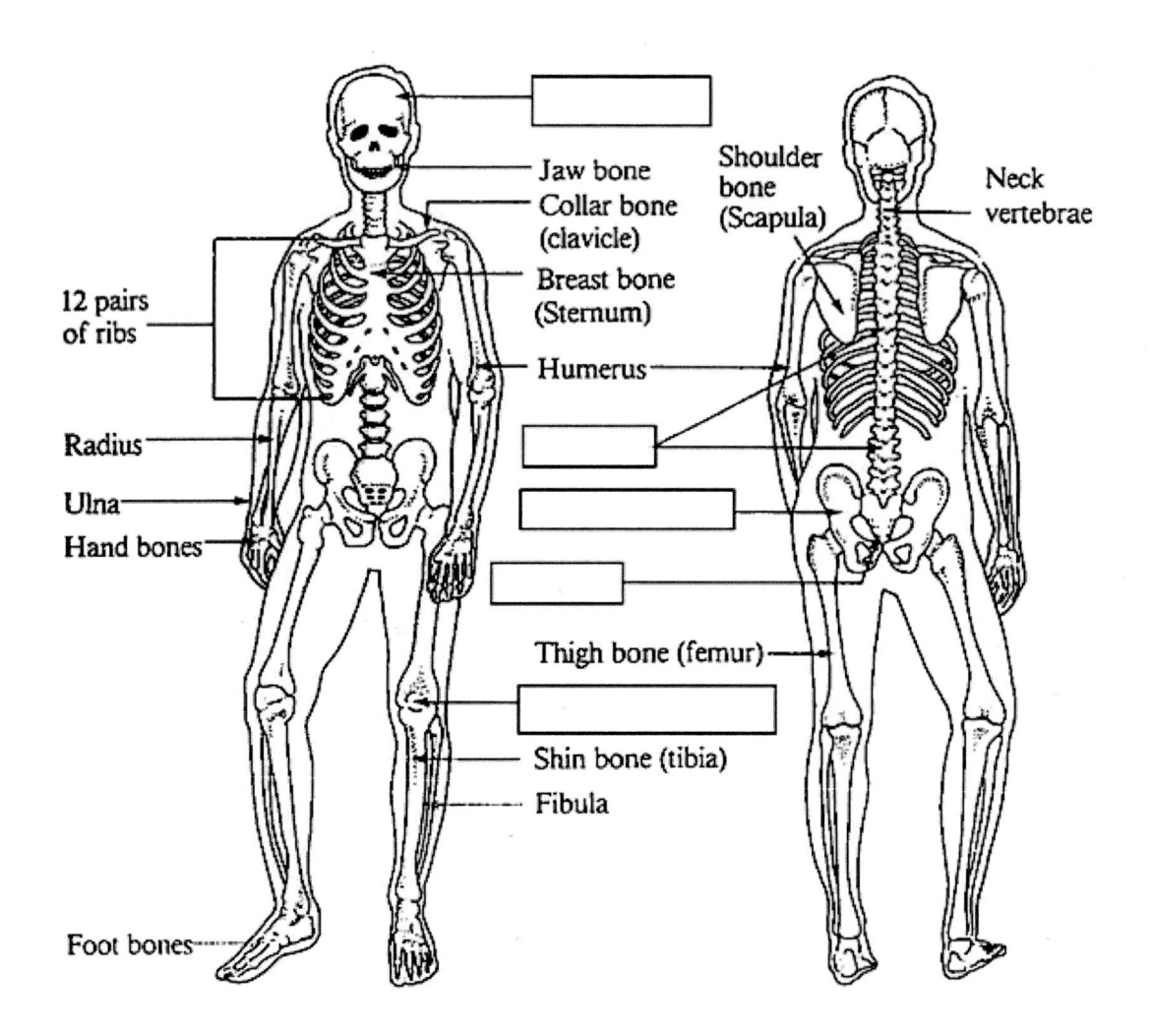

Jaw bone
Collar bone (clavicle)
Shoulder bone (Scapula)
Neck vertebrae
Breast bone (Sternum)
12 pairs of ribs
Humerus
Radius
Ulna
Hand bones
Thigh bone (femur)
Shin bone (tibia)
Fibula
Foot bones

Medical Terminology Study Tools

Nervous System

Five Key Points (FUNCTION):

1. _____

2. _____

3. _____

4. _____

5. _____

Common Problems:

Common Procedures:

Medical Specialists:

Nervous System Word Bank

1. Retina	5. Vitreous Humor
2. Cornea	6. Iris
3. Lens muscle	7. Optic Nerve
4. Pupil	8. Aqueous Humor

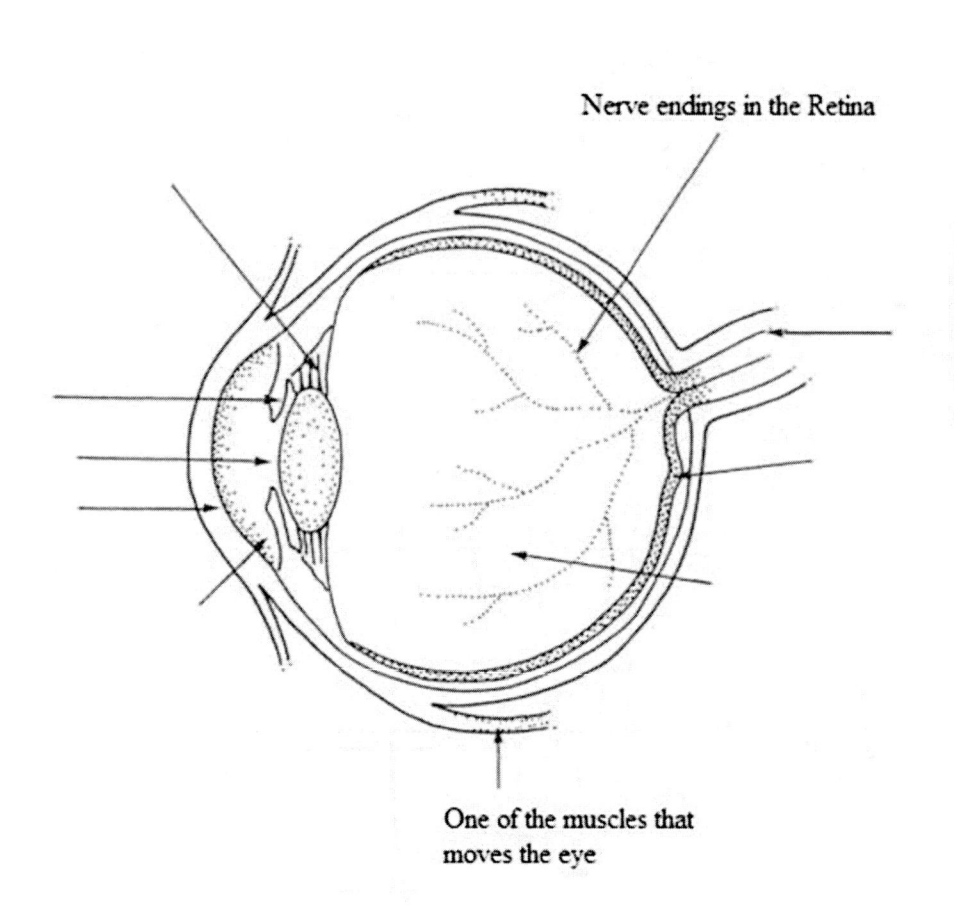

Nerve endings in the Retina

One of the muscles that moves the eye

Respiratory System

Five Key Points (FUNCTION):

1. _____

2. _____

3. _____

4. _____

5. _____

Common Problems:

Common Procedures:

Medical Specialists:

Respiratory System Word Bank

1. Nose passage	6. Lungs
2. Trachea	7. Mouth
3. Esophagus	8. Pleura
4. Diaphragm	9. Larynx
5. Epiglottis	10. Sinuses

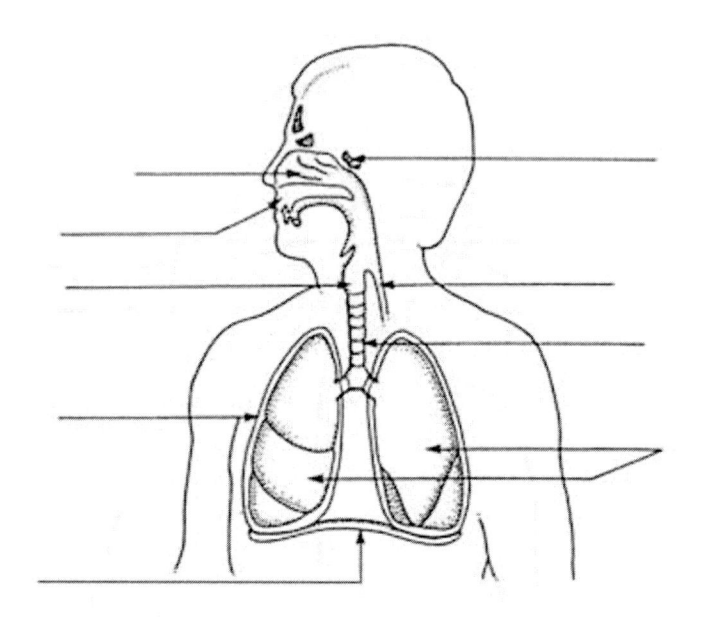

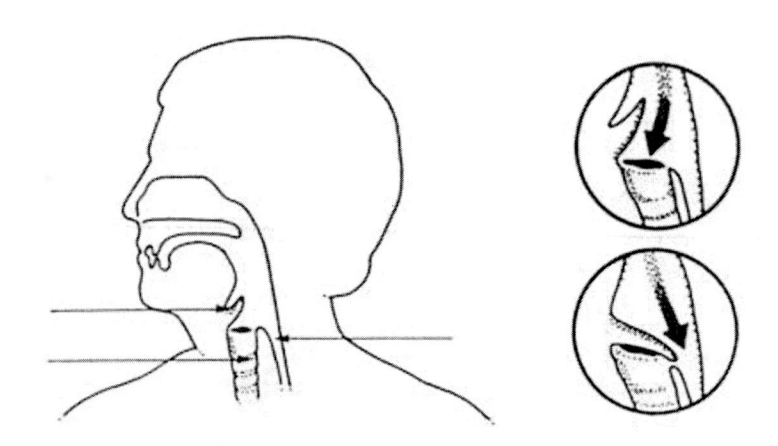

Medical Terminology Study Tools

Skin System

Five Key Points (FUNCTION):

1. _____

2. _____

3. _____

4. _____

5. _____

Common Problems:

Common Procedures:

Medical Specialists:

Skin System Word Bank

1. Epidermis	4. Dermis
2. Blood Vessels	5. Nerves
3. Sweat Glands	6. Hair Follicles (Sacs)

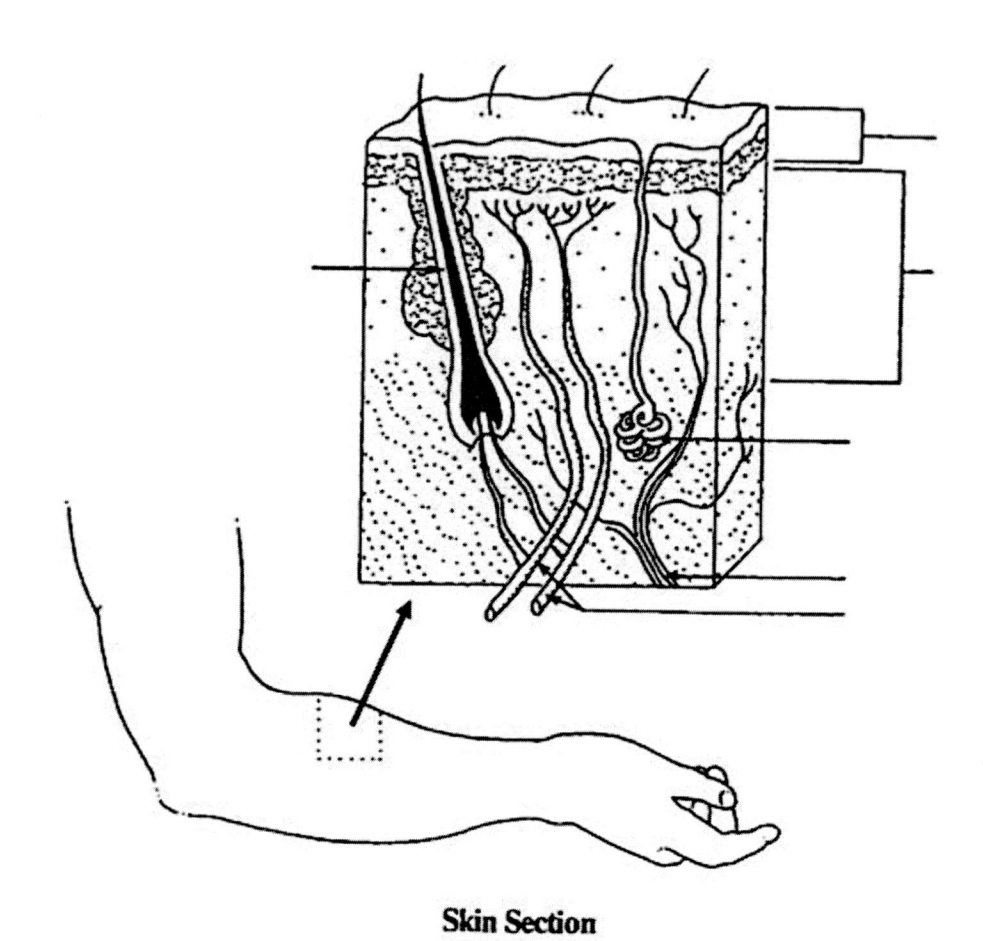

Skin Section

Urinary System

Five Key Points (FUNCTION):

1. _____

2. _____

3. _____

4. _____

5. _____

Common Problems:

Common Procedures:

Medical Specialists:

Urinary System Word Bank

Male	Female
1. Urethra	1. Bladder
2. Kidney	2. Ureter
3. Testicles	3. Fallopian Tubes
4. Bladder	4. Urethra
5. Ureter	5. Kidney
6. Vas Deferens	6. Ovary

Male Urinary System

Female Urinary System

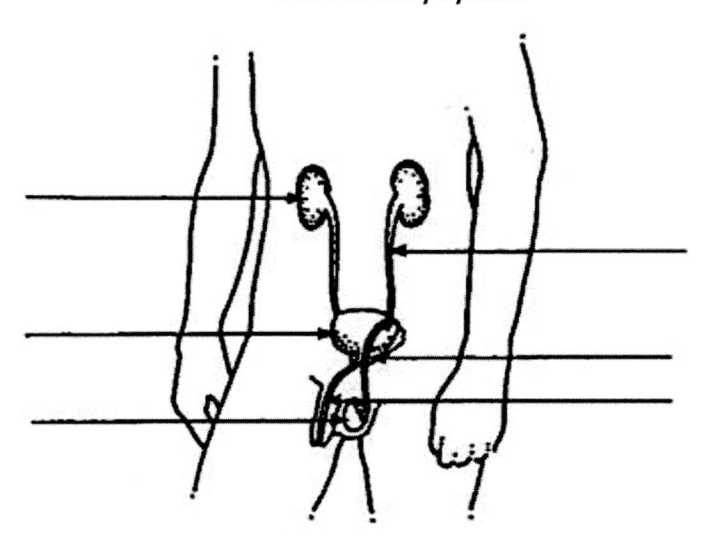

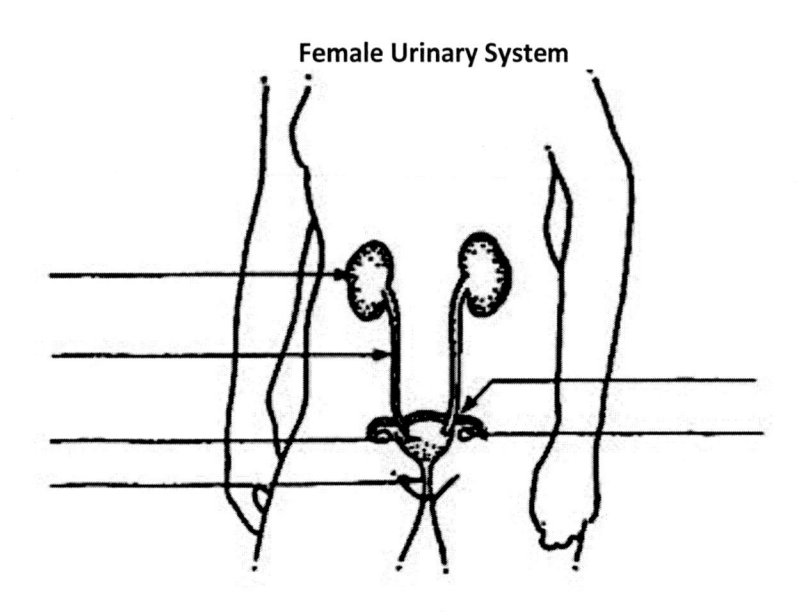

Medical Terminology Study Tools

Female Reproductive System

Five Key Points (FUNCTION):

1. _____

2. _____

3. _____

4. _____

5. _____

Common Problems:

Common Procedures:

Medical Specialists:

Female Reproductive System Word Bank

1. Vulva	5. Uterus
2. Fallopian Tubes	6. Cervix
3. Egg	7. Ovary
4. Vagina	

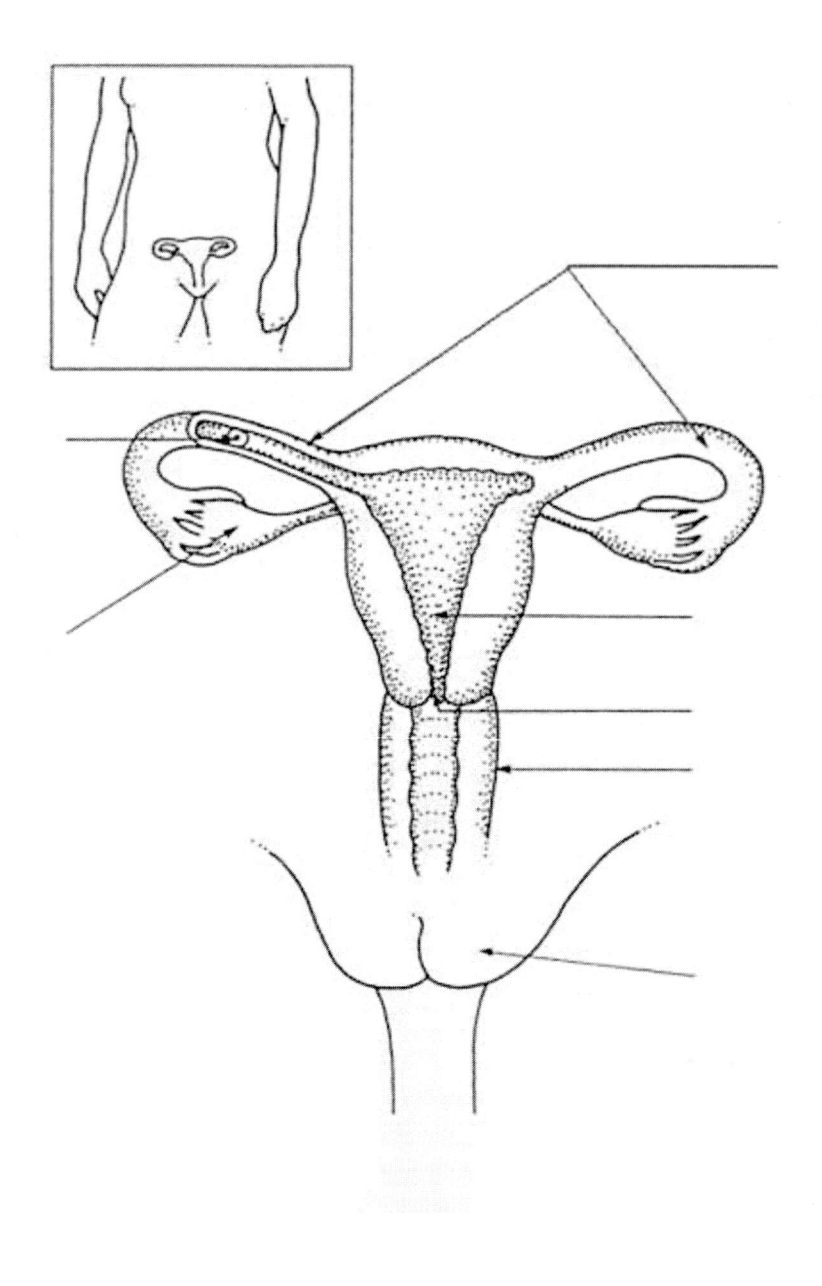

Male Reproductive System

Five Key Points (FUNCTION):

1. _____

2. _____

3. _____

4. _____

5. _____

Common Problems:

Common Procedures:

Medical Specialists:

Male Reproductive System Word Bank

1. Bladder	5. Testicles
2. Vas deferens	6. Ureters
3. Penis	7. Prostate Gland
4. Urethra	8. Scrotum

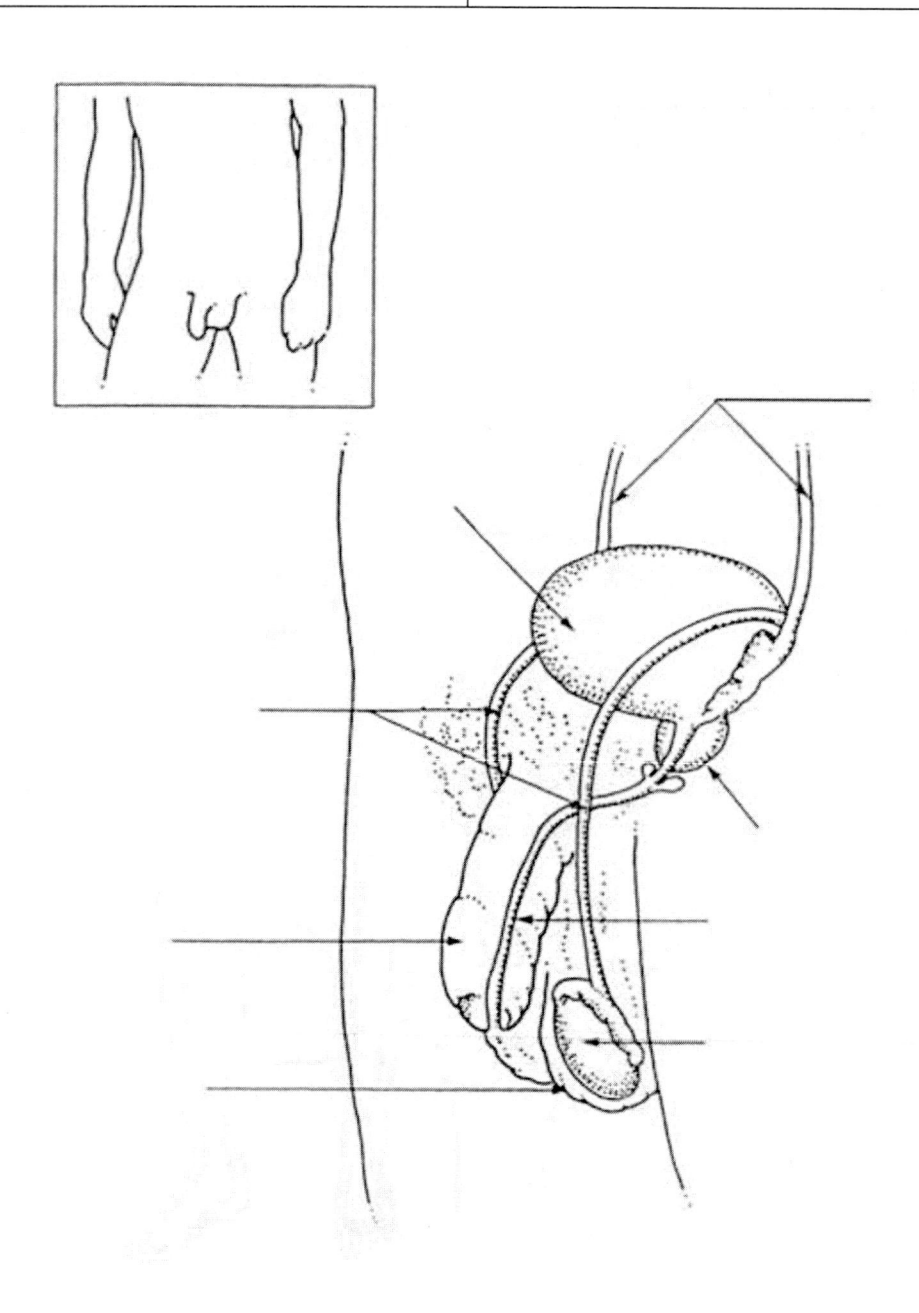

Medical Terminology Study Tools

Medical Procedures Activity

Match the **Group of Procedures** with the appropriate **Body System.**

Identify the purpose of each procedure. Make sure you can explain how a procedure within a group is different from other members of that group.

BODY SYSTEM CATEGORIES   **GROUPS OF PROCEDURES**

1. **Respiratory System**

   Electrocardiogram (EKG)
   Echocardiogram (Echo)
   Blood tests

2. **Nervous System**

   Biopsy   Vasectomy

3. **Digestive System**

   Endoscopy
   Upper GI Series (Barium Swallow)

4. **Cardiovascular System**

5. **Musculoskeletal System**

   Bronchoscopy
   Pulmonary Function Test

6. **Urinary System**

   Pap Smear Test
   Ultrasound   Cystoscopy
   Mammogram   Renal Dialysis

7. **Female Reproductive System**

   X-Ray
   Computed Tomography (CT Scan)
   Magnetic Resonance Imaging (MRI)

8. **Skin System**

   Electroencephalogram (EEG)

9. **Male Reproductive System**

Medical Specialists Activity

PART A: Match the **Medical Specialist(s)** with the appropriate **Body System**. Be sure that you can identify how each specialist within a group is different from other members of that group.

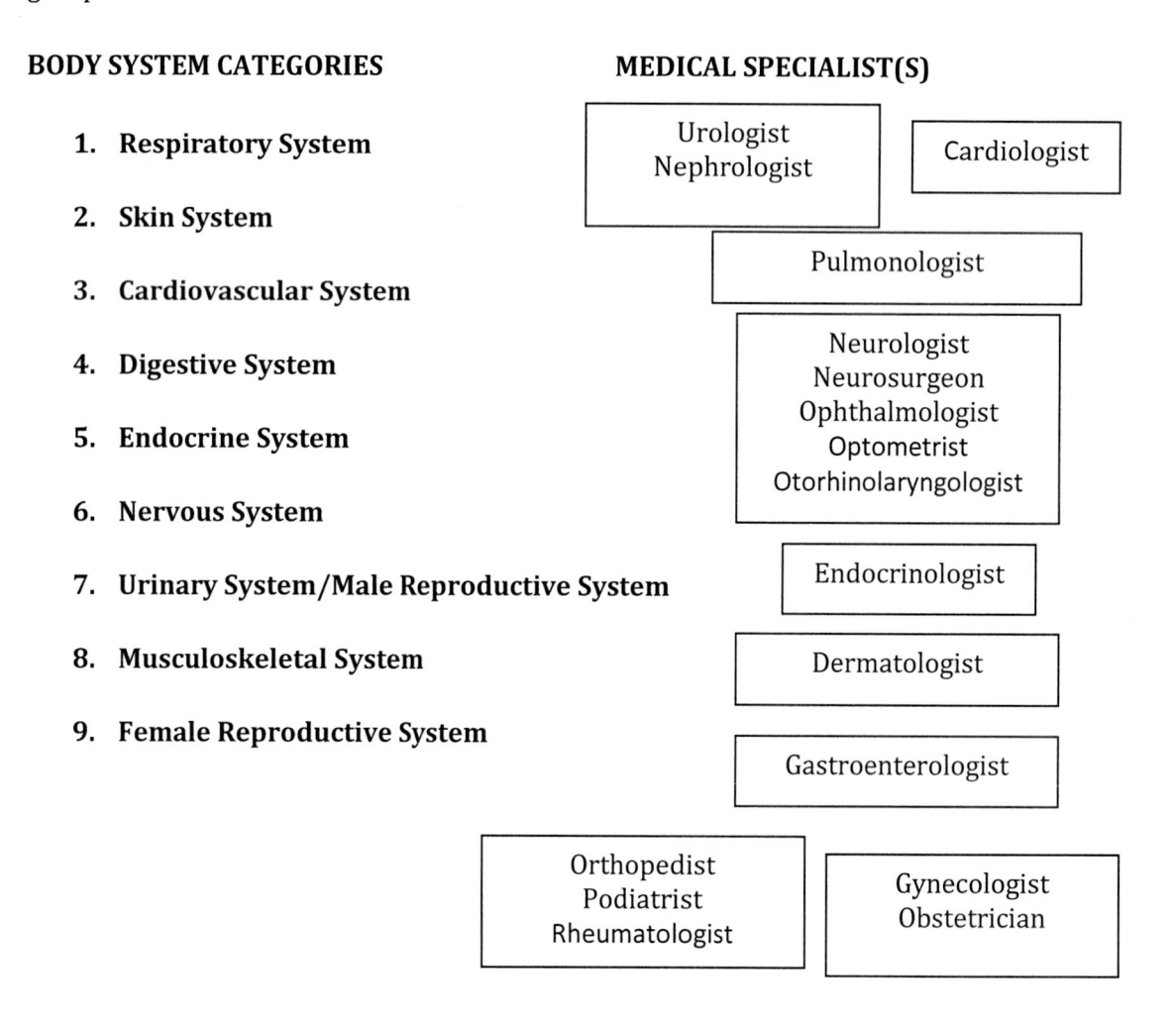

BODY SYSTEM CATEGORIES | **MEDICAL SPECIALIST(S)**

1. Respiratory System
2. Skin System
3. Cardiovascular System
4. Digestive System
5. Endocrine System
6. Nervous System
7. Urinary System/Male Reproductive System
8. Musculoskeletal System
9. Female Reproductive System

Medical Specialists:
- Urologist / Nephrologist
- Cardiologist
- Pulmonologist
- Neurologist / Neurosurgeon / Ophthalmologist / Optometrist / Otorhinolaryngologist
- Endocrinologist
- Dermatologist
- Gastroenterologist
- Orthopedist / Podiatrist / Rheumatologist
- Gynecologist / Obstetrician

PART B: Some medical specialists have specialties that are not directly related to any specific body system. Their specialties can be categorized by the diseases they treat, the procedures they perform or the specific populations they treat.

Using your knowledge of roots, prefixes, and suffixes and outside sources of information, define the specialty of each of the following medical specialists:

1. Allergist	5. Internist
2. Oncologist	6. Anesthesiologist
3. Pediatrician	7. Radiologist
4. Psychiatrist	8. Surgeon

Medical Terminology Crossword Puzzle Review

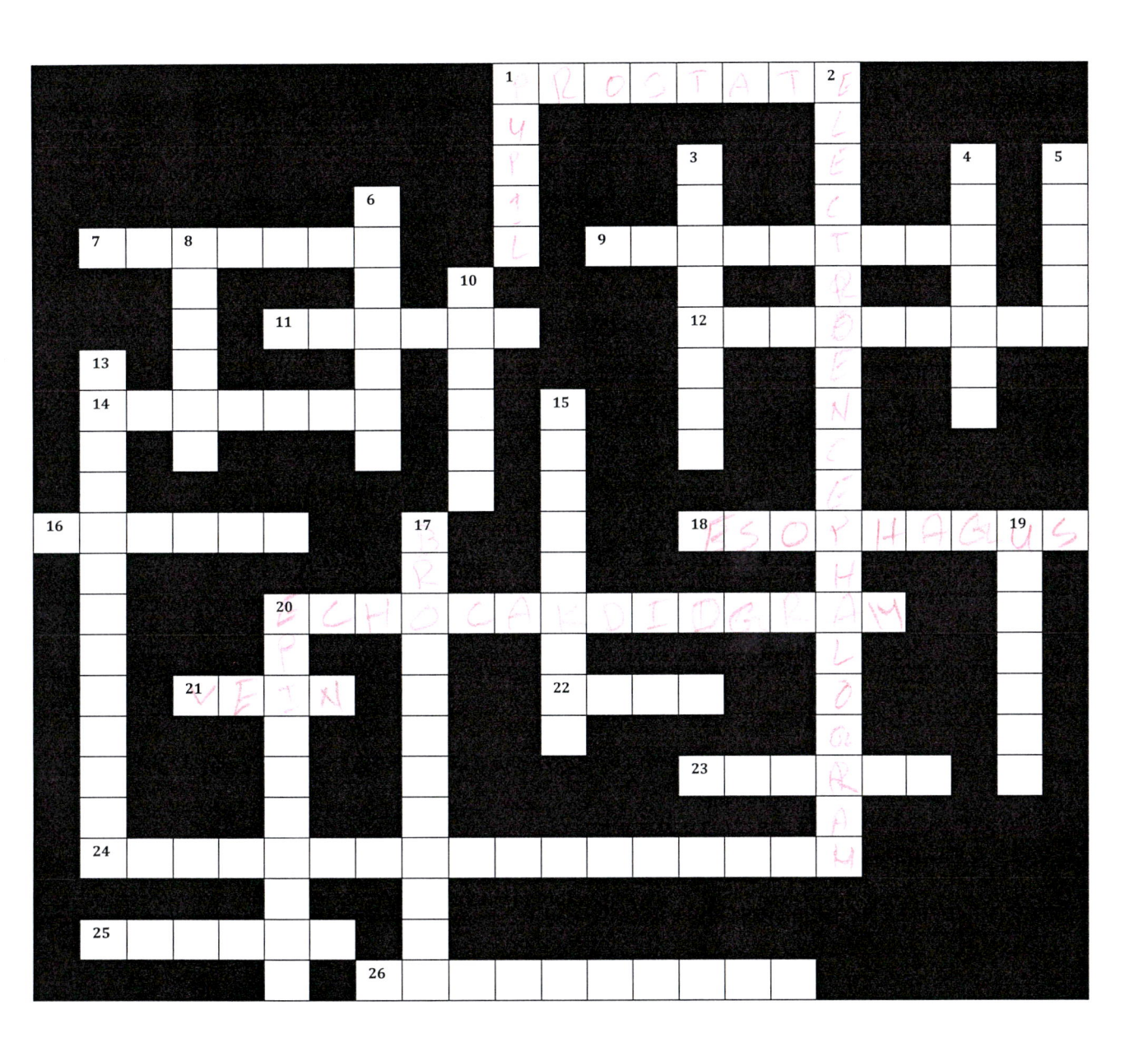

ACROSS

1. In the male reproductive system, the seminal vesicles and the _____ gland add fluid to the semen.
7. This is the tube leading from the mouth to the lungs (also known as the windpipe).
9. This gland makes hormones that control how the kidneys work and how we grow.
11. This is the name given to the smooth, thin lining that holds each lung.
12. During this procedure a fiber optic tube used to create visual images is inserted into the digestive system.
14. This gland produces hormones that control our heart rate, blood pressure, salt content throughout our body, and the development of our sexual organs.
16. This part of the eye is transparent; it covers the lens muscle, iris, and pupil.
18. This is the tube leading from the mouth to the stomach (also known as the food pipe).
20. This procedure uses ultrasound waves to learn about the structure and movement of a person's heart.
21. This type of blood vessel carries blood from the capillaries back to the heart.
22. This part of the eye controls the amount of light that can enter the eye.
23. This is the part of the female reproductive system where the egg, once fertilized, can develop into a baby.
24. This procedure measures the electricity flowing through a person's heart.
25. This bone is commonly known as the hip bone.
26. During this procedure a tube is inserted through the urethra and lights and mirrors are used to examine the inside of the bladder.

DOWN

1. This part of the human eye opens wider in dim light and smaller in bright light.
2. This procedure measures the electricity flowing through the brain.
3. Aqueous humor and _____ humor are the two kinds of fluid found in the eye that help the eye stay clean and maintain shape.
4. This gland controls our metabolic rate.
5. This is the part of the female reproductive system where an egg is released.
6. This bone is commonly known as the knee cap.
8. This type of blood vessel carries blood away from the heart.
10. This tube in the urinary system passes urine from the kidney to the bladder.
13. This is the part of the female reproductive system where an egg is usually fertilized.
15. The skin is made up of two layers. The lower layer is called the dermis and the upper layer is called the _____.
17. During this procedure a fiber optic tube used to create visual images is inserted through the nose, throat, larynx and trachea and into the lungs.
19. This tube in the urinary system passes urine from the bladder to the outside of the body.
20. This flap of skin controlled by the brain ensures that food travels to the stomach and air travels to the lungs through the right pipes.